Innovations in Psychosocial Interventions and Their Delivery

Innovations in Psychosocial Interventions and Their Delivery

Leveraging Cutting-Edge Science to Improve the World's Mental Health

ALAN E. KAZDIN

OXFORD
UNIVERSITY PRESS

OXFORD
UNIVERSITY PRESS

Oxford University Press is a department of the University of Oxford. It furthers the University's objective of excellence in research, scholarship, and education by publishing worldwide. Oxford is a registered trade mark of Oxford University Press in the UK and certain other countries.

Published in the United States of America by Oxford University Press
198 Madison Avenue, New York, NY 10016, United States of America.

CIP data is on file at the Library of Congress
ISBN 978-0-19-046328-1

To my family and the daily and enduring joys they bring

CONTENTS

PREFACE

Mental illness is an enormous burden worldwide, as reflected in the number of individuals who suffer from a mental disorder, the personal pain and suffering they and their families experience, the exorbitant costs of providing but also of failing to provide services, and the spillover of mental health problems into physical health (e.g., many physical maladies and earlier-than-expected deaths associated with mental illness) and functioning in everyday life (e.g., in social relations, employment, happiness, and quality of life). The size of the problem is not news, although contemporary research has elaborated the scope and burden of mental illness in more detail than ever before. Yet, as I will elucidate in this book, the mental health profession has at this moment in time unprecedented potential to embrace new ways to solve the world's mental health problems.

The book brings together current developments that could make an enormous difference. Three broad themes are discussed. First, and most familiar, from contemporary research, we now have many evidence-based psychosocial treatments that provide an array of options for treating mental disorders. Some of these, such as cognitive behavior therapy and mindfulness-based interventions, have seeped into the media and are now somewhat familiar to the public. But there are scores of other interventions available now, much less well known or familiar even to professionals involved in clinical practice. If these interventions only could reach people in need.

Second, the traditional means of providing psychological services, whether evidence based or not, is individual therapy of some kind, delivered by a mental health professional in an office. This model still dominates treatment research and clinical practice and is quite familiar to the public, as portrayed in the media (e.g., cartoons, movies, TV shows). Unfortunately, this model is not likely to be of much help by itself in reaching most people in need of psychological services in the United States and worldwide. Multiple models of delivering treatment are now available, although they are not very familiar or routinely included in the training of mental health professionals. With these models, for the first time we can provide mental health services in many different ways and could have a remarkable impact on mental illness.

Finally, there are new ways of thinking about both the burdens of mental illness and what is needed to have a significant impact. For example, physical and mental health care priorities are mobilized under the rubric of grand challenges with the goal of addressing critical problems in ways that can have a palpable impact. Grand challenges are one way, and are a critical way of considering how to have an impact. If we take as our challenge the goal of reducing the burdens of mental illness, that could greatly alter the nature of intervention research, characteristics of the interventions themselves, and ways of reaching people in need of services. Overall, we know enough to have a significant impact now, in part by doing some new things and by building on promising projects already in place.

The focus of this book is on reducing the burdens of mental illness and related sources of psychological impairment. *Mental illness* usually refers to meeting the criteria for a psychiatric diagnosis, as specified by psychiatric manuals that delineate various disorders. Yet we know from research and clinical practice, and indeed sometimes from personal experience, that many people suffer whether or not they meet the formal and somewhat arbitrary diagnostic criteria. I will focus on reducing the burdens of psychological sources of impairment in its many different forms, even though the emphasis is on mental disorders.

The book is divided into four parts. The first part is *Background and The Mental Health Crisis*. Chapters 1, 2, and 3 in this part convey the domain of our focus and the challenge, namely, reducing the burdens of mental illness. Chapter 1 reviews the current mental health crisis and the need to devise new ways of intervening to have an impact. This chapter also defines the domain of the book and its focus on psychosocial rather than medical interventions, and overviews remaining chapters. Chapter 2 conveys in more detail the scope of mental disorders, subclinical disorders, and other forms of impairment. In addition, the chapter considers the burdens of mental illness in relation to individuals, families, and society at large. Chapter 3 focuses on the treatment gap, namely, the huge chasm between the number of people who are in need of mental health services and the number who actually receive them. In addition, I discuss key barriers to providing and receiving mental health services.

The second part of the book is the *Current Status and Advances in Psychosocial Interventions*. Chapter 4 considers evidence-based psychosocial interventions that now include a very large set of techniques. The chapter poses questions about these interventions in relation to what can and cannot be said about their impact and what we know about how they work. Chapter 5 focuses on current trends in psychosocial intervention research that have a direct impact on providing mental health services. I discuss four such trends, including dissemination of evidence-based interventions, the integration of physical and mental health care services, development of treatments (transtreatments) that can be extended across multiple disorders or domains of dysfunction, and the use of technology as a basis for delivering interventions.

The third part of the book is *Expansion of Interventions and Models of Their Delivery*. In Chapter 6, I discuss the dominant model of delivering psychosocial interventions and its limitations in reaching the vast majority of individuals in need of services. The chapter also elaborates criteria of what we would want in a model of treatment delivery so that the interventions we deliver could be scaled up to reach larger groups of individuals (e.g., ethnic minorities, individuals with lower income, children, older adults) who suffer the greatest neglect in receiving services. Chapter 7 is one of two chapters that provides novel models of treatment delivery that meet the criteria discussed in the previous chapter and that can be scaled up. Models are described, illustrated, and examined in relation to the delivery of interventions for mental disorders. Chapter 8 presents an additional set of novel models of delivery. In this chapter, models of delivery, as well as the interventions themselves, vary from traditional psychotherapeutic treatments.

The fourth and final part of the book is *Extending Our Conceptual Views of Treatment, Research, and Interventions*. Chapter 9 focuses on novel foci in treatment research and delivery and on ways to expand how we think about, investigate, and provide treatment. Stepped care is introduced in the chapter not only in the familiar way of using such care to provide interventions but also in relation to models of delivery and how they are sequenced. Chapter 10 is aimed at moving toward solutions and begins with conceptual views of the challenge of reducing the burdens of mental illness and what different conceptual views offer. Within these views, illustrations are provided about models and programs that are in place to help improve physical and mental health generally as well as to reduce the burdens of mental illness. Chapter 11, the final chapter, highlights key issues about the current status of what we have reviewed. There, I address whether we can intervene to have an impact, whether we should, where to start, how we will know whether we have had an impact, and what changes in health care might be needed beyond the focus of mental illness.

In addition to the chapters, the book includes a list of frequently used abbreviations and a glossary of key terms. Both of these are useful adjuncts because the book draws on multiple disciplines and concepts and methods they use. Indeed, reducing the burdens of mental illness, as will be evident, is a collaborative enterprise involving multiple disciplines, including business, economics, nursing, psychology, psychiatry, public health, social policy, social work, and law and government and nongovernment agencies. The list of abbreviations and glossary will ensure that unfamiliar concepts are easily illuminated.

Overall, the chapters move in a systematic way from discussing and documenting the problem, presenting advances in intervention research, elaborating novel models of delivering interventions that could have an impact, pointing to ways of conceptualizing the challenge of reducing the burdens, and identifying partial solutions ongoing right now. The tragedy of mental illness is that so many individuals are suffering with disabling conditions needlessly, with any treatment, including evidence-based treatments, out of reach. Millions and millions of people are affected in the United States and worldwide, yet few receive any services at all. With this book, I hope to show that we have options—options that are sufficiently available and tested and that have the potential to substantially reduce mental illness and its many burdens. What I propose to be missing is a unified social, governmental, and professional commitment to reject the business-as-usual approach and instead apply what we already know in accountable ways. This book is not a call for more funding for mental health services but instead is a call for a paradigm shift in how services are conceptualized and delivered. This book is an effort to move us forward.

Completion of this book was facilitated by many different colleagues, friends, and others whose contributions to understanding and improving physical and mental health are well known. The individuals to whom I am especially grateful include Kelly Brownell, David Clark, Adam Glick, Elizabeth Hoo, Bradley Karlin, Ronald Kessler, Laura Murray, Vikram Patel, and Angela McGowan. Each of them took the time to guide me on critical questions related to the focus of the book. Two former doctoral students and now quite successful professionals, Stacey Blase and Sarah Rabbitt, helped me work on the challenges and solutions that are included in the book, and I am grateful to them as well. I am also grateful to Leonard Bickman, an internationally recognized scholar in mental health services, social policy, program evaluation, and intervention research, who reviewed an early draft of the book and provided valuable comments. Finally, Sarah Harrington, Senior Editor at Oxford University Press, played a very special role in initiating the project and contributed greatly to both the substance and style of the final result. I have a long-standing relation with the Press and continue to profit from the quality of the senior editorial staff in guiding the entire process from conceptualization to completion.

While writing this book I was extremely fortunate to have research support from the National Institute of Mental Health, the National Institute of Child Health and Human Development, the Laura J. Niles Foundation, the Humane Society of America, the Morris Animal Foundation and Human-Animal Bond Research Initiative Foundation, The Jack Parker Corporation, and the Blue Guitar Foundation. None of the views in this book has been fostered or endorsed by these organizations, but their support and participation in my professional life have made this work possible. Occasionally, in the book I make references to commercial products that illustrate a novel point about interventions or assessment. I have no commercial interest in any products that are mentioned and (somewhat lamentably) do not profit or benefit in any way from their success. Finally, I am grateful to Yale University, which has provided an extremely supportive environment. The University has facilitated this work in part by the ease with which collaboration and informal sharing of ideas are possible and promoted.

Alan E. Kazdin
New Haven, Connecticut

PART I

Background and the Mental Health Crisis

1

Introduction

THE CRISIS

A mental health crisis exists worldwide in both developing and developed countries. In the United States, millions of children, adolescents, and adults experience significant mental health problems and receive no help whatsoever. Approximately 50 percent of people in the United States will experience a form of mental illness during their lifetime. Although much more will be said about that later, it is worth pausing on just that facet of the crisis. With a US population of approximately 325 million, 50 percent is a staggering number. Perhaps with that enormous number, it is understandable that most people in need of psychological services receive no professional help at all. They receive no form of psychotherapy, nor medication, nor do they even connect with the physician who helps manage their physical health and who would be in a position to assist with mental health needs. Certainly there are others who could provide care (e.g., religious leaders, healers, designated "life coaches" of various kinds) and who might also be consulted, and a range of practitioners who provide various interventions (e.g., acupuncture, spa and massage treatments) that are related to mental health care (e.g., alleviate stress, depression). This does not change the overall conclusion: most people in need receive nothing formalized to "treat" or alleviate their mental disorders.

THE SCOPE OF THE PROBLEM

The scope of mental illness and the paucity of treatment services can be broken down into parts (subcrises) to convey the size of the problem and challenges. Consider three facets of the overall crisis to convey the point. First, mental health care simply is unavailable for one reason or another for most people in the United States. Lack of insurance or health coverage of some kind is one part of this. Even when people can afford mental health care or have insurance coverage, they often do not have access to services that are convenient and available near them. Certain groups are especially unlikely to receive mental health services, and among them are children, older adults, members of ethnic minority groups, people at or below poverty levels, single parents, victims of violence (child abuse, sexual abuse, domestic violence, rape), people who are homeless, people who are in prison, and surprisingly many of those in college!

Second, there is often stigma associated with traditional mental health services (seeing a therapist or being hospitalized for a brief period). For some, going to therapy for psychological problems represents a failure or weakness of some kind—one could not take care of one's problems and "had to" seek help. Antiquated conceptualizations of mental illness and of those who suffer from them linger—that mental disorder is the result of a weakness of character, for instance, or the result of a lack of self-control, or possession of evil. Few of us want to consider the fact that we are not "normal" in some way (except for the genius and talents we have that the Nobel Committee continues to ignore). Going to "therapy" for "help" coping with life can easily be seen as a hard-to-deny sign that one is not "normal," that one is unable to take care of things on one's own. This stigma, perceived and real, and the impediments it provides contribute to the problem of people not obtaining services.

Third, many conditions in society (poverty, poor diet, homelessness, ongoing daily life stress) exacerbate existing mental health problems or increase the risk that such problems will emerge. Though such conditions may or may not "cause" mental illness, they nonetheless can precipitate or increase the likelihood that a mental disorder or psychological symptoms (such as bouts of anxiety or depression) may emerge. This is not all that different from physical health diseases (e.g., cancer, heart disease), which, though there may be a genetic component, may have many precipitants in the environment (e.g., air and water pollutants, cigarette smoking, exposure to radiation) that can lead to the disorder. In relation to psychological disorders, many conditions of life (e.g., having a baby, loss of a loved one) can contribute to clinical dysfunction (e.g., postpartum depression in women but also in men, posttraumatic stress disorder). Life's many conditions might also precipitate the need for formal treatment or help when the usual influences that buffer us against disorder (e.g., support of friends and relatives, spirituality) are unavailable or insufficient. Seeking treatment may not be the only option, but options indeed *seem* to be scarce. For example, in the United States there is no formal support network in neighborhoods that could serve as a safety net to check on or connect with families with young children and children with special needs in ways that could reduce parental stress and fatigue or prevent or limit mental health problems. I will have more to say about the crisis further on, and will provide requisite details, but even within these introductory comments the unmet need is evident. This book will also convey that in fact there are numerous options available for help. That is, the need can be met.

WHY CARE ABOUT MENTAL DISORDERS?

Why should we care about the mental disorders and psychological dysfunction more generally, which is "merely" one of many crises facing society (e.g., climate change, natural disasters, crime, violence, sex trafficking)? Of course, I am not suggesting mental health issues are the only challenge facing us today. And yet there are many reasons to care about this particular challenge. Moreover, I shall connect this particular challenge to others (e.g., including climate change and natural disasters, and crime) and in ways that may be helpful in having an impact on and beyond mental health. Before that, we ought to care about mental illness for multiple reasons.

Moral, altruistic, humane, self-interest, and societal interests align to argue for the importance of attending to mental illness as a critical challenge. Moral and altruistic reasons are involved because helping people who are distressed is the right thing to do. Few religious codes, moral philosophies, and cultural values begin with a guiding principle that recommends "neglect those in need." Humane reasons emerge because people are suffering with psychological symptoms, so much so that many complete suicide, think about suicide as a viable option, or harm themselves and their families in other ways (e.g., violence, bankruptcy resulting from use of funds for gambling or substance use); some abandon or even kill their children. Self-interest emerges because psychological dysfunction is likely to touch—or more likely grab—us all in some way. We ourselves may suffer some dysfunction (depression, anxiety); or perhaps a relative, partner, child, or friend is in need of care. We may also suffer personally through the acts of others (e.g., violence, criminal behavior) when those acts have mental illness as a possible contributing factor.

Another reason to care about the mental illness crisis has to do with their staggering cost to society, and how that spending could be put to benefit elsewhere. As discussed later, the financial burdens of mental illness to society are enormous, as reflected in lost years of work by those who suffer impairment, the direct costs of treatment services (e.g., outpatient or inpatient care) for the relatively few who receive care, and a lengthy list of related services stemming from mental illness (e.g., emergency department visits, contact with the courts and prisons, care for the homeless). The economic impact of mental illness overall has increased the involvement of banking and business leaders; the costs of mental illness deplete funds that could be better used in society.

Finally, another reason for concern is that mental illness and physical illness are inextricably intertwined, a topic to which I will return in force later in the book. Individuals with *physical* health problems like diabetes and asthma are at greater risk for mental health problems, and individuals with *mental* health problems are much more likely to die sooner than their peers without disorders (by an average of 15 to 20 years). We often think of the psychological consequences of stress, but the effects are far broader. Prolonged stress in particular not only can promote and precipitate psychological problems such as depression but also can accelerate aging, impair one's immune system, and change the structures and functioning of the brain (e.g., Conrad, 2011; Nordentoft et al., 2013). Thus, if we care about physical health we also must care about mental health (Prince et al., 2007; World Health Organization [WHO], 2005).

The connection of physical and mental health speaks to the critical role of and need for psychological care beyond the boundaries to which we have become accustomed. That is, individuals with physical health problems may well need much more in the way of psychological services than they now receive. This is not a luxury item. For example, individuals with HIV/AIDS have a two-fold greater rate of clinical depression than matched controls without HIV/AIDS (Ciesla & Roberts, 2014). Clinically depressed patients are much less likely to take their medication and are therefore more likely to die of HIV/AIDS and to spread HIV to uninfected individuals. As another example, in the United States and worldwide, the number of older adults is growing because of increased longevity. In the United States, approximately 10,000 people per day turn 65 years old, and this is projected to continue until 2030 (Cohn & Taylor, 2010; Social Security Administration, 2011). With this demographic shift comes increases in physical disability and many conditions associated with it, including social isolation, depression, and suicidality. Here, too, physical and mental health are intertwined. In short, mental health is critical to physical health (and vice versa) for individuals and society and for the world more generally.

REMEDIES AND INTERVENTIONS

I have highlighted the crises in mental health, and I will provide more detail and context later. But the focus of this book is on remedies and how we can reverse the crises. It turns out that there is a great deal that can be done, but that much of what we have in our collective mental health toolboxes is not being applied to help people. In this book I will explain all of this in detail and offer upbeat news about the range of options beyond what mental health professionals like me usually consider.[1]

Many different types of efforts have been put toward alleviating stress and helping people handle life challenges and sources of physical and psychological impairment. There is no recognized list of such efforts, nor is there a universal classification system to convey all the different types of interventions. Yet consider the full domain of interventions devoted to helping individuals with some type of psychological dysfunction or source of distress (e.g., reaction to a natural or human-made disaster such as war). Here I delineate five broad domains of interventions that help people with psychological problems in everyday life. They blend into each other and overlap, but I find this list to be helpful in conveying some of the options on which we draw for help. The notion of drawing on different options will also be very helpful later in the book.

First, *informal interventions* in everyday life are a first line of attack when we experience some form of impairment. I refer to them as "informal" not only to mean casual but also to reflect the fact that interventions in this category are not systematic or formalized, or formally recognized, or even well-studied procedures. These include our contacts with family, friends, pets, and others (e.g., coworkers, neighbors). These contacts help with "treatment" and "prevention." I put these words in quotes because the focuses are on handling a current problem or crisis and on better coping with a future or impending problem, respectively; but they are not conceived of as treatment or prevention in the more formal sense in which these terms are used by mental health professionals.

One's own efforts to control stressors and strains of life fall into the informal intervention strategy as well. Those efforts may be self-medication (e.g., use of medications, alcohol, illicit substances, or other substances) to help negotiate the world, taking a vacation, dropping out for a little while (work, school), or ending a situation (relationship, job) that contributes to one's woes. Some self-coping techniques may be maladaptive and dangerous (including nonsuicidal self-injury, such as cutting oneself, as a way of reducing anxiety; not eating; or repetitive induced vomiting to cope with fear of gaining weight), but that is beyond the purpose here. I only wish to note that for help with psychological adaptation, with anxiety, depression, mood swings, stressors, and more, we already naturally draw on an array of interventions that are not part of mental health professions or not seen formally as a form of treatment.

Second, more formalized interventions that are still not part of recognized mental health professions constitute another category of treatment. Many institutionalized and more formalized activities can provide direct aid for psychological problems. Belonging to and participating in religious, spiritual, or related activities (organized religion, meditation, yoga, spas) and visiting sacred places (ashrams, retreats, religious pilgrimage sites) are examples. These activities often may be directed toward improving life broadly and are often targeted toward specific psychological dysfunctions or psychiatric conditions. For example, exorcism as part of some religions has long been used to overcome psychological as well as physical health problems, and currently is still in use. Exorcism is the process or act of expelling or ridding a person of evil spirits (possession of the devil) by various religious acts, ceremonies, and rituals specially designed for that person (Levack, 2013). This second category of interventions for many is likely to include nonreligious but still spiritual and reflective activities such as meditation and a variety of Eastern practices that connect mind and body through activities, exercises, and mastery, control, or regulation of one's cognitive and emotional processes. What leads me to delineate this second domain is that the interventions are more institutionalized than the day-to-day informal contact with relatives, friends, and peers. Yet, as with the informal interventions I mentioned first, these institutionalized interventions usually are not considered by mental health professions as part of treatments that have been developed and designed to ameliorate psychological symptoms or psychiatric disorders.

Third, many interventions include complementary and alternative components. Interventions in this category, for both physical and mental health, include diverse procedures, many of which do not stem from traditional Western health care.[2] They include herbs, dietary supplements, mind-body exercises, vitamins, and therapies like massage and acupuncture. Such interventions might be considered as part of the domains I mentioned previously. Yet these are worth delineating because complementary interventions represent an important bridge. Many of the procedures (e.g., mindfulness, biofeedback, hypnosis, tai chi, micronutrients) blur into and include formal treatments that are used by mental health professionals and evaluated in the context of physical and mental health.

Fourth, many formalized interventions are designed specifically to treat psychological dysfunctions, and these are practices developed and implemented by mental health and physical health professionals more generally. These interventions are conceptualized as treatment for some conditions and fall broadly within a medical practice model of diagnosing that condition and providing treatment specifically for it. These are the familiar interventions for psychological dysfunction and include psychotherapy, medication, and psychiatric hospitalization. Research, training, and clinical practice in the mental health professions (psychology, psychiatry, social work, family and marital therapy, psychiatric nursing) develop, teach, and implement these interventions for clients or patients who are referred for and seen in the context of formal treatment service. If one asked a mental health professional what the primary treatments are for psychological problems, these interventions would come to mind.

Fifth, many interventions for mental disorders are population based and are not the usual psychosocial therapy treatments delivered on a one-to-one basis. These interventions may draw on policy, regulations, and laws to control or limit behavior. Examples are familiar and include such interventions as taxes on cigarettes or alcohol to reduce overall use of these substances, calorie counts on foods and menus to reduce obesity, and national campaigns to engage in health-enhancing lifestyle activities such as exercise. Some of these interventions draw on cognitive psychology ("nudging" people to make healthy decisions) but still are usually population based and not taught within mental health professions as interventions for psychological problems.

I have delineated five domains only to help outline the range of interventions directed toward helping, improving, and treating psychological problems. As I mentioned, the domains blend. For example, among various cultures, shamans or religious leaders are called in specifically to treat a condition that would be considered psychological, or perhaps more likely spiritual. Exorcism, too, is a practice designed to treat problems both of mental and of physical health. That is, many interventions that mental health professionals may or may not regard as formal treatments are in fact recognized as such in different cultures, and by leaders in those cultures designated as providers of care. Also, interventions that would be considered complementary and alternative interventions by most formally trained mental health professionals, such as meditation and mindfulness, are used as formal treatments for psychological dysfunction and fall within different domains depending on how they are used.

The five domains I have delineated alert us to the scope, range, and types of interventions available to us. There is virtue in capitalizing on these options and in drawing on the benefits that each of the domains represents. Consider a key question that underlies this book: What are the interventions that we can use to treat psychological problems and mental illness and that will have impact? The "will have impact" part for our purposes will rely on scientific evidence, so certainly some "interventions" will be disqualified from our discussion. Even so, we ought to be open to the broadest range of approaches, including the more "traditional" interventions such as psychological treatment, medication, and hospitalization. But we can help individuals and society at large if we open the faucet a bit, perhaps more than a bit, to examine what can be done to help. A lot. This book is all about that, and moves into novel areas. And I will even add to the overall domains new types of interventions that could and perhaps even ought to be used to reduce mental illness and related disorders.

There are enormous unmet needs for psychological care that will ameliorate the impairment and suffering brought by mental illness in its many gradations and forms. The term *mental illness* suggests extreme conditions that depart from what any of us individually may have. Yet the term encompasses psychological functioning in relation to emotions, thoughts, and actions that are associated with impairment. *Impairment* refers to the consequences or associated features that interfere with or impede functioning in everyday life and can include difficulties in managing one's own personal life, meeting expectations and responsibilities with one's family or at work, and negotiating everyday routines. These include anxiety, depression, violent acts, substance abuse, suicidal thoughts and attempts, and severe limits in relating to others and in participating in work and other activities. Definitions in the next section will clarify precisely what the domain and foci are when I speak of psychological problems or dysfunction.

There is widespread recognition that current services for mental health are not up to the many challenges. Leaving aside the data and science behind this, we learn from tragic stories in the media of endless missed opportunities for someone in need of it to receive care, someone who also happened to be prone to violence and who then committed some heinous act. A seeming regular flow of violent acts make the news, including shootings in schools, shopping malls, churches, and movie theaters, and targeted killings of law enforcement officers. Not all such instances can be traced to a cause like "the person was mentally ill," which is not much of an explanation anyway. Even so, there are too few mechanisms in place to provide assessments needed to "pick up" individuals with psychological problems or those who might be especially prone to violence. Even if these individuals are identified, the options for treatment and the likelihood of getting into treatment are rather minute, as discussed further in Chapter 2.

All of this can be improved, in principle and in practice. We have at our disposal the means to more effectively identify individuals in need of help, and to provide services with a strong scientific base that are available to us right now. These means can serve as the basis of providing services to improve mental health not just for those dramatic cases that make it to the news but also for all of us—our relatives, siblings, friends, and fellow citizens.

What are all the means we might use that are scientifically based (have evidence) to reduce the personal and social burdens of mental illness? This book provides a rich set of available solutions. These solutions come from focusing on the question rather than on any particular mental health profession or circumscribed set of treatments and what it can contribute. That approach tends to be limiting. For example, clinical psychology is likely to emphasize psychotherapy, psychiatry is likely to emphasize medication, social work is likely to emphasize family therapy—each profession offers more but begins with a limited view about suitable interventions. In truth we need all of the interventions that all professions can provide. Yet arguably the most significant breakthroughs in reducing the burdens of mental illness will come from drawing on a wide range of professions and disciplines (business, entertainment, social policy, and others), as I will elaborate later. Indeed, I will soon make the case that we got ourselves into this mess in part because of limitations in conceptualizing and providing treatment among the mental health professions.

Definitions, Foci, and Guiding Concepts

It is important to address several terms and concepts, some of which are familiar and relatively standard and others less so. These terms serve as a critical reference point related both to the types of problems we are focusing on and the interventions to be applied to them.[3]

PSYCHOLOGICAL DYSFUNCTION: WHAT ARE WE TRYING TO TREAT OR PREVENT?

This book is about interventions, but it is useful to clarify the domain of what we are trying to change, treat, or prevent. At the broadest level, we are focusing on emotions (affect), thought processes (cognitions), and actions (behaviors) that are associated with impairment in daily life. There are many forms this can take, and it is easiest to convey the most familiar type within this broad definition, namely, *psychiatric disorders*. In keeping with diagnostic terminology, I will use this term synonymously with *mental disorders*.

Mental disorders refer to formally recognized symptom patterns that are delineated in the *International Statistical Classification of Diseases and Related Health*

Problems (ICD-10; WHO, 2010) and the *Diagnostic and Statistical Manual of Mental Disorders* (DSM-5; American Psychiatric Association, 2013). These documents codify the criteria for meeting a formally recognized psychiatric diagnosis. Each psychiatric diagnosis requires that the individual client show a specific set of symptoms and usually for a specific duration. There are a few hundred disorders—more than 400 actually, depending a bit on how disorders and subdisorders are counted. This total includes various broad categories (depression, anxiety) and many subtypes or variations within the category. Many of the terms are familiar because they have been popularized by the media, including news and movies in particular (e.g., major depression, autism spectrum disorder, and schizophrenia); most others are much less familiar (e.g., delusional disorder, child-onset fluency disorder [stuttering]). Substance use and abuse disorders are part of mental disorders as reflected in the diagnostic manuals referred to previously. These disorders consist of recurrent use of alcohol and legal and illegal drugs, such as hallucinogens, stimulants, and opioids, that leads to significant impairment. The domains covered in this book include the treatment of psychiatric disorders and substance use and abuse, and I will say more about them in Chapter 2.

The criteria for meeting a disorder have a significant degree of arbitrariness about them. Yet the diagnoses and their criteria are defensible in the following way. We know that individuals who meet criteria for a diagnosis are likely to suffer impairment; that is, some domain of functioning in their everyday lives or their enjoyment of life is interfered with in a significant way. Many of the disorders have been well studied, so that once we know that someone meets criteria for a disorder, we often can say much more about the person's history (the disorder may run in families), his or her future (the likely course of the disorder, such as whether it continues, remits; whether some additional or other mental or physical disorder is likely to emerge), and whether some form of treatment is likely to be helpful. Thus, although there is some arbitrariness of the diagnoses in terms of which criteria are critical and the exact amount of time a given symptom or set of symptoms must be present, it still helps to know whether a person meets certain diagnostic criteria.

This arbitrariness may be most obvious with regard to the cutoff criteria. We know that having symptoms that do not qualify for a specific disorder like major depression, or having many symptoms spanning different disorders while qualifying for no single disorder, still can lead to problems of functioning in daily life and have a long-term poor prognosis. Psychological dysfunction can impair daily living whether or not it rises to the level of or meets criteria for a formal psychiatric diagnosis. Many disorders are on a "spectrum," which means that they vary in degrees. Spectrum also means that one's symptoms may not meet formal requirements for a psychiatric disorder but still cause significant problems. Sometimes the terms *subclinical* dysfunction and *subsyndrome* or *subsyndromal* disorder are used to denote that the symptoms and impairment do not rise to the level of a formal psychiatric diagnosis.[4]

The terms *psychological dysfunction* and *psychological problems* will be used in this book to encompass not just psychiatric disorders but also all psychological domains that can interfere with functioning in daily life. Maladaptive thoughts (cognitions), difficult to control emotions (affect), and actions (behaviors) alone and in combinations can lead to problems in our lives. For example, people may have repeated suicidal thoughts or paranoia, may be a bit too impulsive, or may engage in violent acts. Also, in the face of great stressors (a loved one's death, natural disaster, health scares), coping can readily break down. Functioning in everyday life can be seriously affected, and the informal resources of family and friends may not be sufficient.

There is no single way to encapsulate all of the psychological conditions (indeed, it is likely that trying to do so is in itself problematic), but identifying domains that affect impairment is one unifying concept. Five signs can be delineated to identify a mental health problem:

1. Personality changes (sudden or gradual changes in the way someone behaves);
2. Being agitated (uncharacteristic anger, anxiety, and related states);
3. Being withdrawn (more isolated and disengaged from usual activities);
4. Poor self-care (regarding personal care, decision making, and risky behavior); and
5. Hopelessness (prolonged grief, change from being optimistic, feelings of worthlessness).

These are not formally researched signs but rather are designed to provide a rule of thumb of sorts when it comes to psychological dysfunction (see Campaign to Change Directions, www.changedirections.org/). The focus of the book is on reducing the burdens of psychological conditions broadly, and conditions that meet the five criteria qualify whether or not any instance meets the bar of a formal psychiatric disorder.

In short, my focus with this book is broad. If we want to reduce the burdens of mental illness we should not be limited to formal psychiatric diagnoses but rather ought to include the full range of psychological conditions that lead to impairment or that make life miserable for so many. I certainly do not mean to imply that "everything" constitutes a mental health problem, or that we all ought to be in treatment. Not at all. Rather the point is that many sources of psychological dysfunction impede our functioning and interfere with important activities like jobs and the responsibilities of family life. Most people handle life challenges fine to well, with normal perturbations as crises and tragedies emerge. Again, though, the scope of dysfunction goes well beyond formally recognized psychiatric diagnosis.

To improve the mental health of individuals and of a nation, we must be concerned with the full range of sources of impairment. Yes, it would be a huge breakthrough to, say, eliminate major depression with a single vaccine, as we do with smallpox. This is highly unlikely, but even if it did happen, there remain multiple sources of psychological dysfunction that place a burden on individuals and on society. We need to think big and broad.

PSYCHOSOCIAL INTERVENTIONS

Definition

There is no universal, standard definition of psychosocial or psychological interventions, but one that is a useful point of departure emerged from an Institute of Medicine (IOM) report specifically evaluating psychosocial interventions for mental and substance use disorders (England et al., 2015). Psychosocial interventions are defined as,

> interpersonal or informational activities, techniques, or strategies that target biological, behavioral, cognitive, emotional, interpersonal, social, or environmental factors with the aim of reducing symptoms of these disorders and improving functioning or well-being. These interventions include psychotherapies (e.g., psychodynamic therapy, cognitive-behavioral therapy, interpersonal psychotherapy, problem solving therapy), community-based treatments (e.g., community homes, community-based support groups), vocational rehabilitation, peer support services, and integrated-care interventions (that provide services for physical and mental health and substance use). Interventions can be delivered in a variety of settings (such as outpatient clinics, individual provider offices, primary care clinics, schools, hospitals, community settings, and virtual settings such as telephone and video conferencing). Interventions occur in different formats (such as individual, family, group, computer-based) and can be administered by a variety of providers, from social workers, psychiatrists, and psychologists to religious leaders and peer providers. (England et al., 2015, p. S-4)

A broad definition is needed to accommodate the range of interventions that can be administered to reduce the burdens of mental illness. As the definition conveys, we want to include very traditional interventions (e.g., forms of psychotherapy), advances related to their administration (e.g., use of technology), and population- and policy-based strategies. At the same time, we want to be open to many different interventions and how they are delivered. In fact, all sorts of exciting and innovative intervention options are available, as will be detailed later, that are in keeping with the broad definition of what is applied, by whom, and in what settings.

Goals and Means of Achieving Them

The purpose of psychosocial interventions is to treat or prevent psychological dysfunction as previously described and improve adjustment and adaptive functioning. The broader goal is to address problems that impair functioning of individuals in everyday life. Both treatment and prevention are included as goals. Typically, treatment focuses on a current and identifiable problem; prevention means intervening to avert a problem before it occurs or to lessen the impact. Treatment and prevention can easily be distinguished: a person has a problem and undergoes an intervention to ameliorate it; or a person does not yet have a problem but is at risk for one, and so undergoes an intervention to decrease or eliminate the likelihood of that problem emerging. But treatment and prevention can also blur together. Treatment and prevention go together in other ways and across individuals, as illustrated in the concept referred to as "treatment as prevention" (e.g., Cohen, 2015b, p. 227). For example, medication for individuals who have HIV/AIDS is obviously designed to treat the disease (reduce or eliminate symptoms, prolong life). This is also treatment as prevention because individuals who do not adhere to their medication are more likely to spread HIV to others. Thus treatment of one individual can relate to prevention of disorder among others.

The concept of treatment as prevention arises in psychological problems as well. For example, maternal depression has an enormous impact on child-rearing practices and places the child at risk for later psychiatric disorder (Goodman et al., 2011). We want to treat maternal depression because it is important in its own right. But successful treatment can serve preventive goals, too, by improving child-rearing practices and reducing the likelihood that the child will develop a psychiatric disorder. In any case, the goal of psychosocial interventions is both treatment and prevention. I will emphasize treatment and psychological problems that interfere with functioning. Impaired functioning might be evident in various settings (e.g., school, work, family responsibilities) and types of relations (e.g., family, friends, but also strangers). Prevention certainly is part of the solution in reducing the burdens of mental illness, but the primary emphasis on treatment allows detailed presentation of novel models of care to help individuals in need now.

We could adopt even broader goals for psychosocial interventions beyond reducing psychological impairment. For example, rather than "simply" overcoming depression, anxiety, posttraumatic stress disorder, and other clinical disorders, we might focus on positive domains such as improving mental and physical health and happiness (e.g., Lynn, O'Donohoe, & Lilienfeld, 2015). That is, we would like people to have fulfilling lives and not just an absence of symptoms or conditions that lead to impairment. I will return to this later because it is relevant to the challenge of this book. Even in the treatment research that focuses on psychological problems, there is growing interest in expanding the usual treatment evaluation criteria focusing on symptom reduction to encompass more positive functioning in various spheres of life (e.g., relationships and purposeful and fulfilling activities).

The *means* by which psychosocial interventions achieve change draw on psychological and interpersonal processes. Typically, these means include the use of talk, feedback, modeling of new behaviors, altered decision making, altered cognitions, coping, and emotion regulation, as well as problem-solving strategies, practice and rehearsal, and engagement in specific activities outside of the sessions, often to apply what was learned or practiced in the session. The means can include public health appeals (e.g., pleas to stop smoking cigarettes or driving while intoxicated) or even policy interventions (e.g., increasing taxes on cigarettes, encouraging exercise). In general, the means draw on theory, research, and techniques that can influence human affect (emotions), cognitions (thoughts, attributions, and beliefs), and behavior (actions or what a person actually does).

Psychotherapy is the dominant and most familiar psychosocial intervention even though it is often presented to the public in a stereotypical form that is not quite accurate. Cartoons online and in magazines, newspapers, and greeting cards are omnipresent and invariably depict scenes in which a client is on a couch speaking to a seated therapist. That therapist often is in the image of Sigmund Freud (1856–1939), who founded psychoanalysis, a conceptual view of human functioning as well as a form of therapy. His often-present image is a carryover from yesteryear, and in fact psychoanalysis is not how most therapy works or is conducted, but it is true that current psychotherapy is usually practiced by a mental health professional with a client individually and in person. The goal of the interaction is to help with some sphere of dysfunction.

As for a general definition, psychotherapy consists of a special interaction between two (or more) individuals in which one person (the patient or client) has sought help for a particular problem and in which another person (the therapist) provides conditions to alleviate that person's distress and to improve functioning in everyday life (Garfield, 1980; Walrond-Skinner, 1986). The interaction is designed to alter the feelings, thoughts, attitudes, or actions of the person who has sought or has been brought to treatment. Typically, very special conditions define the interactions of therapist and client.[5] The client usually describes his or her difficulties and life circumstances and the reasons for seeking help. The therapist provides support, acceptance, and encouragement aimed at fostering the interpersonal relationship, as well as systematic experiences (e.g., new ways of behaving through practice, role-playing, homework assignments, advice) designed to produce change. The definition is necessarily general because of the range of approaches and dizzying list of techniques—several hundred—that need to be accommodated, as discussed later. Thus the hundreds of specific treatments (including but not limited to client-centered therapy, multisystemic therapy, graduated exposure, dialectical behavior therapy, mindfulness) occasionally are subsumed under more general rubrics such as individual, group, family, insight-oriented, behavioral, cognitive therapies, humanistic and existential therapies, and others. Many forms of psychotherapy have strong evidence in their behalf and will be discussed and evaluated later.

Psychotherapies are the most commonly used psychosocial intervention for clinical problems. However, it is important to keep in mind the broader focus on psychosocial interventions of which psychotherapy is only a part. The reason has to do with the goal. If we wish to reduce the burdens of psychological impairment to individuals and society, psychotherapy is part of the solution, but probably only a very small part, at least as currently conceived and administered. We begin with the goal of reducing the burdens and pause there. We now ask, "What options are available that might have a scientific base?" We need a definition of *psychosocial interventions* that is open and inclusive, and not restricted to psychotherapies alone.

WHAT IS EXCLUDED FROM PSYCHOSOCIAL INTERVENTIONS?

Excluded from the definition are interventions that use biological and medical means of producing change, such as medication, psychosurgery, electroconvulsive shock therapy, and brain implants and stimulation. These interventions are directed toward psychological functioning (e.g., medication to control hyperactivity, deep brain stimulation or electroconvulsive shock therapy to alter depression). Certainly the most familiar is the use of medication to control symptoms of a large set of disorders and to help people function in everyday life.

Medications for depression, anxiety, and attention deficits and hyperactivity are part of everyday life and in widespread use. Approximately one in five adult Americans takes at least one psychotropic medication. Among women the statistic is one in four (Medco, 2011). Moreover, it appears that the majority of individuals (approximately 68 percent) who receive such medication do not meet criteria for a psychiatric diagnosis (Wiechers et al., 2013). The medications typically are provided by general practice physicians rather than psychiatrists or psychologists licensed to administer medications and trained in mental health. Clearly, medication and other biologically based interventions play an important role in treating mental disorders and are definitely part of the solution to reduce the burdens of mental illness, but I am not taking up medication and other biological interventions here in order to allow more in-depth elaboration of psychosocial interventions, their unique issues, and the range of novel options that are not well known and are rarely used in the United States.

Also excluded from discussion here are interventions directed toward academic and educational objectives. This would include various school and counseling programs and special individual educational programs and experiences aimed at enhancing achievement and school performance. Academic functioning among children and adolescents overlaps with psychiatric disorders in at least two ways. First, psychiatric diagnostic systems specifically include as disorders deficiencies in reading and math, dyslexia, and intellectual disability (e.g., DSM-5, ICD-10). These have been designated as *mental disorders* and can lead to impairment in everyday life. Second, academic functioning overlaps with physical and mental health more generally insofar as they are correlated and predictive. Academic problems (e.g., reading, language, communication) early in life increase the risk for later mental disorder and psychological impairment; mental disorders early in life predict academic dysfunction (e.g., Klein et al., 2012; Mitchel et al., 2006; Robst & Weinberg, 2010). Even so, interventions that focus on education (e.g., improving test scores, grades, achievement in school) as a primary goal will not be covered here, again to allow in-depth discussion of the issues associated with psychosocial interventions and mental disorders.

Psychosocial interventions, especially as considered in this book, reflect a large class of methods that can be used to change clinical dysfunction. They raise special issues and present opportunities that could not be detailed if the book also covered the full range of medications and other biologically based and educationally based procedures. Even so, I will make exceptions by wandering into complementary and alternative interventions (from the standard therapies) as illustrated by comments on diet and exercise, two broad interventions that might well be argued are biologically based. Exceptions will be made to bring in treatments for psychiatric disorders that are not well recognized, prescribed, or used, but could be, and that have supportive evidence arguing for their use.

Purpose of This Book

The purpose of this book is to examine what can be done to reduce the personal and social burdens of mental illness. I have defined two broad domains to achieve that focus. *Psychological problems* are a broad domain that includes mental illnesses that meet formal (well-specified) criteria of psychiatric disorder, but also subclinical dysfunction, that falls below that bar, as well as any facet of affect, cognition, or behavior that impairs functioning in daily life. *Psychosocial interventions* is a broad term to allow us to cover a range of novel interventions that can address those clinical problems. Psychotherapy is a large set of interventions within that broad domain and will be discussed. Yet the book moves well beyond traditional treatments and how they are delivered. Despite remarkable advances in developing psychotherapies, their impact on the overall burdens of mental illness is minimal, a statement I lament, discuss, and support later.

Above and beyond psychotherapy, there are other remarkable opportunities for helping people to overcome impairing conditions, as well as to improve life. These opportunities are held back by various sources of inertia, including conceptualization of both the problems and solutions, professional boundaries and efforts to protect them, and policy limitations. For example, understandably, various mental health professions (primarily psychology, psychiatry, and social work) approach how to provide treatment within the confines and dictates of their disciplines with the tacit question that is equivalent to, "What within my discipline can be used to alleviate the burdens of mental illness for my patients or even for the population of patients in need of care?" In clinical psychology and social work, that can often mean what form of psychotherapy, family therapy, or case work is to be applied? In psychiatry, that can mean what form of medication can be used to help people? There are many exceptions, and the simplification here is merely to convey the point: sometimes professionally dictated formulations of a solution to a problem can be extremely restrictive in what is considered as a viable option for helping people. Also, one can readily justify a given approach. For example, the recommendation of psychotherapy for many problems is reasonable in light of supportive evidence that such treatments can help people. So I do not quibble with the standard treatments one would expect from the mental health professions. Yet more, different, and better interventions are needed if we are to reach people effectively.

This book approaches mental health care from a different point of departure by focusing on the problem rather than on the point of view of a particular profession. That is, given all those who are in need of or who could profit from mental health care, what can be brought to bear to help them? By starting out with the problem rather than with a discipline or profession, one is open to a vast array of interventions from multiple disciplines. This book begins with what we are trying to accomplish and then brings in a range of solutions that go far beyond what is currently being done to help people in need.

The emphasis of the book is on interventions that can be used and that have some evidence on their behalf. Given the range of remedies I mentioned earlier, we need a way to sort out hoaxes, fake treatments, and persuasive gurus who might promote techniques that that have no evidence or that actually violate what we know about interventions and change. Scientific evidence is never perfect, and conclusions we reach from that evidence do not always lead to "do this but not that" guidelines. Nevertheless, evidence accumulates, and based on multiple studies we often learn what treatments are effective or better than standard treatments currently in use. Whatever the flaws of science, the results more reliably surpass opinions, arguments from authority, and fads that may come and go in relation to how to treat problems of mental and physical health. And yet if we only look at evidence, we leave out possible interventions that might be effective but have not been studied. All of this will be taken up with the goal of answering the question: What can be done to reduce the burdens of psychological impairment? The question opens us to a broad range of possibilities, including those that have not emanated from the mental health professions.

2

Scope and Burdens of Psychological Dysfunction

This chapter addresses several key background topics, including the range and types of psychological dysfunctions we experience, the scope of the problems in terms of incidence and prevalence of cases, and the burdens these place on individuals as well as society at large. Essentially, this chapter conveys core features of the mental health crisis and why innovation in developing remedies is so critical.

A simple model that has guided treatment research on psychological dysfunction has four interrelated steps: identify the clinical problem (e.g., anxiety, depression), develop a model of the underpinnings (e.g., causes, bases) of the dysfunction, identify effective treatments, and deliver them to resolve the problem or maintain some level of stability if the problem cannot be resolved. The application of this model is easily seen in the context of physical health for special instances in which causes, treatments, and outcomes are fairly clear. Several examples of physical health maladies (e.g., rabies, broken bones, strep throat) allow for the application of a relatively simple model of diagnosis. These examples make relatively clear the four-step model I have noted. Not all physical health problems follow this, but at least there are clear instances in which the model can be easily applied.

Both the nature of psychological dysfunction and the treatments make this simple model rarely applicable. Diagnosing problems is not so simple; abstract conceptualization of disorders is relatively easy, but proving that the conceptualization actually accounts for the problem is less so. Then, deciding what the treatment ought to be, getting that treatment to people in need, and achieving a particular, predictable, or clear outcome is fuzzy at best. The ambiguities begin with delineating what is to be treated (the diagnosis part) because the range of dysfunctions formally and not formally recognized as mental disorders is vast. Let us delve into the nature of the problems because this will better convey the scope of what we must do to affect the burdens of mental illness, and on what scale we must apply our actions in order to make a difference.

TYPES AND SOURCES OF PSYCHOLOGICAL IMPAIRMENT

Our mental health is challenged in many ways that vary in degrees and duration from the many minor annoyances of everyday life (e.g., transient stressors from our smartphone, incorrect bill for something, temporarily lost keys), to matters more significant (e.g., resolvable misunderstanding in a relationship or at work, move to a new city), and to extremes of dramatic and life-changing experiences (e.g., major relationship break up, loss of a loved one, natural or human-made disasters such as a hurricane or war). These may vary in the extent to which they are enduring in their physical and mental health impact. For many disturbances related to our emotions, thoughts, and actions (e.g., depression, anxiety, substance abuse), often external events can be identified that precipitated the reaction. Yet these disturbances can be and often are enduring.

There is no accepted or single organizing principle to capture the scope of psychological challenges and their impact. For purposes of this book, the primary focus is on psychological characteristics that impede our functioning in everyday life. That could include any trait or characteristic—those of us with annoying social skills or unusually bad manners (or breath) certainly have characteristics that hold us back (e.g., from relationships, jobs, promotions), but this is not the level of impairment that is the focus of this book. Rather, the focus is on mental illness and disorders and closely related domains that impede meeting expectations and carrying out roles. For purposes of presentation, I have grouped the sources of psychological dysfunction into three domains: mental disorders, subclinical dysfunction, and other sources that lead to impairment. Although these are overlapping categories, they are useful in conveying the domains of interest. Further, when it comes to developing and implementing interventions to have broad impact, we want to be sure not to neglect any of the domains that can impair functioning.

Mental Disorders

An Overview

Mental disorders refer to specific patterns of symptoms associated with problems in functioning in daily life and what usually is meant in professional circles when one refers to mental illness. The diagnostic system of the *International Statistical*

Classification of Diseases and Related Health Problems (ICD-10; World Health Organization [WHO], 2010) is the dominant diagnostic system in use worldwide to codify both physical and mental illness.[1] Within that diagnostic system, a *mental disorder* refers to a set of symptoms associated with distress that interferes with or impairs a person's daily functioning. A set of symptoms that appear together is referred to as a *syndrome*. Each of us is familiar with what a syndrome is from our bouts with common physical illnesses. For example, a cold or flu does not usually include one symptom (e.g., I have a runny nose, you have a sore throat, and someone only gets a fever). A cold and the flu (and various diseases, infections, and insults or injuries more generally) have a set of symptoms that go together (syndrome). In fact, accurate diagnoses often depend on identifying the full set of symptoms and hopefully something unique in that pattern that reveals precisely what the syndrome is (and is not). The syndrome can be very important to identify because so many symptoms (e.g., nausea, headache, feeling blah) are common to many disorders; if one sees the full set of symptoms, an accurate diagnosis is much more likely. And in many cases, an accurate diagnosis directly helps in guiding treatment.

The concept of *disorder* is sometimes used to go beyond syndrome by implying more information. With a disorder we know more about it than just a collection of symptoms. Mental "disorders" in this sense are a good illustration. For example, depression includes a set of symptoms that go together (syndrome). Yet depression can be considered a disorder because we know more about it than just co-occurring symptoms. When a person is depressed clinically, we know there is a higher than usual likelihood that depression is in the family history, that the individual may have a higher risk for suicide, that symptoms of the disorder are very likely to remit (go away or be reduced) within a year but then return, and that certain treatments (e.g., some forms of cognitive therapy, some medications) are likely to be effective, as well as many other features. That is, beyond the collection of symptoms (syndrome), we have information about many other features such as likely history, course or pattern of change, and outcome.

A key feature of mental disorders is that they are defined and identified in part because they are associated with significant impairment. That means the symptoms interfere with functioning in various spheres of one's life. That impairment may include distress in social, occupational, or other important activities or increased risk for suffering in some way (e.g., death, pain, or loss of freedom). One can easily see the use of the same term in ways that might or might not count as a disorder. Someone might be depressed today for whatever reason (e.g., weather, horrible night's sleep, his or her partner or significant other began the day with the phrase "we have to talk"). This depression is likely to be transient and may make the person mopey and perhaps irritable. The person gets through the day and feels better tomorrow. At the other extreme is clinical depression (e.g., major depression), the formal diagnosis, in which a person might be virtually immobilized by sadness, stay in bed rather than go to work, and have very negative cognitions and emotions about oneself and the future. This does not turn around in a day or two. This latter level of depression is likely to lead to impairment in many domains (social, work, school). As another example, a person might occasionally use an illicit substance that alters mood, emotions, and behavior. That might be readily distinguished from a substance abuse disorder, in which there is significant dependence on the substance, the substance or obtaining that substance guides or dictates behavior, and there is significant impairment.[2]

Broad groupings are used to encompass various psychiatric disorders. Box 2.1 provides several of the main categories of the ICD-10. Each of these is divided into several categories and then subcategories of different disorders and subtypes leading to more than 400 recognized disorders. Box 2.1 does not convey the level of specificity needed to see how diagnoses "work," or the symptom requirements. Consider one category, mood disorders, listed in Box 2.1. Within that category there are several types of disorders (e.g., manic episode, bipolar disorder, major depressive disorder [single episode or recurrent], and others). Box 2.2 illustrates a description of major depressive disorder to further convey what the syndrome or set of symptoms entails. Finally, I have listed even more concretely the diagnostic criteria that are met for the disorder, along with its varying degrees.

Illustrating one disorder in detail in Boxes 2.1 to 2.3 conveys some of the challenges and arbitrariness of the diagnoses. I have mentioned the cutoff point, which is clearly a salient issue—where should the line be drawn between a mental

---

Box 2.1

Categories That Encompass Mental, Behavioral, and Neurodevelopmental Disorders in the International Classification of Diseases (ICD-10, Version 2016)

- Mental disorders due to known physiological conditions;
- Mental and behavioral disorders due to psychoactive substance use;
- Schizophrenia, schizotypal, delusional, and other nonmood psychotic disorders;
- Mood [affective] disorders;
- Anxiety, dissociative, stress-related, somatoform, and other nonpsychotic mental disorders;
- Behavioral syndromes associated with physiological disturbances and physical factors;
- Disorders of adult personality and behavior;
- Intellectual disabilities;
- Pervasive and specific developmental disorders;
- Behavioral and emotional disorders with onset usually occurring in childhood and adolescence; and
- Unspecified mental disorder.

Note: These are only the broad categories that encompass many subcategories, specific disorders, and subtypes of disorder totaling more than 400 diagnoses in all. A list can be found for the revised (2016) version at http://apps.who.int/classifications/icd10/browse/2016/en.

Box 2.2

Characteristics of Major Depressive Disorder (Single Episode)

Clinical Information

- Depression is a mental disorder characterized by melancholic feelings of grief or unhappiness. It is a mental condition marked by ongoing feelings of sadness, despair, loss of energy, and difficulty dealing with normal daily life. Other symptoms of depression include feelings of worthlessness and hopelessness, loss of pleasure in activities, changes in eating or sleeping habits, and thoughts of death or suicide. Depression can affect anyone and can be successfully treated. Depression affects 15 to 25 percent of cancer patients.
- Depression is an affective disorder marked by dysphoric mood, inactivity, lack of interest, insomnia, feelings of worthlessness, diminished ability to think, and thoughts of suicide. The mood disturbance is prominent and relatively persistent. The term *depression* (emotion) is also used for nonclinical depression.
- Depression is a serious medical illness that involves the brain. It is more than just a feeling of being "down in the dumps" or "blue" for a few days. The feelings associated with depression do not go away; they persist and interfere with the person's everyday life. Symptoms can include:
  - sadness;
  - loss of interest or pleasure in activities you used to enjoy;
  - change in weight;
  - difficulty sleeping or oversleeping;
  - energy loss;
  - feelings of worthlessness; and
  - thoughts of death or suicide.
- Depression is a disorder of the brain. There are a variety of causes, including genetic, environmental, psychological, and biochemical factors.
- Depression usually starts between the ages of 15 and 30 years, and is much more common in women. Women can also get postpartum depression after the birth of a baby. Some people get seasonal affective disorder in the winter. Depression is one part of bipolar disorder.
- Depressive states are usually of moderate intensity, in contrast with major depression present in neurotic and psychotic disorders.
- Marked depression appears in the involution period and is characterized by hallucinations, delusions, paranoia, and agitation.
- Mild depression is not considered clinical depression. For clinical depression, the term *major depression* is used.
- One or more periods of depression may occur in the absence of history of manic or hypomanic episodes; the chronic type lasts two or more years;

and the melancholic type is more severe, has vegetative signs, and responds well to somatic therapy.
- An unpleasant, but not necessarily irrational or pathological, mood state can be characterized by sadness, despair, or discouragement ("the blues"); depression may also involve low self-esteem, social withdrawal, and somatic symptoms such as eating and sleep disturbance.

Source: This information is available in the public domain at www.icd10data.com/ICD10CM/Codes/F01-F99/F30-F39/F32-/F32.9.

Box 2.3

Criteria for Meeting the ICD-10 Diagnosis for Major Depressive Disorder

Key Symptoms

At least one of these, most days, most of the time for at least two weeks:

- Persistent sadness or low mood;
- Loss of interests or pleasure; and
- Fatigue or low energy.

If any of the above is present, ask about associated symptoms:

- Disturbed sleep;
- Poor concentration or indecisiveness;
- Low self-confidence;
- Poor or increased appetite;
- Suicidal thoughts or acts;
- Agitation or slowing of movements; and
- Guilt or self-blame.

The 10 symptoms then define the degree of depression, and management is based on the particular degree:

- Not depressed (fewer than four symptoms);
- Mild depression (four symptoms);
- Moderate depression (five to six symptoms); and
- Severe depression (seven or more symptoms, with or without psychotic symptoms).

Symptoms should be present for a month or more, and every symptom should be present for most of every day.

Source: General Practice Notebook: http://www.gpnotebook.co.uk/simplepage.cfm?ID=x2009112315220 518 2440.

disorder and distress that is not to be considered a disorder? How many symptoms for what duration and how much impairment "count" to meet criteria for a diagnosis? At the margins (absolutely no symptoms at all versus many of the symptoms that are severe and on a daily basis) "having" or not having a diagnosis is clear. Most of the patterns of symptoms people have are not at these margins.

Whether a given individual meets these criteria can be measured by standardized interviews that have been developed specifically for this purpose.[3] A trained mental health professional interviews the client (or child and parent of a child) and identifies whether the individual meets criteria for a particular symptom as well as the severity and duration of the symptom. The interview covers multiple disorders and the symptoms of which they are comprised. At the end of the interview, one can decide whether the client meets criteria for no, one, or multiple disorders. All of this can be very systematic but still weak, in part because of the reliance on subjective reporting. (At some distant point these will be confirmable and complemented by laboratory tests, the way many physical diseases are evaluated.) Often in clinical work, as opposed to research, diagnostic labels are applied informally and without suitable documentation or systematic assessment. The diagnostic labels are not trivial and may even determine whether treatment will be reimbursed by insurance or other third-party payer.

The key point is that there are numerous identifiable mental disorders—hundreds as I noted previously. One can immediately see the challenge; if there are hundreds of different disorders and subtypes, do we have treatments to address them all? Of course, we are not looking for just any treatments but for ones with some evidence that they can make a difference. The main message is that many disorders have been identified and require intervention.

Critical Issues and Challenges

Many disorders (e.g., schizophrenia, major depression, anxiety disorders) and their subtypes and variations have been well studied. Even so, many basic issues remain to be resolved. I note six such issues briefly because they have implications for developing interventions and deciding what to treat.

First, what are "mental disorders" and what does "mental" even mean? If nothing biological in nature (brain assault or injury) can be found to explain one's psychological symptoms, that must mean the problems emerge from another source, namely, psychological or interpersonal processes. These processes can include conflicts, unexpressed emotions, or various deficiencies in one's psychological development that express themselves as symptoms of mental disorders (e.g., delusions, anxiety, aggression). We know now that not finding biological factors does not mean such factors are absent. Decades ago, before the availability of fine-grained analyses of the brain and genome, many differences among individuals with and without psychological disorders could not be detected. Also, environmental influences (e.g., related to parenting, exposure to domestic violence, poor diet) can have both biological and psychological effects. Fast-forward to current science: we now recognize that "mental" (or psychological) versus "physical" is a difficult distinction to maintain and that many nuanced differences in biological structures and functions can distinguish mental states and disorders.

Psychological and biological characteristics blend, influence each other, and so on. We know this from everyday life—having a cold or flu (physical condition) is associated with being grumpy and irritable (psychological condition). Being stressed from daily life (psychological condition) can really interrupt sleep and, if enduring, can even speed up aging (e.g., physical condition). Scientific advances reveal that multiple characteristics of the brain (structure and functioning), hormones, neurotransmitters, and genetics are among physical characteristics that are associated with mental disorders. Now there is clear recognition that mental disorders have underlying biological and psychological processes and that these processes relate to each other. There is some effort to even replace the term *mental disorders* with *brain disorders* or *brain circuit disorders* (Insel & Cuthbert, 2015). The latter terms are far from catching on, but they convey an effort to shift the focus from "mental" and to better recognize the integration of psychological and biological processes.

Second, the disorders as currently formulated in diagnostic systems are not validated by well-studied objective laboratory tests that go beyond delineating symptoms. Consider physical disorders as a comparison. We can say that polio, breast cancer, and stroke are distinct conditions that can be readily evaluated by laboratory tests to make the diagnosis (e.g., blood tests, biopsy, neurological examination). True, laboratory tests are far from perfect. Occasionally, tests indicate that people have an illness when in fact they do not (false positives), or the reverse (false negatives). Many different disorders can have overlapping or common symptoms (e.g., headache, fever, nausea, diarrhea), necessitating further laboratory tests to straighten out their underlying bases (e.g., cause) or subtype, and to rule out other possible disorders along the way.

In contrast, for mental disorders, there is a common set of labels (diagnoses) but no set of laboratory tests to delineate the various disorders and their subtypes (Insel, 2013). Self-report or other-report (e.g., relatives), questionnaires, and interviews are commonly used for psychiatric diagnosis, if a systematic measure is used at all. These have enormous limitations. Questionnaires and interviews are too blunt an instrument and are limited by "normal" perceptual, cognitive, and memory biases. We need more objective measures (e.g., psychological tests of perception, cognition, brain functioning and circuitry, neurotransmitter function, genome data) to clarify diagnoses and the various subtypes that might exist.

Third, saying that a disorder is a syndrome or group of symptoms that go together masks a curious dilemma. Many individuals with the "same" disorder may barely resemble one another. The reason is that to meet criteria for a diagnosis, one usually must experience a few symptoms from a longer list of symptoms. This means that two individuals could have the diagnosis but no overlapping symptoms. For example, for posttraumatic stress disorder (PTSD; DSM-5), over 20 symptoms are delineated and form more than 10,000 combinations to meet the diagnosis. For conduct disorder (aggressive and antisocial behavior), more than 32,000 symptom combinations are possible for individuals to meet the diagnosis. That means a small football stadium filled with children diagnosed with conduct disorder might include thousands who do not share the same symptom pattern! In general, diagnoses may allow too much heterogeneity or may not be the most meaningful or useful way to classify symptom groupings.

Fourth, for years, disorders have been viewed as distinct. That is, various subtypes of depression are separate from one another, as are larger designations such as depression and anxiety. Two major lines of work have challenged this. To begin, many disorders go together, a phenomenon referred to as *comorbidity*. If a person has one disorder, it is very likely that he or she will have another disorder, too (e.g., Kessler et al., 1994; Wichstrøm et al., 2012). Second, specific patterns are evident, so some disorders seem to be connected or go together (e.g., depression and anxiety; anorexia and bulimia; attention-deficit hyperactivity disorder and conduct disorder). That means that meeting criteria for one of these disorders increases the likelihood of also meeting criteria for the other one. And one can have multiple disorders. For example, at an outpatient clinic where I have worked, approximately 70 percent of the children meet criteria for two or more psychiatric disorders (range of 0 to 5 disorders; Kazdin, 2017a). Having one disorder does not mean a person inevitably will have the other disorder, but many disorders are comorbid. That suggests that perhaps disorders are not so separate after all or maybe that we are not delineating them in ways that make the most sense.

Fifth, for many years, disorders have been regarded as all or nothing—one does or does not have that disorder. That is, a person is clinically depressed or not based on qualifying criteria. Over the years, the continuity and dimensional nature of diagnoses have begun to dominate our views (e.g., Kotov et al., 2017). Disorders now are regarded as being on a spectrum or continuum. In the public media, this has been prominent in relation to the diagnosis of *autism spectrum disorder* (ASD), a term substituted for what used to be called autism. For many other disorders, there are varying degrees in severity and number of symptoms. Major depression (Box 2.3) shows this nicely with an effort to include what is needed for the diagnosis (must have these symptoms) while also recognizing varying degrees of them. The acknowledgment of a spectrum is important but also raises others issues for us in relation to who is in need of or could profit from treatment.

A final challenge to mention is the role of culture, ethnicity, and sex in relation to diagnosis. Here, the question is whether a diagnosis or the criteria for a diagnosis are universal or if they vary as a function of one of these variables. In fact, symptoms and impairment can vary as a function of cultural norms and values (Alarcón, 2009; Lewis-Fernández & Aggarwal, 2013). Also, the rates of dysfunction for a given disorder can vary greatly across cultures (Kessler et al., 2009), as mentioned later in the chapter. Even so, there are many common symptoms, risk factors, and impairments associated with a given disorder across ethnic and cultural groups (e.g., Kessler & Bromet, 2013). Certainly, a challenge in providing services begins with identifying what is to be "treated," who has what sort of problem, and how individuals view what we might label as "problems" or "symptoms."

Researchers are actively investigating diverse facets of mental disorders using the latest technologies to evaluate the brain and genes, and at increasingly fine-grained analyses (e.g., molecular changes, brain networks, and circuits and how they develop to produce clinical dysfunction). There is also some interest in moving away from traditional diagnostic classification as reflected by the ICD-10 and DSM-5. A relatively new and increasingly dominant diagnostic model of elaborating mental disorders is referred to as *Research Domain Criteria* (RDoC; Cuthbert & Insel, 2013). RDoC has the goal of identifying core psychological and biological processes that result in clinical dysfunction. RDoC takes a basic science approach, asking what the underlying psychological (e.g., perception, memory, learning) and biological (e.g., genetic, brain circuitry, neurohumor) processes are that characterize, predict, and may be causally related to mental illness. While the ICD-10 and DSM-5 are used often in research, they are most heavily relied on in clinical work and patient care. Indeed, diagnosis in clinical work often is essential for reimbursement from insurance companies. Currently, RDoC is not used to diagnose disorders in the context of research (e.g., describing participants in a study, selecting cases for comparing one group to another) or in clinical practice. Rather, the goal of RDoC is to develop a stronger scientific base for understanding disorders; this might well change the way domains of dysfunction or disorders are delineated, eradicating many of the problems I have highlighted with current diagnostic systems.

I mention key challenges in the context of this chapter because of their implications for identifying effective interventions that can reach people in need. Traditionally, treatment has focused on devising specific interventions for specific disorders. Yet, if rates of comorbidity are high, maybe such targeted efforts are misplaced. Anyone we treat may have some other disorder, too. Do we target both illnesses at the same time, or one after the other? And which one first? Similarly, if there are common or overlapping symptoms or underlying features (e.g., etiology, risk, genetic and environmental factors), do we want treatments that focus on these commonalities? That, too, would move us away from specific treatments for specific disorders. Finally, if disorders are on a spectrum, that means more individuals than we thought might be in need of treatment or might be experiencing disability of some kind. Perhaps we are underestimating the range of individuals in need of treatment. The treatment implications of these kinds of diagnostic issues are of central concern to us here.

Although fundamental questions about mental disorders and their diagnoses remain, the immediate task before us is clear. Millions of individuals in the United States and millions more worldwide experience mental disorders as delineated in the standard diagnostic systems. Our challenge is two-fold: to understand the nature of the disorders and to develop interventions to ameliorate them. While basic research is underway to better understand disorders, we can effectively treat and prevent many of them.

Other Sources of Dysfunction

Subclinical Disorders

Mental disorders that are formally recognized in diagnostic systems are not the only source of dysfunctions that warrant intervention. Sources of dysfunction that do not meet the criteria for a formal psychiatric diagnosis are sometimes referred to, somewhat oxymoronically, as *subclinical disorders* (if we know "sub" clinical disorders are associated with dysfunction, then we ought to include them in formal diagnoses and call them "clinical," not subclinical, mental disorders). If they do not really lead to dysfunction in everyday life, then why are we calling them "clinical"? These are reasonable questions.

The fact is that people often meet some or many, but not all, of the criteria for a particular diagnosis. Yet that does not mean they are free of dysfunction. Missing one or two criteria for a formal diagnosis may still be associated with current and long-term impairment. The term *subsyndromal* also is used in these cases, and I find this term somewhat more informative. Diagnoses reflect a collection of symptoms that go together—a *syndrome,* a term used with both mental and physical disorders. Understandably, patterns of dysfunction that do not include all the symptoms or to a required degree of severity fall "under" formal diagnoses (hence "sub" syndromes). Nevertheless, I will use the broader term *subclinical* here, in part because the utility and validity of the "syndromes" are in question, and there is no need to perpetuate them here.

Subclinical conditions are common, even though everyday use of the term is usually not. For example, in medicine, the prefix "pre" is sometimes used to denote a condition for which one has symptoms or laboratory test results that depart or differ from "normal" levels, but not enough to meet criteria for the diagnosis. Pre-diabetes is one example, pre-cancerous is another. In each case, one is either above or below "normal" on critical measures, but does not have the full-fledged disorder. These conditions are important to identify because they put people at risk for the full-fledged disorder; it should be monitored closely in case conditions or test results draw closer to a formal diagnosis.

To return to mental disorders, we already discussed the notion of disorders being on a spectrum or a continuum. As an illustration, consider the diagnosis of major depression (Box 2.3). We can see that degrees of depressive symptoms are acknowledged and receive different labels, but the cutoffs for the different labels themselves can be challenged. If someone has depressive symptoms for two rather than three months, or five rather than six symptoms, are these meaningful differences? The distinctions do not have a defensible evidence base—they are arbitrary. That may be helpful in some way: for example, insurance companies will reimburse the costs of treatment only if one qualifies formally for a disorder; in that case, strict qualifications for what is or is not to be reimbursed is understandable, whether or not the cutoff makes any sense scientifically. At the same time, if we are to succeed in reducing the burdens of psychological dysfunction on a large scale, we must shake off such arbitrary systems of classification and focus on who really needs help.

Subclinical can mean one is experiencing dysfunction in everyday life. For example, subclinical levels of depression are associated with unique brain activation patterns related to depression (processing of emotions), decreases in the quality of life, more thoughts about committing suicide, increased death rates, greater use of health care services, and greater costs to society, when contrasted with individuals who do not have these levels of depression (e.g., Modinos et al.,

2013; Rodríguez et al., 2012). Similarly, many individuals may experience subclinical levels of eating disorders (anorexia nervosa, bulimia, and binge-eating disorder). Such individuals may display other sources of dysfunction, including symptoms of anxiety and depression, subclinical or otherwise (e.g., Touchette et al., 2011).

There is no need to elaborate multiple subclinical dysfunctions except to convey that missing the cutoff or diagnostic criteria for a disorder is no guarantee of very much, and one's condition can still be associated with short- and long-term consequences and impairment. In the short-term, many people are miserable who do not meet criteria for a disorder. Meeting or not meeting the criteria is moot if one experiences impairment in daily functioning (e.g., relationships, meeting role expectations). Some form of intervention could make a difference. Moreover, we should be providing treatment broadly because of long-term issues. Subclinical dysfunction can predict the onset of formal psychiatric diagnosis (e.g., subclinical schizophrenia to schizophrenia; subclinical depression to major depression) and can predict other diagnoses (e.g., subclinical anxiety to Bulimia) (e.g., Pine et al., 1999; Wolitzky-Taylor et al., 2014). Clearly, we must begin providing interventions for subclinical levels of disorders. Some research has already been done in this area (e.g., Cuijpers et al., 2014), but we still do not know long-term benefits (for instance, whether early treatment prevents later dysfunction and prevents earlier than expected death, another characteristic of mental disorders).

Leaving aside psychiatric diagnosis and so-called subclinical variations of these diagnoses, there are still other sources of dysfunction. I use "other sources" as a catchall to capture problems that can impede functioning in everyday life. They are familiar concepts, but the range of impairments with which they are associated often is less so. Familiar or not—they can lead to significant problems, whether or not they are mental disorders or almost mental (subclinical) disorders.

Stress and Distress

Stress is ubiquitous in everyday life and can vary in degree, duration, and severity. Researchers make fine-grained distinctions to classify different components of stress and a variety of types and degrees (see Wheaton & Montazer, 2010). Stressors, stress, and distress are three related and intertwined concepts. *Stressors* are those conditions that pose threats, challenges, and demands to the individual. Often these are unpredictable or uncontrollable events or conditions and can include natural disasters and family catastrophe, as well as more mundane events such as examinations, fender benders, break up of relationships). Large and small alike, stressors tax one's coping abilities.

Stress refers to the psychological and biological reactions to stressors, which can vary in many ways that are adaptive or maladaptive. Temporary worry, loss of sleep for night or two, and engaging with one's support system are common reactions. They are short lived and usually do not impede our functioning. *Distress* often is reserved for maladaptive consequences, including the presence of symptoms such as anxiety and depression.[4] Distress is a reaction that does interfere with functioning in some way. As with other concepts, stress and distress are on a continuum, and whether and when one's functioning is impaired is a judgment call if not extreme. Yet stress can be readily distinguished from distress. This can be dramatically illustrated by the impact of traumatic stressors (e.g., rape, exposure to war or to a natural disaster), exposure to which can precipitate the onset of PTSD, a formally recognized psychiatric diagnosis with a variety of symptoms (e.g., severe emotional distress; re-experiencing the traumatic event through flashbacks and dreams; avoiding all reminders of the event, including places and people). *Adjustment disorder* can also be a reaction to stress, and this term is used occasionally when symptoms associated with some other disorder (like anxiety or depression) can be traced to a particular event and the reaction is likely to be transient.

The point in noting these diagnoses is to convey that stress is already included in psychiatric diagnosis (see Maercker et al., 2013). I introduce stress here because less extreme forms that do not precipitate a formal psychiatric disorder can nevertheless have a significant impact on physical and mental health and can lead to distress. For example, enduring stress reactions can harm the immune system such that people are less able to ward off infection and inflammation. This is not minor; inflammation is a key factor in many diseases (arthritis, diabetes, heart disease, cancer, Alzheimer's disease, and others). Apart from the immune system, enduring stress can speed up the process of aging at the cellular and chromosomal levels (e.g., Shalev et al., 2013). Stress is also strongly associated with earlier than expected death (Forman-Hoffman et al., 2014).

In short, distress can be such that individuals meet criteria for some psychiatric disorder. The stress I mention here falls into the category of subclinical disorders, but is broader because it extends well beyond all disorders. I treat it separately in part because it is well studied, and the extent to which people experience stress is somewhat surprising. Also, stress reactions increase risk for a formal psychiatric disorder and can indeed precipitate depression and suicide. Thus, in the context of reducing the burdens of mental illness, alleviating stress should play an important role.

Loneliness

Loneliness is a well-studied topic even though it is not usually considered in the context of psychological conditions worthy of intervention (see Cacioppo & Patrick, 2008). Yet loneliness can have significant mental and physical health consequences and hence lead to impairment. *Loneliness* refers to the subjective experience of being socially isolated. It is important to clarify that this is not necessarily *being* socially isolated or having no or just a few number of social contacts. Rather, loneliness is how people experience the world and how they feel—not objectively whether they are socializing or socially isolated, are in a relationship, or have many contacts with others. If loneliness is enduring, all sorts of other consequences follow.

In passing, it is worth noting that social isolation, which is the objective fact that an individual does not have social contacts, also has untoward long-term consequences (e.g., increased rates of death earlier than life expectancy) (Holt-Lunstad et al., 2015). So experiencing loneliness and in fact being socially isolated would be a particularly onerous combination in relation to health. Yet the distinction is important to maintain. Perhaps the distinction is most poignantly illustrated by a decades-long marriage in which two people are objectively in a relationship even though one feels lonely and isolated and has felt that way for some time.

As with stress, a brief bout of loneliness is not necessarily a problem. Enduring loneliness is the critical state, though there is no exact way to define "enduring" because it may vary from individual to individual. Yet one can say a lot about the characteristics of individuals who are lonely. To begin, people who are lonely have physiological characteristics that are indicative of stress or being in a state of alert or responding to threat (e.g., measures of cortisol and epinephrine in saliva and urine) (see Cacioppo, Capitanio, & Cacioppo, 2014). Brain characteristics associated with loneliness include diminished responsiveness or less activation in the reward circuits (ventral striatum) in response to positive social cues (smiling faces), and reduced executive function (prefontal cortex). Genetic studies show that loneliness has a heritable component. This does not mean it is inevitable, but parent history of loneliness merely places offspring at greater risk for being lonely themselves. Of course, environmental characteristics contribute to loneliness. For example, college first-year students are at higher risk for loneliness. Students who begin college are away from their families and friends and have yet to connect with others who would reduce or halt the duration of loneliness (Wei, Russell, & Zakallik, 2005). Here is a case where subjective experience (loneliness) and objective facts (few real social contacts) converge. Colleges and universities do not usually focus on "loneliness," but still offer support (e.g., provide precollege experiences weeks before first-year students begin their initial term, pair new students with upper classmates to have someone close by, have various welcoming gatherings, parties, and events with free food, plastic cups, and other rah-rah university identity paraphernalia) to foster connections and opportunities to meet one's peers, all designed to enmesh new students with others right away and help with the transition.

Perhaps the most dramatic and unexpected findings on social isolation might be those related to physical health. People who are lonely show gene activity that diminishes their ability to respond to inflammation and to defend against viruses. This is a huge disability and may explain why the lonely are more susceptible to viruses (from the common cold to HIV) and cardiovascular disease (which is related to inflammation). It should be no surprise, then, that longitudinal research evaluating people as they age shows earlier than expected death among those who are lonely (Luo et al., 2012). The impact of loneliness on risk for death is estimated to be equal to that of cigarette smoking and more than that associated with obesity or physical inactivity. Being lonely, it turns out, is bad for one's physical health. Perhaps it does not come as a surprise that loneliness has consequences associated with mental health, too. As one example of many available, depression, anxiety, aggression, and suicidality (thoughts and attempts) are all much greater among individuals who are lonely (Cacioppo et al., 2015; Lasgaard et al., 2011; Schinka et al., 2013; Stravynski & Boyer, 2001).

The impact of loneliness on both physical and mental health supports the notion that in considering the mental health needs of a nation, the burdens and challenges of psychological dysfunction extend well beyond formally delineated psychiatric disorders or even subclinical disorders. Misery and impairment need not result in a formal diagnosis of mental disorder or a subclinical counterpart. Stress and loneliness may be associated with other disorders and may even play a role in bringing on a disorder, yet they represent sources of impairment in their own right because of their physical and mental health consequences, huge personal costs (misery, lost days of health and work), and monetary costs to society (e.g., physical health care that increased vulnerability to serious disease).

Suicide

Suicide is a huge problem in the United States and worldwide. The WHO estimates that by the year 2020, approximately 1.5 million individuals will complete suicide annually, with 10 to 20 times more than that attempting suicide. This translates to one suicide occurring in the world every 20 seconds and one attempt every two seconds (Bertolote & Fleischmann, 2015; WHO, 2014b). These numbers are particularly noteworthy because suicide as a cause of death is estimated to be greatly underreported, by 20 to 100 percent. Suicide attempt is included in diagnostic systems as a complication or symptom of other disorders (mostly mood disorders and less often as a complication of schizophrenia and substance use disorder) and as a diagnosis in its own right.

Although suicide is included in diagnostic systems, it is not covered well and not agreed on as a mental disorder. Many individuals (mean across multiple countries is about 37 percent) who complete suicide have no history of mental disorder, but the percentage varies widely among different countries (Milner, Svetcic, & De Leo, 2013). We will focus on psychosocial interventions with the goal of addressing multiple sources of dysfunction, impairment, and conditions leading to injury and death. Reducing the personal misery and conditions leading to suicide attempt certainly qualifies as a critical focus.

General Comments

My purpose here has been to demonstrate that not all conditions associated with psychological impairment fall squarely within psychiatric diagnoses in their clinical and subclinical ranges. Our goal as a society must be to reduce the burdens that psychological conditions can cause. Central to that is to focus not only on well-studied mental disorders (e.g., depression, schizophrenia) but also on other impairing conditions. Many of these other conditions lead to impairment in daily functioning and also increase the risk for the emergence of mental disorders that are more formally recognized.

Co-occurring Mental and Physical Dysfunction

Mental and physical health are inextricably related. A Latin phrase derived from the Roman poet Juvenal of the late first and early second century is a familiar way

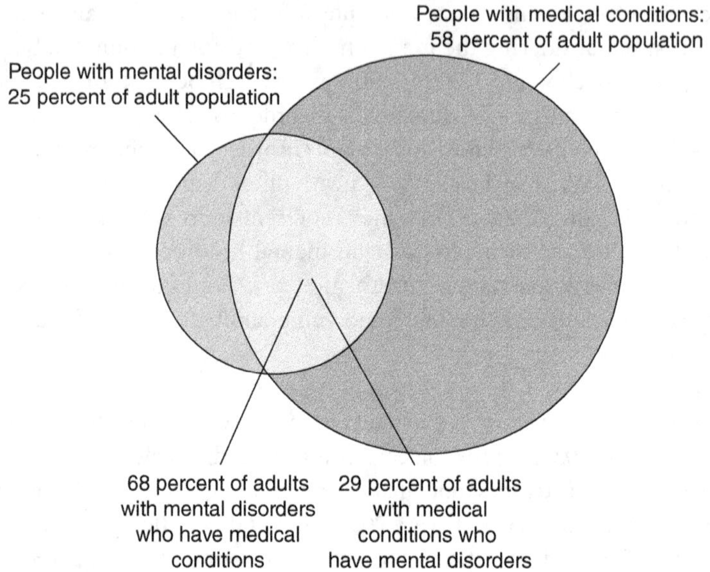

Figure 2.1 Percentage of adults with medical disorders and/or medical conditions.
SOURCE: Alegria M, Jackson JS, Kessler RC, Takeuchi D. National Comorbidity Survey Replication (NCS-R), 2001–2003. Ann Arbor, MI: Interuniversity Consortium for Political and Social Research, 2003. Reprinted with permission.

in which this relationship is summarized, "*Mens sana in corpore sano*" (Juvenal, *The Satires*, #10). Often this is translated as "a sound mind in a sound body" and then interpreted to reflect the idea that both go together. It is easy to make the scientific case that mental and physical health go together, but that does not appear to be Juvenal's meaning by the phrase.[5]

Figure 2.1 provides an excellent summary of the large-scale characterization of health in the United States (Alegria et al., 2003; Goodell, Druss, & Walker, 2011). As one can see from the left side of the figure, approximately 25 percent of the population (12-month prevalence) meet criteria for at least one psychiatric disorder, a point we will discuss further in this chapter. Of those individuals, 68 percent also have medical conditions. Consider the larger circle (on the right side) that conveys 58 percent of individuals in the United States have a medical condition. Of these, 29 percent also have mental disorders. Clearly, on a large scale, one can see that, in fact, having one type of disorder (mental or medical) is linked to an increased likelihood of having another.

The relationship between mental disorders and physical health is perhaps most poignantly illuminated by their relation to mortality. Large-scale studies involving thousands of participants have shown that people with a mental disorder die much earlier than their life expectancy (compared with those who have no disorder; Nordentoft et al., 2013). The reduction in life expectancy was 15 years for women and 20 years for men. To build on the data presented in Figure 2.1, clearly not only do individuals with mental disorders have higher rates of physical disorders, they are also likely to die much earlier than otherwise would be expected.

I am focusing on people with mental disorders and their physical health and mortality, but we could also begin with physical conditions and examine their mental health consequences and associated features. For example, a national survey in the United States revealed that an estimated 25.3 million adults (11.2 percent of the population) experience daily pain and have had that pain for at least the preceding 3 months (National Institutes of Health, 2015). We know from rather extensive research in the United States and across several nations that individuals with pain have higher rates of mental disorders (e.g., Demyttenaere et al., 2007; McWilliams, Goodwin, & Cox, 2004). Research has gone beyond establishing the general association; for example, depression and pain often go together: one increases the likelihood of the other, and both conditions share common biological pathways and neurotransmitters (Bair et al., 2003).

What is it about having a mental disorder that leads to physical illness and early death? No doubt multiple factors can explain the connection. For example, we know that people with a mental disorder are much more likely to smoke cigarettes and that alone could be one critical connection (e.g., Stanton et al., 2015). Other factors could be involved as well, such as not adhering to medical treatment regimens, engaging in behaviors (such as substance use and abuse) that carry their own risks (like overdose, becoming infected by dirty needles, higher rates of suicide), and having a weakened immune system; these are all associated with having a mental disorder and could help explain early mortality.

Consider the example of a single disorder, depression, to understand how intertwined physical and mental disorders can be. Among people with a physical illness, depression is the most common form of psychiatric disorder (Steptoe, 2007). Moreover, depression can exacerbate many other conditions. For instance, individuals who have HIV, diabetes, and other chronic diseases are much less likely to take their medications if they are depressed, which could also help explain why they die earlier than expected (e.g., Gonzalez et al., 2008, 2011). Women who have breast cancer have a lower rate of survival (over the next 5 years) if they have a prior history of depression (Suppli et al., 2016). The basis for this correlation is not known, but it could be that depression is associated with not carrying out treatment (e.g., missing treatment, not taking medications) or suicidal thoughts that may also interfere with seeking or adhering to treatment.

A robust set of findings also connects depression and heart disease. Individuals who are depressed are much more likely to have a heart attack than are those who are not depressed (Lichtman et al., 2014; Nemeroff & Goldschmidt-Clermont, 2012). And among individuals who have a heart attack, those who are also depressed are approximately three times more likely to die from a future heart attack than those who had an attack but are not depressed (Bush et al., 2005). This example reveals not only the connection between physical and mental health but also that connection's bidirectional nature—each exerts some influence on the other. The connection between depression and heart disease has feasible bases in specific areas of the brain and in hormone functioning that could affect both, although this is not yet firmly established (see Adelborg et al., 2016).

In the health care of a nation, it is clear that mental and physical health often must be considered together. It is likely that those who have mental health problems as their dominant source of impairment, and who are in a mental health care system, are likely to have their physical health needs less well attended to, merely by virtue of the system in which they are seen. Similarly, individuals with physical illness are less likely to have their mental health needs met. Of course, there are important exceptions (e.g., most cancer treatment involves opportunities for mental health care, including support groups, psychotherapy, and antidepressant or antianxiety medication). Mental health care may warrant much greater attention in medical cases in which psychological symptoms (like depression or anxiety) might reduce adherence to recommended treatments, increase the likelihood of engaging in risky behaviors (cigarette smoking, alcohol abuse), or have untoward effects on other lifestyle habits (e.g., poor diet, not exercising) that might exacerbate the medical conditions.

SCOPE OF CLINICAL DYSFUNCTION

As discussed, there are the hundreds of formally recognized psychiatric disorders, subclinical sources of dysfunction, and many other instances in which psychological functioning is associated with impairment in daily functioning. Another critical question to address is, How many people are experiencing psychological dysfunction? Obviously, if the number and proportion of people suffering within a given population is small, our challenge in providing services is commensurately small. But in reality the number and proportion of the population with the sources of dysfunction I have described is enormous, and there are more than enough data to support this.

Mental Disorders

Research has shown us the prevalence of mental disorders. Two common metrics are prevalence within a given period of time (often within the past year) and over the course of one's life. Over the past approximately 50 years, surveys have evaluated prevalence of mental disorders throughout the world (Steel et al., 2014). Changes in the diagnostic criteria for many disorders, the emergence of newly defined disorders and elimination of others, different methods of assessment (in-person versus phone interviews; retrospective versus prospective studies), and the actual instruments (questionnaires) that many of the surveys use mean that there is no single definitive number. Nevertheless, one finding is consistent: mental disorders are highly prevalent in the United States and worldwide.

A series of ongoing studies, part of the World Mental Health Survey, an initiative from the WHO, periodically assesses mental, substance use, and behavioral problems in multiple countries (see www.hcp.med.harvard.edu/wmh/). As an example, in one report, 12-month and lifetime prevalence rates of mental disorder were evaluated among 28 countries (e.g., United States, Mexico, Nigeria, South Africa, France, Ukraine, Japan, New Zealand) from multiple regions of the world. Within a one-year period, prevalence ranged from 6 percent (Nigeria) to 27 percent (United States). Lifetime prevalence ranged from a low of 12 percent to a high of 47.4 percent (same countries, respectively) (Kessler et al., 2007, 2009). In general, prevalence of disorders was generally higher in Western developed countries than in developing countries.

In addition to the WHO surveys, there have been others. In the United States, the most visible has been an ongoing program of research known as the National Comorbidity Studies.[6] Multiple studies within this project have examined the prevalence of specific disorders and severity and impairment, as well as prevalence by sex, age group, and other factors. For example, according to two reports on the US population, the 12-month prevalence of any disorder was 26 percent (Kessler, Chiu, et al., 2005). Lifetime prevalence was 46 percent, again close to one-half of the population (Kessler, Berglund, et al., 2005). The breakdown of prevalence by disorders is as follows: anxiety disorders, 28.8 percent; mood disorders, 20.8 percent; impulse-control disorders, 24.8 percent; substance use disorders, 14.6 percent; any disorder, 46.4 percent. (Of course, these percentages for individual disorders surpass lifetime rates because an individual can meet criteria for more than one disorder.) Median age of onset is much earlier for anxiety (11 years) and impulse-control (11 years) disorders than for substance use (20 years) and mood (30 years) disorders. Half of all lifetime cases (persons with a disorder) start by age 14 years, and 75 percent start by age 24 years.

Other large-scale surveys have been completed as well, and they vary in many ways (e.g., area of the world that is sampled, type of disorder that is studied, and diagnostic system used [versions of DSM, ICD]). As two illustrations, a large-scale evaluation in the European Union (EU) included data from all member states ($N = 27$) plus Switzerland, Iceland, and Norway (Wittchen et al., 2011). In a given year, 38.2 percent of the EU population suffered from a mental disorder. That corresponded to approximately 165 million people, from children to older adults.

Many studies focus on particular types of disorders rather than the full range. The purpose is often to identify characteristics (e.g., age, sociodemographic variables, age of onset) unique to the disorders. For example, an ongoing large-scale study in the United States is referred to as the National Epidemiological Survey, which provides periodic reports on mental and substance use disorders and draws on a nationally representative sample of thousands of adults (18 years and older). In one report from the survey, prevalence rates for major depressive disorders were 5.3 percent and 13.2 percent for 12-month and lifetime disorders, respectively (Hasin et al., 2005). Higher rates of depression were associated with being female, Native American, middle-aged, widowed, or separated or divorced, or having a low income. Lower rates were associated with being Asian, Hispanic, or African American. Both current and lifetime major depressive disorders were significantly associated with other psychiatric disorders, notably substance dependence, panic and generalized anxiety disorder, and several personality disorders. Another report from the same survey focused on alcohol use disorders. Among adults in the United States, 13.9 percent of the population met criteria for the disorder during a 12-month period; for lifetime this climbed to 29.1 percent (Grant et al., 2015). These numbers do not include all substance abuse (drugs, tobacco) but rather *just* alcohol abuse.

The programs of research in the United States and worldwide that study prevalence have generated remarkable data sets, with my illustrations sampling only a few. The purpose here is to make the case that many people at a given point in time and over the course of their lives will meet criteria for at least one psychiatric disorder. The percentages are astounding, and given the US population of more than 325 million (as I write this; see http://www.census.gov/popclock/), approximately 81 million people in any given year (25 percent of the population) and 163 million over the course of their life (50 percent of the population) meet criteria for a psychiatric disorder—and these are conservative estimates; some disorders (e.g., schizophrenia) often are left out of the surveys, and subclinical disorders usually are omitted. Some of the reports even show higher lifetime rates (www.hcp.med.harvard.edu/ncs/ftpdir/NCS-R_Lifetime_Prevalence_Estimates.pdf).

One must exercise caution in citing statistics like these because diagnostic systems, the number of disorders within them, how individual disorders are defined, and methods of assessment all can influence the numbers; so can whether one asks individuals retrospectively what their problems were or monitors these prospectively over time (Moffitt et al., 2010). Nevertheless, the conclusion is clear: the prevalence data are astounding whether addressing current disorders (e.g., 12 months) or those experienced over a lifetime. Variations in diagnostic systems and methods of assessment cannot detract from that conclusion.

Additional Sources of Dysfunction

Large-scale epidemiological studies have focused on mental disorders and substance use disorders. Less work has focused on quantifying subclinical disorders or other psychological sources of dysfunction that can cause impairment. Even so, some data exist indicating that many of us could use some help whether or not we meet criteria for a disorder.

Stress and Distress

I mentioned that stress can be a source of psychosocial dysfunction, apart from its presence in psychiatric disorders. There are many ways to measure stress in everyday life, but there is no cutoff that consistently defines when it leads to impairment. But we do have data on the how many people experience stress and to what extent.

For the past approximately 10 years, the American Psychological Association (APA) has sponsored a national survey of stress of more than 3,000 adults in the United States. Key findings (APA, 2015) include the following:

- Seventy-five percent of Americans report experiencing at least one symptom of stress in the past month;
- Twenty-five percent of Americans state that stress has a very strong or strong impact on their physical or mental health. The most commonly reported signs of stress include feeling irritable/angry, being nervous/anxious, having a lack of interest/motivation, feeling fatigued, feeling overwhelmed and being depressed/sad (32 percent), and that stress has interfered with exercising (29 percent);
- Many people noted that they engage in unhealthy behaviors because of stress, such as lying awake at night (42 percent) or eating too much/eating unhealthy foods (33 percent);
- Social relations appear to be adversely affected: 41 percent of adults who are married or living with a partner report they lost patience or yelled at their spouse or partner due to stress; and 18 percent of those who are employed say they snapped at or were short with a coworker; and
- People who state they have someone to ask for emotional support report less stress and less depression than those who do not have someone. Yet 21 percent of the sample reported they have no one to rely on for support.

Another national survey with a sample of just more than 2,500 individuals 18 years and older in the United States provided similar results (Blendon et al., 2014). For example, among the findings was that 49 percent of individuals surveyed said they had a major stressful event in the past year. Individuals who experienced a great deal of stress identify too many responsibilities, finances, and work problems as main sources of stress. Also, they report that stress influences their family life, health, work life, and social life with friends.

The surveys show variations in the experience of stress as a function of region of the country, income level, sex, and age group. For example, general reports of stress and its impact are worse for individuals of lower income, women, and individuals born from 1960s to the 1980s (Generation X) and the 1980s to the 2000s (Millennials) (APA, 2015). Stressors and stress reactions do not invariably lead to distress (symptoms and impairment), but they can, and people often report that they do. I mentioned surveys in the United States, but stressors and their impact on mental and physical health is a worldwide concern. Especially relevant are individuals living in war zones and being displaced because of conflicts and natural disasters.

Clearly, many people report distress, that is, problems related to mental and physical health and interpersonal relations. Distress can fall squarely in the realm of psychiatric diagnosis (such as PTSD) by precipitating or contributing to one of the recognized diagnoses or key symptoms even if the formal criteria for the diagnosis are not met (Maercker et al., 2013). Distress can be more circumscribed with one or a few symptoms or actions that impede functioning (ceasing to exercise, eating poorly, sleeping poorly, increasing alcohol consumption or cigarette smoking) that can interfere with physical health. Distress reactions are in need of attention and could profit from psychosocial interventions if suitable interventions were more readily available.

Loneliness

As noted, loneliness is another example of psychological dysfunction that can be impairing. How many individuals experience loneliness beyond a transient state (e.g., on a given day or week in response to some transition)? We do not have good data on this, although existing data have led several writers to refer to loneliness as an epidemic (e.g., Doman & Le Roux, 2012; Killeen, 1998; Wood, 2014).

The rates of loneliness vary. A study across 12 countries in Europe sampled 8,787 individuals 65 years and older (Sundström et al., 2009). Prevalence was based on self-reported loneliness "all or most of the time." The prevalence rate of loneliness overall for all countries combined was 12.2 percent, with a range from 3.8 percent (Switzerland) to 20.5 percent (Greece). This work focuses on an older adult sample and cannot be assumed to characterize the broader population of adults.

Another study with a broader age range included approximately 1,200 individuals (aged 15 to 97 years) in the United Kingdom (Victor & Yang, 2012). For the entire sample, 6 percent of the participants were lonely (all or most of the time). Women tended to have higher rates of loneliness than men. Individuals with depression had particularly high rates of loneliness (38 percent). This study included a review of other epidemiological studies and loneliness rates across several of these, spanning ages 15 to 65 years and older. Across all studies and age groups loneliness rates were in the upper teens (about 16 to 18 percent), with a range of 13 to 30 percent.

These numbers come with important caveats. Perhaps the main one is that methods of measurement can be challenged. For example, in several studies only one self-report item may be used to measure loneliness, which is problematic (there is usually no established reliability or validity, there are inherent biases of response sets). Also, more often than not, studies have focused on older adults (>65 years of age), because of the view that this is the group most likely to experience loneliness and isolation and in light of living conditions and physical limits on the activities in which many can participate. Interestingly, there is a curvilinear (inverted U shaped) relation in which both younger (<25 years) and older (>55 years) people show low rates of loneliness and the ages in between show a higher rate (Victor & Yang, 2012). Summing across age groups and taking lower bound estimates (e.g., 6 percent from one study I mentioned or 16 to 18 percent summing from a review), many people experience loneliness.

GENERAL COMMENTS

In general, the problems I have discussed represent misery for individuals and often those in contact with them and reflect a public health problem. A public health problem would be a condition in which the problem or characteristic

- Occurs at a high rate and might place individuals at risk for other more severe problems;
- Is associated with impairment;
- Creates a burden for individuals or others (family, society); and
- For which an intervention might be possible.

The rates of mental illness and other impairing and risky conditions (e.g., loneliness, high stress) individually meet more than one of the previous criteria. In this book, we are addressing the full range of problem domains I have delineated because each includes an important public health problem and is worthy of intervention.

BURDENS OF PSYCHOLOGICAL DYSFUNCTION

Overview

The need for effective intervention is reflected in the large proportion of individuals (prevalence) who experience dysfunction. This need is further heightened by the actual impact these sources of dysfunction have for the many individuals who experience them. I refer to impact by the term "burden" that is commonly used in this context.

Burden refers broadly to the deleterious consequences that clinical dysfunction has for individuals, families, societies and countries, and the world. A goal of psychological interventions is to reduce the burdens for the individual, but at each of the other levels as well. The burdens of mental and physical illness are many and can be looked at from different perspectives and with different metrics.

For the individual with a mental disorder, the burdens include the limits that the symptoms place on functioning in multiple spheres of life. Depending on the type and severity of symptoms, this could include difficulty in developing or maintaining interpersonal relationships, remaining in school, holding down a job, or experiencing enjoyment from interests and hobbies, as well as in general impairment, restrictions, and limits on personal freedoms. Psychiatric disorders may be associated with health problems, as I have noted (see Figure 2.1). For example, for women who experience trauma (e.g., rape), there can be PTSD that places a burden on the individual. Short- and long-term consequences of rape can include physical health problems (e.g., Martin, Macy, & Young, 2011). For some psychiatric disorders (e.g., depression, anxiety) the medication used for treatment can bring on deleterious consequences (e.g., reduced sexual interest and functioning).

Burdens can come in swarms and can readily spill over into multiple spheres of life for the individual with a mental disorder.

For parents, relatives, and families, there are burdens as well. Many know from personal experience with their own families or friends that the tasks and challenges of caring for a child, adult, or elderly parent with a mental disorder are enormous and can last for decades. In years long past, youth with severe mental disorders (e.g., children with autism spectrum disorder or extreme intellectual disability; adolescents and adults with psychoses) were routinely hospitalized. More often now such individuals, especially children, live at home, where parents are responsible for direct care and often for helping to implement interventions to improve their children's lives and skills. Such care can also include dressing, helping with toileting, comforting in times of anxiety, trying to manage uncontrollable bouts of anger or mood swings, or making arrangements for additional care (e.g., scheduling contacts with health professionals, keeping up with doctor visits, medication, and medication changes), just to mention a few. This work can dominate daily life depending on the type and severity of disorder and the intensity and type of intervention, and can itself become a stressor and have direct consequences (distress) in reactions of family members. Many parents and families do this with love and do not frame the tasks as a burden, but that does not alleviate the effects they experience on a daily basis, including psychological consequences (e.g., depression, helplessness) and negative impact on relationships (e.g., marital discord, divorce).

For society, the burdens often are considered in terms of resources and financial costs. These include the costs of providing health care, which include many separate line items such as emergency department visits; inpatient, outpatient, and community mental health services; and developing and staffing country, state or province, and city agencies to administer services. Also, many individuals with mental disorders are involved disproportionately in other systems (e.g., special education, criminal justice and prison, physical health care). These systems are often already understaffed and underfunded. Untreated or uncared for individuals with mental health problems are more likely to have acute and chronic physical disorders, to be homeless, or to be in jail (Greenberg & Rosenheck, 2008; Torrey et al., 2010). Each of these conditions brings wrenching individual and family burdens, apart from the societal level burdens we are discussing.

The costs of mental and physical health disorders are discussed at a global level by governmental and business leaders because health has a far-reaching economic impact on business and industry and society at large (Bloom et al., 2011; WHO, 2011b). The impact is reflected in health care services, loss of productivity, and other expenditures that could be used to support private and public investment and other needed services. And the costs are enormous. In an evaluation of 36 countries (from diverse regions of the world) representing 80 percent of the world's population, the cost of untreated depression and anxiety alone was estimated to be more than $1 trillion (US) per year (Chisholm et al., 2016). This extends to several trillion dollars per year when other mental disorders and substance use are included (Bloom et al., 2011). There are limits on meeting these expenses both in developing and developed countries given other social problems (e.g., food insecurity, lack of access to safe water, lack of sanitation, poverty, homelessness).[7] A potential solution is not to cut spending on health care but rather to address these problems in more effective and efficient ways that reduce the burdens of mental illness for individuals and society.

In short, the burdens of mental disorders are enormous and at multiple levels, including individuals, groups (families), and nations. The burdens can be enduring, too. Mental disorders often run in families, and many risk factors for poor mental and physical health (poverty, poor prenatal nutrition, loss of homes, victims of abuse or sex trafficking) endure for generations. One would like to think that intervening effectively with individuals or at a societal level could interrupt the cycles and the onset of new cases in generations yet to come.

How to Measure the Burdens of Mental Illness

There are numerous ways in which burdens of mental illness can be systematically evaluated. I highlight three because of their extensive use and because they elaborate the goals and targets of our interventions.

Questionnaires and Interviews

Many measures or scales directly evaluate impairment or how a given disorder or set of symptoms interferes with a person's functioning; I will discuss two that are frequently used. First, the World Health Organization Disability Schedule (WHODAS, Version 2.0; WHO, 2014a) is a scale that measures functioning in six domains:

- Cognition—understanding and communicating;
- Mobility—moving and getting around;
- Self-care—hygiene, dressing, eating, and staying alone;
- Getting along—interacting with other people;
- Life activities—domestic responsibilities, leisure, work and school; and
- Participation—joining in community activities.

Among the advantages of this scale is that it is used across all diseases (physical, mental, neurological, and addictive disorders) and is applicable across cultures and all adult populations. Indeed, this measure has been adopted as the official international standard measure of health and disability among WHO member nations (191 at the time of adoption in 2001).

An obvious advantage of the WHODAS is that it enables us to assess disability at the individual and population levels. Consequently, we can compare various types of disorders and their impact within and among countries and cultures. There are different versions (e.g., 12, 26 items) and formats for administration (self-report, interview, or by proxy wherein a family member or other person completes the measure). The measure has been developed through an international collaboration and is readily available for use (www.who.int/classifications/icf/more_whodas/en/).[8]

Another measure is the frequently used Sheehan Disability Scale (SDS), which is designed to assess functional impairment in three domains: work/school, social, and family functioning (Sheehan, 1983; Sheehan & Sheehan, 2008). This is a self-report scale that can be administered in interview format or as a questionnaire. The measure is simple and brief (three visual analogue scales that individuals can use to note their impairment). As a self-report measure, individuals are asked to fill in a circle on a visual scale from 0 (not at all) to 10 (extremely). The SRS is used to evaluate impairment for a range of disorders (e.g., multiple anxiety disorders, schizophrenia, depression, pathological gambling) and has been translated into 48 languages (Sheehan & Sheehan, 2008). The SRS has enjoyed widespread use because of its brevity and utility both in clinical practice and research trials on the effectiveness of treatment.

Costs

The burden of mental disorders often is expressed in terms of financial costs. For a given state, government, or country, how much do mental disorders cost in monetary terms? And as another way of evaluating cost data, what are the costs and relative costs of various disorders or types of disorders? Overall, costs and domains (e.g., disorders, special populations) where costs are particularly great can be critical for allocation of resources such as efforts at treatment and prevention as well as policy decisions (e.g., taxing use of substances).

Although cost itself seems a relatively straightforward concept (dollars or currency of a given country), calculating costs is not so simple. World and local economic shifts (e.g., value of the currency, inflation) might be challenging enough. However, the estimation of costs of mental disorders has special problems. Specifically, mental disorders overlap with all sorts of other domains and contacts with other systems (e.g., physical health care, the legal system, special education, community services as reflected in shelters or meals for homeless individuals). Pricing each of these and deciding what to attribute to mental disorder, in what proportion, and at different points in time over the course of development (costs vary with childhood, adolescence, and adulthood and course of specific disorders) are just some of the inherent challenges in assigning cost.

Costs often are classified as direct and indirect. *Direct* costs refer to those incurred by the care required for the disorder such as all treatment or contacts with health services and payments for those services. These include medication, clinic visits, hospitalization, and payment for care by insurance or government providers. *Indirect* costs include the costs of a reduced number of people in the workforce who pay taxes, public (financial) support of care of individuals through social service programs, costs resulting from reduced educational attainment, and costs associated with other consequences of mental and substance use disorders such as homelessness and incarceration. Another kind of indirect cost results from the high rate of medical complications associated with serious mental illness, leading to high rates of emergency department visits, physical disease, and early mortality. For example, there is a high rate of pulmonary disease among individuals with a mental disorder. Persons with mental illness smoke 44 percent of all cigarettes smoked in the United States. The cost of treating that disease and what facet of that cost relates to mental illness are not straightforward. The broad and sweeping indirect effects of mental illness can lead some families to poverty and to a continued cycle and connection of mental and physical disability and poverty (Alderman, 2011; Patel & Kleinman, 2003). Poverty has its own sequence of potential consequences that are not only personally devastating but also costly in light of services (social, health, legal), and these consequences are likely only to increase. From all of this we can say there are many indirect costs, but their estimation is obviously difficult.

While indirect costs have been challenging to quantify, they are critical for informing public policy. After we assess the key components of the economic burden of mental disorders, we can have a more informed discussion about what should be invested to prevent and treat these illnesses and, indeed, what priorities may be considered in light of the relative magnitude of the burden of different disorders. Needless to say, there is no definitive way to capture indirect costs. Add to that the issue of cost over time; costs and impairment depend on the onset (e.g., childhood, adolescence, or adulthood) and the course of the disorder (does it end, wax and wane, become more or less severe). Most mental disorders have an onset in childhood or adolescence (e.g., de Girolamo et al., 2012; Kessler & Wang, 2008). Yet the disorders and their costs vary as a function of severity and comorbidities with physical health and other mental disorders. Thus knowing the onset of a disorder is not sufficient for precisely estimating costs.

Even direct costs can be challenging to compute. Direct treatment services (e.g., psychotherapy, medication, and monitoring of medication) that are costly are not equally available to those with a given clinical problem (e.g., Druss & Rosenheck, 2014; Knapp, Mangalore, & Simon, 2004). That is, there are no costs or perhaps very expensive hidden costs because services are simply unavailable or available but never accessed. Consider this analogy: there is no cost for shoes in a family that does not have access to purchasing them, so the cost of shoes = $0, but all of the children and parents are barefoot. Depending on where they live, buying no shoes could end up being very costly because of resulting injuries, diseases, and resulting disabilities (Bethony et al., 2006). For this and other reasons we cannot easily put an exact price on a given disorder, multiply that by the number of people with the disorder, and end up with an accurate figure.

Thankfully, that level of precision is not necessary for addressing the approximate burden. We can use estimates of costs, relative costs, and changes in costs over time to guide decision making and evaluation of progress or lack thereof. Also, one can make comparisons of the estimated costs of different disorders and diseases (e.g., depression, alcohol use, cancer, heart disease) or broader categories of disorders (e.g., psychoses, substance use and abuse). One of the reasons that mental disorders are so costly and are costlier than physical disorders is that their onset is often early in life. In contrast, many physical disorders (e.g., most cancers, heart disease, Alzheimer's disease) come on much later and have a shorter course until the end of life.

Disability Measures

A third and widely used measure has emerged in an effort to describe and evaluate the burdens of physical diseases and injuries in a consistent way across countries (WHO, 2013). That measure has been extended to mental disorders as well. Beginning in the 1990s, an extensive study began to look at more than 100 different diseases and sources of injury that led to premature death, loss of health, and disability. A common metric or index is referred to as *disability-adjusted life year* (DALY).

DALY refers to one year of a healthy life that is lost because of some impairment (e.g., cancer, stroke). Stated another way, the measure is the difference or gap between current health status and an ideal situation based on how long one would be likely to live into old age, free of disease and disability (WHO, 2013). With this measure, one can evaluate the burden or impact of diverse sources of injury and disease and do this across countries. This information can be extremely useful for prioritizing health care services and resources and for tracking changes over time.

Using DALY as a measure of the burden, mental disorders can be more impairing than many common chronic medical disorders, with particularly greater impairment in the domains of home, social, and close-relationship functioning (Druss et al., 2009). As a dramatic illustration, in 2004, the burden of depressive disorders (DALY) was ranked third among the list of mental and physical diseases worldwide (World Federation for Mental Health, 2011). By 2030, depression is projected to be the number one cause of disability in the world, ahead of cardiovascular disease, traffic accidents, chronic pulmonary disease, and HIV/AIDS (WHO, 2008a).

Many studies have used DALY, and it has become a standard way of making judgments about the impact of dysfunction. In addition, there are measures to quantify duration and quality of life that are related to DALY.[9] As with cost, DALY and related measures are not simple calculations; assumptions and judgments are needed. Yet the measures provide a consistent metric that can be used worldwide and across multiple domains (e.g., mental and physical illness, injury, violence).

Impact of Mental Disorders

Thanks to measures such as those I have sampled and many of their variations, we have extensive data on the burdens of mental disorders. Studies vary on whether several or some subset of all of the disorders are covered, age of the sample (e.g., children, adults), countries (several versus some smaller number), the specific measures that are used (e.g., cost, DALY), and precisely what is included if cost is estimated. I sample a few studies to address the broad conclusion about the impact of mental disorders.

Cost

I begin with the cost of mental illness. A report of data on the most costly medical conditions nicely sums up the financial burden of mental illness (Soni, 2015a). Figure 2.2 illustrates the costs of various disorders and diseases (heart disease,

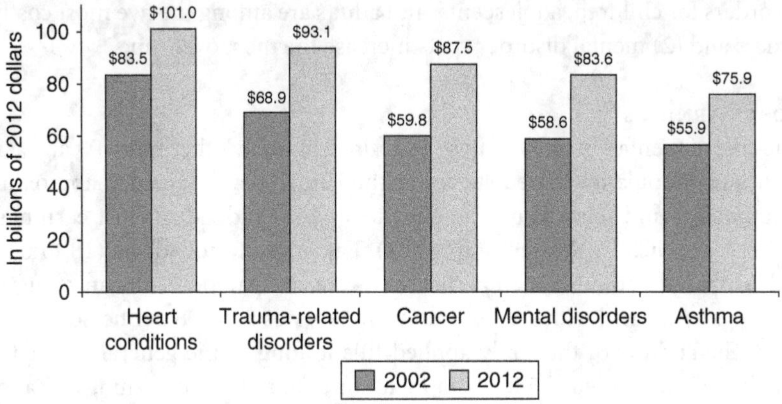

Figure 2.2 Expenditures of the Five Most Costly Conditions, Assessed for Two Years, 2002 and 2012.
SOURCES: MEPS Statistical Brief #470 (April 2015). *Trends in the five most costly conditions among the U.S. civilian noninstitutionalized populations, 2002 and 2012.* Retrieved from https://meps.ahrq.gov/data_files/publications/st470/stat470.shtml; Center for Financing, Access, and Cost Trends; Agency for Healthcare Research and Quality. Household Component of the Medical Expenditure Panel Survey, 2012. Reprinted with permission from AHRQ.

trauma-related disorders, cancers, mental disorders, and asthma), in 2002 and again in 2012, among adults. The costs are in constant dollars (adjusted to 2012 dollars) to take into account inflation.

Costs are what was paid for health care services and include the sum of direct payments for care provided during a one-year period, including out-of-pocket payments and payments by private insurance, government agencies, and other sources. As is evident in the figure, mental disorders are the fourth most costly among the five conditions in 2002 and 2012. Where they are placed is less important perhaps than the staggering costs. In addition (but not in the figure), the number of people accounting for expenses for mental disorders increased from 31.1 million to 45.2 million from 2002 to 2012, and that increase in percentage and absolute numbers was greater than for any of the other conditions.

Extension of this work to children and adolescents (<18 years) again included the five most costly conditions. From most to least expensive were mental disorders, asthma and chronic obstructive pulmonary disease, trauma-related disorders, acute bronchitis and upper respiratory infections, and infectious diseases (Soni, 2015b). Overall, the treatment of mental disorders in children cost $13.9 billion in a one-year period. Interestingly, of these five most costly conditions, mental disorders had the highest cost per child.

The two studies were of health care services in a given year and do not measure costs over time and how a given problem spills into other domains (the prison system, care for the homeless, and so on) or is associated with lost time from work (earnings, paying taxes). As I mentioned previously, these indirect costs are especially difficult to estimate but are real. Even so, one can see that (1) mental disorders for children, adolescents, and adults are among the five most costly disorders and (2) mental disorder costs increase the most over time.

Lost Earnings

The cost of mental disorders can be examined in many other ways. As an example, a national population-based survey in the United States included approximately 5,000 adults and focused on the extent to which individuals lost earnings in a given year (NCS-R; Kessler et al., 2008). Earnings of individuals (18 to 64 years old) with and without a mental disorder were compared. The mean reduction in earnings associated with serious mental illness was $16,306 per person in a given year. The authors of the study applied this finding to the general population of individuals with mental illness to yield an annual loss of earnings of approximately $193 billion. Even this is likely to be an underestimate because two impairing disorders (schizophrenia, autism spectrum disorders) were not included in the study. Also not evaluated was loss associated with missed work of family members to attend to individuals with mental disorders.

These and other studies show that the costs of mental illness are enormous, yet there is no single figure to represent total cost. One review based on several studies in the United States summed a few major components of these costs, including health care expenditures, loss of earnings, and government disability benefits, with results equaling approximately $318 billion in a given year (Insel, 2008). That figure, arrived at in 2002, when adjusted for inflation would translate to approximately $429 billion in 2017.

Disability

Considering disability as a measure of burden conveys the problem in yet another way. A large and comprehensive evaluation of disability is the Global Burden of Disease study (http://www.healthdata.org/gbd). This is an ongoing evaluation of diseases worldwide. In a recent iteration, disability associated with 20 mental and substance abuse disorders was evaluated across 187 countries (Whiteford et al., 2013). Three disability measures were used, including DALY, YLL, and YLD. Mental and substance use disorders accounted for 183.9 million DALYs (or 7.4 percent of all DALYs worldwide). These disorders together accounted for 8.6 million YLLs (or 5 percent all YLLs) and 175.3 million YLDs (or 22.9 percent). Mental and substance use disorders were the leading cause of YLDs worldwide. Depressive disorders, anxiety disorders, illicit drug use disorders, alcohol use disorders, and schizophrenia were the top five sources of disorders accounting for DALYs.

These numbers may be difficult to integrate because they are more abstract than metrics like financial cost. But consider how momentous these indices are. Years of life lost by premature death is 8.6 million. The lives of individuals with mental disorder are on average reduced by 15 to 20 years compared with those without such disorders. Think about this in the context of real people that we knew and have lost (a parent, sibling, or child) to an early death because of mental illness (Nordentoft et al., 2013).

Depression has received special attention in relation to cost and DALY given the pervasiveness of the disorder. Research has repeatedly shown that depression is a leading cause of the burden of disease in the world in terms of DALY (Ferrari et al., 2013). For treatment of depression alone, the annual cost in the United States is estimated to be more than $71 billion (Dieleman et al., 2016).

Depression is useful in other ways for evaluating the impact of mental disorders beyond cost and DALY. Individuals with depression are at much greater risk for heart disease, suicide, and earlier than expected death from all causes (referred to as *all-cause mortality*) (Diniz et al., 2014; Zivin et al., 2015). For example, adults with depression are more than 20 times more likely to commit suicide than are individuals in the general population.

The burdens of formally recognized mental disorders reveal an enormous problem, but notice that I have left out the subclinical and subsyndromal disorders. As discussed previously, these can also be impairing. For example, subsyndromal depression is associated with interpersonal problems at home, financial problems, impairments in job functioning, restricted activities, and poor health status (e.g., Judd et al., 1996; Lyness et al., 2007). Moreover, the level of impairment can match that of depression that *does* meet criteria for a disorder. Similar results have been found for other domains of dysfunction that do not meet some diagnostic threshold. For example, subsyndromal PTSD, anxiety disorder, and gambling disorder are associated with significant current impairment in multiple domains of functioning and put people at risk for other disorders (e.g., McLaughlin et al., 2015; Mendlowicz & Stein, 2014; Parhami, et al., 2014). It is likely that estimates of the scope and burdens of dysfunction are lower bound approximations in light of the exclusion of subthreshold sources of dysfunction.

Mental disorders rank among the costliest disorders in the United States, and the costs associated with mental illness appear to be increasing more rapidly than the costs of other disorders. I have emphasized data from the United States, but worldwide the situation appears to be similar. In addition, the burden of mental disorders is underestimated for a plethora of reasons. Various efforts to evaluate costs and disability over time, across nations, and among diverse disorders have painted a clear picture of where mental disorders fall in the costs to individuals and society. This is enormously important when considering how to allocate resources, and the scope of the problem (e.g., prevalence) and burden (e.g., cost, DALY) means we need to reconsider what services are provided and how they are delivered. A business-as-usual approach, providing more of the same resources (funds, clinics, mental health professionals) to do more of the same work, will have very little impact. Further on I will propose and discuss needed changes to the services that can be provided and how they should be delivered in order to have the broadest impact possible.

SUMMARY AND CONCLUSIONS

The chapter discussed the range of dysfunctions and how many people have them. Just focusing on mental disorders, leaving aside subclinical disorders and other domains of dysfunction, conveys that the problem is huge. Even without those additions it would be readily understandable why we cannot provide treatment to reach the millions in need. The chapter ended with a discussion of the burdens of psychological dysfunction. The burdens can be measured in many ways, including measures of impairment, costs, disability, and lost days. What can be concluded from research is that the costs and lost days of adequate functioning and lost days of life are enormous as a result of mental illness. The impact of mental illness is difficult to state precisely because the direct costs (providing treatment and services) are accompanied by indirect costs that result from consequences and associated features of having a mental disorder (e.g., costs of services for homelessness, emergency department visits, incarceration; lost days of work of caretakers; hospital care resulting from physical maladies). Yet we do not need the precise estimates to know that in the United States, billions of dollars are spent annually as a result of mental disorders and substance use disorders. Again, these costs omit many sources of dysfunction I reviewed that fall outside of formal mental disorders.

My aim with this chapter was to establish the need for more effective interventions in light of the range of dysfunctions, the high number of people who experience them, and the burdens these dysfunctions cause. There is a second part that has yet to be addressed, namely: How are we doing in providing treatment and clinical services? For that we turn to Chapter 3.

3

Treatment Gap

Barriers to Providing and Receiving Services

Clearly, mental disorders are relatively common, with approximately 50 percent of people in the United States expected to experience a diagnosable psychiatric disorder during their lifetime—and remember that this omits subclinical dysfunction, which does not qualify for formal diagnosis, as well as other conditions (e.g., stress, loneliness) that impair everyday functioning. One might expect that the attention and resources allocated to providing care for these disorders would be on par with their scope and impact on individuals and society. Alas, no. Resources provided for mental health care are paltry; there are too few resources, too few people delivering services, two few services available where treatment is needed most, and too many treatments that are of questionable value (effectiveness) even when they are delivered. (Other than that, things are great!)

This chapter will expose the gap between treatment services that are needed and those that are provided, as well as barriers to providing and receiving services. Before moving on to my primary goal of proposing and promoting novel strategies and solutions to reduce the burdens of mental illness, I want to examine key problems and impediments that are firmly in place now because new models of treatment and delivery will need to surmount current barriers to be effective.

TREATMENT GAP: LIMITED CLINICAL SERVICES FOR THOSE IN NEED

Two basic issues are our starting point, namely, the extent to which individuals in need of services actually receive care and precisely what that care is. In an ideal world, we might want all in need of services to actually receive them. We would also want those services to have the benefit of strong evidence showing that they make a difference. In reality, in the United States (and worldwide), conditions depart drastically from these ideals. Let me highlight the evidence to support this claim.

The *treatment gap* refers to the difference between the number of people who have disorders or suffer psychological dysfunction (prevalence) and the number of those who actually receive care (Kohn et al., 2004). The World Health Organization (WHO Mental Health Survey Consortium, 2004) provided extensive data on the treatment gap from surveys of more than 60,000 adults in 14 countries in the Americas, Europe, Middle East, Africa, and Asia. The proportion of respondents who received health care treatment for emotional or substance use disorders during the 12 months preceding the survey ranged from a low of 0.8 percent (Nigeria) to a high of 15.3 percent (United States). These percentages reflect those who received treatment among those in need, and also show that the vast majority of individuals in need (99.2 percent and 84.7 percent, respectively) did not receive treatment.

Perhaps treatment is differentially available as a function of severity of disorders and impairment. In the prior report, disorders were evaluated by severity. Serious disorders were defined largely by individuals reporting that they were totally unable to function for at least 30 days in the past year in light of their disorders. As might be expected, the proportion of individuals who received treatment was much higher among those with severe versions of their disorders (ranging from 14.6 percent [Lebanon] to 64.5 percent [Spain]). In the United States 52.3 percent of individuals with severe dysfunction received mental health services. Of further interest is that in the United States, 8.1 percent of individuals with subclinical dysfunction received treatment. Overall, developed countries provided more services than did developing (low-income) countries, as shown in this study. It is all the more dramatic to confront the limited services provided in the United States, where only 15 percent of those in need received care.

If one looks at specific domains of dysfunction in detail based on data from large surveys, the gap in services is further corroborated. For example, a large survey evaluated more than 46,000 adults in US households and found that 8.4 percent meet criteria for depression (Olfson, Blanco, & Marcus, 2016). Only 28.7 percent of those people actually received treatment for depression. A sample of more than 36,000 adults in the United States revealed a lifetime prevalence of 29.1 percent for alcohol use disorder (Grant et al., 2015), but only 19.8 percent of them ever received any treatment! Similarly, as part of the same sample, 9.9 percent met criteria for a drug use disorder over the course of their lifetime. Yet only 24.6 percent had received any treatment. A 2016 report by the US Surgeon General noted that only 10 percent of people with a substance use disorder receive treatment for their disorder. This is an enormous gap, especially in light of data that drug use, abuse, and overdose and opioid addiction are on the rise (Rudd et al., 2014). Finally, a survey of 50 countries, spanning low-income to upper-middle-income countries, focused on services provided for individuals with schizophrenia (Lora et al., 2012). A median of 31 percent of these individuals received care. This leaves 69 percent with the disorder not receiving treatment. Understandably, as different disorders, countries, locales, sampling methods, and measures change, so do the percentages. Consequently, no percentage serves very well as a single statistic about the treatment gap. Yet, based on all the different numbers, the inevitable conclusion is stark and simple. Most people in need of mental health services receive no treatment.

Important to add here is that there are considerable ethnic and cultural disparities in access to mental health care. For example, in the United States, ethnic minority groups (e.g., African, Hispanic, and Native Americans) have much less access to care than do Americans of European descent (e.g., Holliday et al., 2009; McGuire & Miranda, 2008; Wells et al., 2001). The situation is even worse (lower percentages of people who receive treatment) when ethnic and cultural disparities combine with other factors that hamper care. For example, in general, children are much less likely to receive services for their mental health problems than are adults. They are even less likely to receive treatment if they are minority group members (e.g., Marrast, Himmelstein, & Woolhandler, 2016).

Overall, the lack of available services for most people and systematic disparities among those services underlie the importance of delivering services in ways that can reach many more people and target special groups. I will return to the matter of disparities in mental health services later in the chapter. At this point, it is simply important to acknowledge that the lamentable fact that most people do not receive services is even worse for individuals of nonmajority cultural or ethnic minority status in the United States.

But what of the apparently elite group, namely, the people who did receive services? What exactly did they receive? In the WHO study, "receiving services" was based on whether respondents ever saw any one of a long list of caregivers, either as an outpatient or inpatient, for problems with emotions, nerves, mental health, or use of alcohol or drugs. Included were mental health professionals (e.g., psychiatrist, psychologist), general medical professionals (e.g., general practitioner, occupational therapist), religious counselors (e.g., minister, sheikh), and traditional healers (e.g., herbalist, spiritualist) (World Mental Health Survey Consortium, 2004). The list varied across countries depending on local circumstances where types of healers may vary. The precise service that was provided by these individuals was not identified. Also, the duration of the intervention was not known, but receiving services required at least one contact. This is a low and ambiguous criterion for what qualifies as receiving services. One visit with even a highly trained mental health professional, for someone with major depression, substance abuse, or severe anxiety, is not likely to accomplish very much. So when we say that 15 percent of individuals received treatment, the bar is low and could mean one contact with someone who has absolutely no mental health training.

In the United States, the National Comorbidity Survey Replication (NCS-R) study has provided data on who receives treatment as well as some further information about the nature of that treatment (Wang et al., 2005). More than 9,000 individuals with psychiatric disorders answered questions about their treatment that included who the service provider was (psychiatric, family physical, social worker, spiritual advisor, and others) and the type of treatment (self-help group, medication, hospital admission). Minimally adequate treatment was defined as receiving an intervention (e.g., medication, psychotherapy) that followed evidence-based guidelines for the specific disorder of the individual and included multiple contacts (rather than only one visit).

Overall, across the sample, 17.9 percent received some form of intervention. For individuals with a psychiatric disorder, 21.5 percent received treatment from a mental health specialist, but 41.7 percent received treatment if this is expanded to include contact with any health care person, in addition to those trained in mental health. Regarding individuals who did not meet criteria for a disorder (subclinical or subsyndromal), 4.4 percent received treatment from a mental health specialist and 10.1 percent received treatment if this is expanded to include any contact. Overall, across the entire sample, only 32.7 percent were classified as receiving at least minimally adequate treatment. The investigators concluded that only one-third of treatments provided met minimal standards of adequacy based on evidence-based treatment guidelines.

Other conclusions were noted from this survey. First, treatments were used that have unclear benefits. For example, complementary and alternative treatments accounted for 31.3 percent of all mental health visits despite the absence of evidence attesting to their effectiveness. Second, most services and mental health visits were consumed by individuals without meeting the criteria for disorders (subclinical). They account for almost one-third of all mental health visits. This is striking given the unmet need for services for individuals with well-defined mental disorders.

I have only sampled studies from large literatures on who receives treatment and what counts as treatment (e.g., Becker & Kleinman, 2013; Merikangas et al., 2011). A few points are worth reiterating. First, around the world, the majority of individuals with mental disorders do not receive treatment. Though studies vary and there is no one percentage to be held up as representative of those with unmet needs, it is nevertheless clear that we are not providing treatment to enough people in need of it.

Second, even when care is provided, we generally do not know whether it was a high-quality regimen of treatment specifically aimed at the clinical dysfunction in question. That is, "receiving care" includes basic "contact" and does not necessarily indicate a formalized treatment of any type (psychological treatment, medication, spiritual intervention).

Third, evidence-based treatments are used infrequently for mental disorders for those few individuals who receive care. Epidemiological surveys are not designed to probe precisely what the intervention was, for how long it was administered, whether the treatment was delivered in the way in which it was developed in research, or whether the persons administering the treatment were trained in its use. Beyond the surveys, we know that evidence-based interventions are not being used for mental and substance use disorders as a general rule. This situation has been referred to as a "quality chasm" and reflects the gap between what is known to be effective by researchers and what in fact is actually used in clinical practice. This chasm applies to mental health and substance use disorders as well as physical health and disease (Institute of Medicine [IOM], 2001, 2006). The ideal for individual patients and service providers should not just be to receive and provide any treatment, but rather to receive and provide the best treatments and specifically those that have an evidence base.

Fourth, none of the studies reporting on who receives treatment and what those treatments were evaluated the outcome of treatment. In the end, this is arguably the most critical index. Do people get better whether or not they receive treatment, and does the treatment they receive make any difference in their lives? We cannot even assume that if evidence-based treatment was provided that it actually helped; such treatments are often diluted in clinical work and do not achieve the touted effects proposed in research (Weisz et al., 2014). It is important to keep in mind that treatments, whether medical or psychological, can make people better, or can have no impact, or can make people worse. It would be useful, if not essential and ethical, to know what the outcomes are of the treatments we are using. Receiving treatment is critical, but whether treatments make any difference or actually help is hardly trivial.

There are limitations in the studies I have cited and in the research methods more generally. For instance, in some surveys (e.g., WHO Consortium, NCS-R) certain diagnoses are omitted (such as schizophrenia); whether treatment has been provided is usually examined in the context of a restricted period (often 12 months); and much of the data are based on self-report (and retrospective report at that). Self-report of having received services and actually receiving them could yield different results; people may be reluctant to report on clinical services or may have intended to go but did not. (Yet, in many surveys, self-report is confirmed by face-to-face interviews or phone interviews, so there is attention to this problem at least.) Even with limitations of individual studies and different methods of assessment, samples, time periods, and countries, the overall conclusions are quite similar: (1) most people in need of services are not receiving services, and (2) those who do are receiving an odd array of "services" provided by many people with no training in the care of mental disorders.

The absence of data on improvement and adaptive functioning in everyday life has its own set of ambiguities, namely: How many people improved whether or not they received services, and is the improvement greater (stronger effects, more people affected) among those who received treatment (controlling for severity of dysfunction, impairment, levels of stress, and so on for possible confounds)? It is important to raise these questions here; but later in the book they will be approached as challenges that can in fact be overcome to better provide services that reach people in need.

BARRIERS TO RECEIVING TREATMENT SERVICES

If we are going to reduce the burdens of mental illness, we will need to identify persons in need of treatment and provide services for them, ensure that care consists of more than one contact if needed, and ensure that the treatment has supportive evidence in its behalf, if any such treatment is available. These might be enough challenges for one day, or even constitute an insurmountable obstacle. So let us hold off on the solutions for a bit and instead fill out the picture of obstacles to be overcome.

Receiving services for psychological dysfunction is a process of multiple steps:

1. Experiencing symptoms or some form of dysfunction;
2. Identifying those as symptoms or something in need of help;
3. Deciding whether action is needed to do something about the symptoms;
4. Identifying the options for intervention (e.g., a psychosocial "treatment," medication, or something else);
5. Seeking and actually obtaining treatment if that is the option selected;
6. Beginning the treatment; and
7. Remaining in treatment as needed, with recurrent disorders traversing the process or abbreviated variants again.

There may be numerous obstacles at each of these steps that impede or prohibit a person from moving forward in the sequence and actually receiving care. These are often referred to as *barriers to care* or *barriers to treatment.*

Barriers to care vary in their sources. Two broad categories are often defined: system factors (financial costs, whether a service is available, and government, law, policy issues, and so on) and attitudinal factors (e.g., fear of stigmatization, views that treatment will not be of much help). Table 3.1 lists these two broad categories of barriers to treatment and some examples of each type.

System Factors

By system factors, I refer to factors outside of the individual that typically concern the services themselves and their availability. (The category of system factors is useful for presentation, but most efforts to define barriers outside of the individual and inside the individual are not sufficiently nuanced, as I will discuss shortly.)

Cost of Mental Health Services

Cost of mental health services can influence whether people receive treatment and generally amounts to the cost of providing and obtaining services. Consider a few cost considerations and how they create barriers to treatment. First, we begin with individuals and their families, and their ability to pay for services. In the United States, health care generally is covered (paid for) either through direct

Table 3.1 BARRIERS TO MENTAL HEALTH CARE

Barrier Type	Brief Description
System Factors	
Cost of mental health services	Treatment is not affordable because services are not covered by insurance of the client, services are not completely covered, or the out-of-pocket costs are too expensive. The complexity of understanding what is and is not covered or negotiating all of this (reimbursement forms, appealing after a claim has been refused) can be daunting.
Policy and legal constraints	Government policies (e.g., federal, state, province) and third-party payers may restrict what conditions can be treated and reimbursed or for how long treatment can be provided (e.g., number of sessions, days) and still be reimbursed. These constraints also include limited financial resources as a matter of budget, policy, or law that provides too few services and therefore less accessible services.
Too few providers to deliver services	Mental health professionals are not available in sufficient numbers to provide services to meet the need. This is a worldwide problem in developing (low- and middle-income) and developed (higher-income) countries as well. In the United States, trained professionals are insufficient in number to treat all those in need and are concentrated in urban areas. Too few meet the ethnic demographic of the nation or focus on clinical problems for which the need is the great.
Attitudinal Factors	
Stigma	Stigma refers to negative beliefs and practices by a group about a condition—in this case mental disorders. Concerns among potential clients or consumers of treatment are with being labeled (diagnosed) with a mental disorder or being associated with treatment for a mental disorder. Stigma can lead to genuine discriminatory practices and domains of rejection (e.g., employment, promotion). Also, individuals may view their own dysfunction with stigma (self-stigma), which can interfere with identifying themselves as having a mental disorder and seeking treatment.
Mental health literacy	Mental health literacy refers to information that individuals have and what they know about mental disorders, whether one has symptoms or a disorder that warrants treatment, what the options are for treatment, and how to pursue those options and obtain treatment.
Cultural and ethnic influences	Individuals of cultural and ethnic minorities have less access to services for health care in general, including mental health care. Views about whether psychological problems warrant treatment, about entry into any health care service, or about seeking treatment can vary widely. Some problems (e.g., anxiety, depression) may not be seen as a reason to seek "treatment" or to be involved with a health care system. This is not the same as mental health literacy, which is more about knowing, but rather is more firmly rooted in cultural practices and beliefs.

(*continued*)

Table 3.1 Continued

Barrier Type	Brief Description
Other Factors	
Case identification	Not identifying individuals at risk early in their course toward dysfunction is another barrier to treatment. This includes the absence of systematic assessments early in life that would identify individuals who are at risk and the absence of follow-up with action to help them.
Model of intervention delivery	Psychosocial interventions for mental disorders usually are delivered one to one, in person, with a mental health professional. This inherently limits the number of individuals who can receive treatment and the reach of treatment to the range of populations that need to be served.

payment or partial payment (copay with some insurer) or by a policy provided by one's employer. Even when mental health services are covered through one's job, often payments are required (copayments) because only part of the cost is covered by insurance; often a small portion is paid by the patient. Whether insured or not, the cost of mental health services is for many people a barrier to enrolling in treatment (this goes, incidentally, for physical health treatment, too).

Many individuals in need of services do not have coverage, or the coverage they do have is restricted to services that are not conveniently available where they are living. For example, in the city in which I work, few mental health service providers accept insurance. (Among the reasons are that reimbursement is much lower than the going rates of therapy and that dealing with reimbursement plans can be onerous.) This means that having insurance is not necessarily very helpful, if many services will not accept it. Services that do accept one's insurance plan might be more difficult to find. So, add availability of services as a related barrier.

But let us say a person with insurance has found an agency that will accept that insurance; it is not yet time for relief. Sometimes when insurance claims are submitted for reimbursement of a service, the claims are refused. Some feature of the problem that was treated (e.g., the precise diagnosis), the treatment (e.g., what the therapist used as the treatment), the service provider, or small print on the policy leads to rejection of the claim. These rejections come after the treatment sessions of course, so the patient must bear costs he or she thought were covered. The complexities and the uncertainties of insurance and reimbursement are huge barriers to receiving care.

Treatment even when reimbursed may have *clear* limits. Whether one can be treated and for how many sessions are all potential limitations, at least in the United States. In the usual case, one must meet criteria for a psychiatric disorder or be referred to treatment because of physical health problems exacerbated by mental health problems. Then, there might be some fixed number of sessions and some hoops or obstacles to go through to obtain additional treatment.

Treatment even when reimbursed may have *unclear* limits. For example, individuals who use a service covered by their plan may be surprised to learn that some part of their care was not part of the plan. A doctor or service may be called in or used that the patient mistakenly assumed would be covered, only to receive a big bill later (Cooper & Scott-Morton, 2016).

There is great unevenness in health insurance plans and coverage in the United States. For example, one's status (citizen, immigrant, visitor on a visa, international student) can influence whether services are to be reimbursed. Within a given group (e.g., employees at a given company), insurance plans can vary tremendously, with those variations influencing whether or how much of a service will be reimbursed. All of these are barriers because individuals may refrain from services owing to the costs they will bear, the perceived costs they will bear (plans are not at all clear to many), and real or perceived challenges of negotiating the systems to receive services and reimbursement. System barriers (e.g., financial costs, service-providing constraints) can meld into attitudinal barriers (factors within the individual) when perceptions, beliefs, and worries about what care will be provided and reimbursed have an impact on seeking services. "Insurance is great until you need it," goes the saying, which reflects the concern (at least in the United States) that not all care is covered as thoroughly as one may have imagined and that there are likely to be surprises when it comes to reimbursement.

In short, there are all sorts of nuances, limits, and escape clauses for various reimbursement policies. In the United States, that means that even if one has coverage one might need to be cautious in assuming treatment will be fully covered. And people who enter treatment without insurance are at increased risk for dropping out early (Enlund et al., 2002).

Many of these reimbursement issues are likely to be less evident with medications as treatment rather than psychosocial interventions. For medications, doctors and pharmacies have reasonably informed ideas of what is covered and know the set of plans in a given area. Consequently, patients can be assured more explicitly about what is and is not covered and what their contribution will need to be if anything. Although individuals filling a prescription are surprised by little exceptions here and there (e.g., "I thought there was no copay"), this is not close to the mystery of insurance plans and how they handle mental health reimbursement.

Policy and Legal Constraints

Several barriers to care pertain to laws, policies, and regulations (e.g., McGowan et al., 2016). Within the United States these can be a maze of factors, and among different countries there are varied and rich options pertaining to what services are provided and to whom, as well as the extent to which patients are charged. Let us consider the category generally. Many of the issues are also related to financial barriers and are worth distinguishing.

Government spending has direct implications for whom receives care and ease of access to care. States and cities often cannot afford even to provide services in many areas of the community. For example, in the United States, each of the 50 states has areas classified as rural (often defined as <3,500 residents). Rural areas have very limited access to care. Less dramatic instances can occur in urban cities where care is not evenly provided among sections within the city. One can ask whether services or treatments are available in a given area (e.g., inner city) and if they readily accessible (e.g., known about, welcoming) for prospective clients.

Policy and changes in policy can greatly introduce barriers and do so routinely. In the United States, many mental health services are funded and provided by the individual states and are subject to budget fluctuations. A major evaluation of cuts in mental health services revealed that the need and requests for mental health services in the United States have been rising, but many state governments have cut back on the amount of funds allocated for mental health services (Honberg et al., 2011). Services that are either eliminated or downsized include

- Emergency and long-term hospital treatment;
- Crisis intervention teams;
- Intensive case management services (for children, adolescents, or adults);
- A team approach with home visits to treat and monitor functioning, as needed; and
- Psychiatric medication.

In the United States, Medicaid is a federal source of funding and is the most important source of funding for public mental health services for youth and adults. Added to reductions in state budgets for mental health are reductions in Medicaid for such services (Honberg et al., 2011). Reduced funds mean that treatment is available to fewer people in need of services. A particular service may be eliminated or greatly reduced. Individuals simply would not have access to a service that previously had been available.

The number of hospital beds (inpatient care) for mental disorders is a dramatic illustration of reduction and elimination of services over the past few decades (Bastiampillai, Sharfstein, & Allison, 2016; Sisti, Segal, & Emanuel, 2015). A large movement going back 50 years focused on placing individuals in community settings rather than hospitals and maintaining them with services and medication that had the stigma but not the cost of psychiatric hospitalization. The number of hospital beds has continued to decline, and of those provided, many are for incarcerated people with mental disorders. Of course, the need for inpatient care has not magically declined.

Overall, we have a "perfect storm" in which the need for services is on the rise, most people in need already receive nothing, and services are routinely cut back in times when budgets are strained. The cutback is reflected in cost in another way, with businesses cutting back ever so slightly on health benefits or requiring larger contributions of employees when they seek services.[1] The cutbacks are designed to decrease expenditures, but in fact reduced social services in general are known to be associated with increases in physical health care costs (e.g., from adult obesity, asthma, days with limitations of activity, mortality rates for lung cancer, heart attack, and diabetes) (e.g., Bradley et al., 2016; Bradley & Taylor, 2013).

The paucity of services provided by local and state governments and insurance coverage plans combine to convey the impediments to receiving care. It is quite possible that services are available, but many individuals do not have reimbursement plans to make those accessible. It is also possible that people have adequate reimbursement plans and coverage but services are not readily available. The perfect situation in which services are readily available and individuals in need of care have adequate coverage is not likely to emerge very often. It is important also to keep in mind that in negotiating services, presumably we are talking about a person with mental health problems (e.g., depression, anxiety, suicidality). These conditions are not optimal for negotiating anything, let alone the intricacies of the mental health system and its reimbursement challenges. And if a family member without mental illness is taking up the challenges, there probably is desperation to get help as soon as possible. Here, too, we want access to be as easy as possible when in fact there is a steeplechase of hurdles.

Too Few Providers to Deliver Services

If one wants services, providers are not as readily available as one would imagine. On the world stage, especially in low- or middle-income countries (where 85 percent of the world population resides), there is only a fraction of care professionals needed for providing services (e.g., Bruckner et al., 2011). Perhaps the situation is fine in a developed country such as the United States? Not at all.

There are many mental health professionals but not enough to meet the need for treatment, at least in the way treatment is provided. There is no single definitive survey, method of sampling, or even definition of "mental health professional" in the United States. But as an instructive guide, two estimates have yielded figures of 550,000 and 700,000 individuals providing mental health services (see Health Resources and Services Administration, 2010; Hoge et al., 2007; Substance Abuse and Mental Health Services Administration [SAMHSA], 2013). These figures may be underestimates given the range of providers not usually included, such as other professionals (e.g., nurses, pastoral counselors, art therapists, school counselors) and individuals with various titles (e.g., counselor, personal coach, life coach, healer, therapist). Some of the terms (e.g., counselor, therapist) are only partially and inconsistently regulated, which means they can be used by anyone without special training. In short, the number of individuals who provide therapy with or without formal training in the mental health professions would be hard to count. Even with all of these qualifiers and caveats in mind, it is difficult to envision that a number within this range of the two figures I presented, or indeed less than 1 million service providers, would help sufficiently if 25 percent (or approximately 81 million) of the United States population in any given year or 50 percent over the course of one's life (or approximately 163 million people) meet criteria for a psychiatric disorder, leaving aside the added group of individuals outside of these percentages who evince subclinical disorders.

An initial obvious reaction is that we just need more trained mental health professionals who can provide treatment. That is, this is a "person-power" problem. Actually not. Having more mental health professionals might be valuable but cannot be expected to have a significant impact on reaching palpably more people. The main reasons relate to the geographical distribution, interests, and composition of the professional workforce and a latter barrier I discuss regarding how they usually provide treatment. Consider the limits of delivering care just pertaining to the providers.

First, in the United States mental health professionals are concentrated in highly populated, affluent urban areas and in cities with major universities (Health Resources and Services Administration, 2010). As I mentioned previously, all of the states include rural areas where the concentration of people to square miles of land is low (www.hrsa.gov/ruralhealth/aboutus/definition.html). For these areas and small towns more generally, very few, or more commonly, no mental health professionals may be available.

Second, the majority of mental health professionals do not provide care to populations and clinical problems for which there is an especially great demand (e.g., children and older adults, individuals of minority groups, special populations in need such as victims of violence, single-mothers living below or near the poverty line, and more generally individuals of lower income). Most psychiatric disorders have their onset in childhood and adolescence, but most individuals in the mental health professions are trained in the treatment of adults. At the other end of the age spectrum, the proportion of older adults is expanding rapidly in the United States (and worldwide); this group is underserved and, in light of the expansion, increasingly underserved by mental (and physical) health services (IOM, 2012). Too few mental health professionals are trained to provide services to older adults, even if this group were not expanding so rapidly. Indeed, it would be very unusual for a graduate training program (e.g., clinical psychology, social work) to train therapists specifically in treatment of older adults. Similarly, few internships offer options, let alone supervised training, in the treatment of older adults. Older adults are merely an example of the more general problem; where need is great, services are often especially sparse

Finally, disproportionately few mental health professionals reflect the cultural and ethnic characteristics of many of those in need of care. Individuals do not necessarily have to be treated by persons of the same ethnic and cultural group with which they identify. Yet entering into treatment, forming an alliance with the therapist, being able to communicate in one's primary language, and having a shared view of psychological problems can all depend on a good match of therapist and patient in relation to ethnicity and culture. A mismatch of ethnicity and culture between prospective client and therapist at minimum adds another barrier for receiving services. A mismatch can have a variety of deleterious influences, including not remaining in treatment, lower quality of the therapeutic alliance, and less therapeutic change (e.g., Kim, Ng, & Ahn, 2005; Zane et al., 2005). Even obtaining diagnostic information could be influenced by a mismatch. For example, when interviews are conducted in the native language of the client, rather than their secondary language (e.g., English), clients report more and more severe symptoms (Brown & Weisman de Mamani, 2017). The effects of treatment can also be influenced. In one review, treatment was more effective when ethnically adapted and placed in the native language of the client (i.e., two to four times more effective, as measured by effect size) (Griner & Smith, 2006). In short, having poor ethnic and cultural representation among mental health professionals who can provide services maintains and fosters huge disparities among groups and obstacles for entering treatment.

Overall, adding more mental health professionals to do what they are doing now, including how they provide services, to whom, and where, will not palpably (if at all) reduce the burdens of mental illness. We could use more person-power (and more to come on that topic), but having more people providing the usual treatment to mostly majority-group individuals and mostly in urban areas perpetuates rather than solves a problem.

Attitudinal Factors

By *attitudinal factors* here I refer to influences within the individual that provide obstacles in obtaining or seeking care. These factors are readily distinguished from system factors at the margins, but they can also blend. For instance, services may be available to those in need of care, but perhaps people do not believe they will be reimbursed or reimbursed completely. Beliefs about the system of care are deterrents, too. Attitudinal issues are not minor and indeed are considered to be the main source of barriers to receiving care. Here are salient barriers within this category.

Stigma

Attitudes and perceptions of the public serve as major barriers to providing mental health services. These attitudes encompass views about several aspects of mental illness, including perceptions of psychiatric disorders (what they are and what it means to "have" one), concerns about acceptance by other individuals if they admit to having a disorder, the value of interventions designed to treat mental disorders, views about mental health professionals and others who provide services, and more generally a reluctance to get involved in mental health treatment. Stigma is the most familiar barrier that comprises an attitudinal factor. Stigma means that mental illness tends to be associated with negative attributes such as disgrace, shame, weakness, lack of control, irrationality, and others. Stigma can result in people with mental illness being rejected, shunned, and treated in a discriminatory fashion (Hinshaw & Stier, 2008). Stigma is not limited to mental illness and is also associated with various physical characteristics (disabilities, disease), culture and ethnicity, varied gender identity, homelessness, poverty, and use of illicit substances, to mention major contenders. Regrettably, rejection, discrimination, and attribution of pejorative characteristics have many victims.

Separate facets of stigma can be delineated. First, there are the negative effects on the person who is stigmatized. Stigma includes prejudice, stereotypes, and discrimination against people with mental disorders. That discrimination can be expressed in many ways, including limited opportunities for work, housing, and insurance coverage (because of a preexisting condition). At school and in the workplace, bullying, physical violence, and harassment may result from the stigma against mental illness and any symptoms that suggest psychological problems. Most of us have seen rejection of individuals with seemingly odd emotional, cognitive, or behavioral characteristics.

Second, the stigma individuals hold against themselves can affect their attitudes toward their own mental health problems. This is known as *self-stigma,* or the internalization of the broader view one might hold toward others. Because of self-stigma, individuals may be unlikely to acknowledge a possible mental illness or symptoms, or to seek treatment. Even if one acknowledges symptoms, one would want to avoid certain stereotypic attributes such as being "crazy" or unable to handle everyday life commonly associated with mental illness or treatment.

Stigma is so pervasive that even health care professionals are susceptible to it and can display numerous negative reactions, prejudice, and stereotypes (e.g., about dangerousness) in relation to individuals with mental illness (e.g., Ahmead, Rahhal, & Baker, 2010; Lauber et al., 2004; Nordt, Rössler, & Lauber, 2006; Reavley, Mackinnon et al., 2014; Van Boekel et al., 2013). This is instructive because it demonstrates that education and information do not necessarily protect people from harboring stigma.

Stigma related to mental illness is well studied, with theory and research going back several decades and spanning many different countries (Corrigan et al., 2012; Pescosolido, 2013). National surveys and laboratory studies have evaluated various negative responses to psychiatric disorders and the people who have them. These views include stereotypes about how dangerous people with mental illness are likely to be and the need for coercive and restrictive treatments to contain or control individuals labeled as mentally ill. Efforts to inform the public that mental illness is a disease, with biological bases (in the brain, genetics), were made in part to reduce stigma. Unfortunately, such educational approaches have generally failed to reduce stigma—indeed, they have occasionally increased it—because they introduced a more fatalistic view, namely that not much can be done for individuals with a disorder (e.g., Phelan, 2005; Schnittker, 2008; Stuart et al., 2012).

Stigma and self-stigma can be influenced (moderated) by several other variables, including culture, country, age of the target patient (child, adult), type of disorder, and descriptors used to portray mental illness (e.g., Pescosolido, 2013). These nuances are important, but for present purposes the overall concern is more critical, namely, stigma presents a huge barrier in seeking and providing services. The degree of perceived stigma is inversely related to the likelihood of seeking treatment (Clement et al., 2015).

Many people because of stigma are reticent to label their conditions as mental illness and to enter into mental health systems and services. Obtaining effective treatment and overcoming some impairing condition are weighed against risking stigma and discrimination. The stigma and discrimination risks are real and are associated with all sorts of discriminatory acts, including not being hired, being denied loans, being treated with discourtesy, and being seen as dishonest (e.g., Kessler et al., 1999). Individuals with mental illness or a history of illness may be restricted in other ways, such as the ability to obtain or renew a driver's license, vote, serve on a jury, hold elected office, or maintain custody of children. The discrimination associated with mental illness has its own consequences in terms of emotional and stress reactions that can exacerbate mental health problems (e.g., Capezza et al., 2012). In short, stigma and self-stigma go beyond "beliefs and attitudes." Disclosing one's mental illness or symptoms can have untoward consequences, and even in situations in which there might not be "real" negative consequences, the perception alone that these consequences could or will occur are more than enough to keep people from seeking treatment.

Real or perceived risks of disclosing mental illness are likely to outweigh any gain of disclosing for at least two reasons. First (and as discussed in the next section), public views of psychological treatments and mental health services are not very positive or hopeful. Many people do not see treatment as a viable or effective option, so the advantages of treatment seem paltry when weighed against the seemingly greater costs of stigma and discrimination.

Second, as a general rule, we humans tend to avoid risk—it seems to be a feature of our neurobiological makeup as a species even when there might be a benefit, or greater benefit than can be quantified (e.g., more money earned than money at risk to be lost). Even the neurobiological underpinnings of this risk-averse style have begun to be unraveled (e.g., Macoveanu et al., 2013). One can understand the reticence of participating in any mental health service to minimize the perceived risk that is associated with stigma.

Mental Health Literacy

Another pervasive and multifaceted barrier to seeking treatment is *mental health literacy,* which refers to "knowledge and beliefs about mental disorders which aid their recognition, management, or prevention" (Jorm et al., 1997, p. 182). Mental health literacy includes knowledge about disorders and their treatment and prevention, recognition of the emergence and presence of disorders, and awareness of help-seeking options, including self-help strategies and professional treatment options. Literacy in this context goes beyond simple knowledge but instead indicates the likelihood of actually following through and acting on that knowledge (Jorm, 2012).

Lack of mental health literacy is a barrier to receiving treatment and affects multiple facets of entering treatment. To begin, individuals with a mental disorder may not immediately recognize there is a problem nor seek treatment right away when the problem is recognized. One study found an average total delay of 8.2 years, with 6.9 years passing before recognition of the problem and 1.3 years before obtaining treatment (Thompson, Issakidis, & Hunt, 2008). Similarly, a large-scale survey of people in 28 developed and developing countries revealed that only a fraction of individuals in need of treatment received any (Wang et al., 2007); among those who did receive treatment, the delay in seeking treatment was long (e.g., 1–14 years for mood disorders, 3–30 years for anxiety disorders, and 6–18 years for substance use disorders).[2]

Delays in identifying the need for treatment are due in part to the human tendency to use more normalizing terms (e.g., stress, life problems) rather than more clinically informed and more severe labels (e.g., depression) when referring to symptoms and clinical dysfunction. Of course, such terms tend to minimize the significance of the problem while also classifying it as not requiring professional mental health services. When individuals are given descriptions of mental disorders, they often do not identify them as problems at all (for a review, see Jorm, 2012). Outside of the laboratory, a large percentage of those with a disorder (44.8 percent) do not perceive the need for treatment (Mojtabai et al., 2011). Simply put, people often just prefer to handle their problems on their own.

Mental health literacy may be all the more difficult because of obstacles of identifying disorders in childhood and adolescence. The majority of mental disorders arise during these periods. Yet childhood and adolescence are periods that can show marked changes in emotions, thought processes, and behaviors that are normative. Consequently, in childhood and adolescence, it may not be so easy to distinguish whether something is a problem or signs of a problem and whether that sign is transient or permanent and worthy of intervention. Many problems that can indeed be significant (e.g., tics, stuttering, language delays) often emerge and then just as quickly disappear in childhood. Thus the transient nature of some clinical problems and the fluctuations of "normative" child behavior can make clinical dysfunction difficult to identify unless it is extreme (for instance, the extremes of autism spectrum disorder or intellectual disabilities) and there is clear impairment in key areas (like self-care and school functioning).

With so many mental health disorders, with ambiguity in terms of what is and is not a problem, and with the huge variation in personality and social behaviors among individuals, one might say that identifying mental health problems is inherently difficult. That might well be the case, but a larger problem is worth noting here. When it comes to other types of health issues, including hearing problems, vision problems, and obesity, individuals are not all that good at identifying problems and seeking interventions (Davis et al., 2007; Lydecker & Grilo, 2016; Noertjojo et al., 2006). So, the problem of health literacy is not limited to mental disorders.

Mental health literacy also includes knowing what the range of treatment options are and how to access and enter treatment.[3] Limits in people's views about what viable treatment options exist and attitudes toward the various options provide barriers to obtaining professional help. One study found that in general adults consider parents and family to be their primary sources of support and help, and view these sources more positively than they do a mental health professional (Jorm, 2012). Apart from family and friends, many people consider certain self-help strategies (vitamins, special diets, physical activity, getting out of the house more, and courses on stress management) to be effective means of addressing their mental health problems (sometimes more so than professional mental health treatment). In short, mental health care is not necessarily the first resource people consider. People may question the effectiveness of mental health care. Indeed, a survey in six European countries indicated that one-third of individuals believed that professional mental health care is worse than or equal to no help at all for mental disorders (ten Have et al., 2010).

Educational efforts clearly are needed to inform individuals of the process of identification and how to move from identification to obtaining effective help

(Perry et al., 2014; Reavley, McCann et al., 2014). Yet, by themselves, educational efforts may not be sufficient. Evidence shows that knowledge of mental health is improved after intervention, but it is not clear that this shift would have any impact on actual identification of problems in everyday life, change how the problems are labeled, or be followed by action in obtaining treatment. Knowledge and attitudes on self-report measures are rather easily changed; behavior change usually is much more difficult.

Cultural and Ethnic Influences

In the United States, cultural and ethnic identity can serve as a barrier to receiving services. Well documented is the lower likelihood of receiving mental (or physical) health care for individuals of ethnic minority status (e.g., McGuire et al., 2006; Nelson, Smedley, & Stith, 2002; US Department of Health and Human Services [USDHHS], 2001). This is frequently discussed and referred to as *disparities in health care* and reflects the differences among various groups and their access to care (not attributable to differences in health status, e.g., prevalence of dysfunction) or preferences of the group. For example, if 25 percent of every ethnic and cultural group experienced dysfunction and 20 percent of each group received treatment, there would be no disparities. It is when this proportion varies among groups that disparities arise. In the United States, certain minority groups (e.g., African American, Hispanic American, and Native American) are victims of these disparities.

The factors that contribute to these disparities are many and include characteristics of the services themselves, cultural views of mental health care, and attitudes and bias based on cultural and ethnic stereotypes among those who deliver services (Smedley et al., 2003). Let us consider a few of these factors in more detail. To begin, the availability of services places a limit on receiving care. Minority groups are disproportionately living in poverty in the United States, and services (e.g., clinics, hospitals) for mental health care are less available to the poor (Anderson, 2012). People living in poverty are not likely to have insurance or other sources of funds for physical or mental health care. So, even if one lived next door to an outpatient mental health service (very unlikely), being able to pay for services also is unlikely.

Second, services are not available that are culturally or ethnically congruent with the population in need. For example, treatment rarely is provided in the United States in different languages (e.g., Native American languages, Spanish, Chinese), so individuals with primary fluency in one of these languages might not seek treatment, even if they could communicate sufficiently in English. Those who are not fluent or less fluent in English in the United States might feel even less comfortable discussing psychological problems and participating in the entire process (e.g., intake assessment, therapy of some kind). Too few mental health professionals are available who reflect the cultural and ethnic characteristics of those in need of care (see Commission on Ethnic Minority Recruitment, Retention, and Training, 2008). Finding a practitioner of a given ethnicity who specializes in the problem at hand is difficult; most practitioners in the United

States are European American. In principle, a perfect ethnic match of a therapist and client is not a prerequisite for effective treatment (Miranda et al., 2005), but the lack of available services and professionals that do match one's culture could certainly deter one from seeking and entering into treatment.

Above and beyond the nature of services and providers themselves, key values and characteristics of individual cultures also can derail the processes of defining disorders, identifying what suitable interventions are, and seeking treatment. For example, cultures that emphasize self-reliance and spirituality as a health care option, or that see the family or community as a source of care, would be less likely to pursue "mainstream" (European American) health care or even to consider it relevant. As an example, exorcism and spiritual worship are major and, in some cases, primary means of addressing mental health problems in some non-Western cultures (e.g., Nguyen, 2014; Sabry & Vohra, 2013). Recall that earlier I mentioned that mental health treatments are not the first line of attack for many of those in need of care, and mainstream Western treatments often are not seen as likely to be effective anyway.

The notion of mental health literacy, discussed previously, itself is culturally based because it is based on the view that there is a fixed objective condition that some people can or cannot identify an once identified seek or do not seek treatment for that condition. Yet, many individuals, based on cultural traditions and personal beliefs, do not identify impairment in emotions, thinking, or behaviors as a psychological problem or a "problem" necessarily at all. For people who do not see their problems as psychological, mental health literacy is an irrelevant concept. If one does not see the problem from within the same cultural context in which mental health services have been devised, understandably one would not seek out such services. Overall, there are enormous cultural barriers in diagnosis, assessment, and treatment (Constantine & Sue, 2005; Paniagua & Yamada, 2013).

Providing public information and increasing knowledge are important but less likely to have a direct impact on our goal of reducing the burdens of mental disorders. An assumption of mental health literacy, as with stigma, is that more information and education will reduce that barrier, open the gate, and allow individuals to go to treatment. This remains largely an assumption, with mixed findings at best. Knowing more does not translate to doing something about it or doing something differently. This is not an argument against knowledge, information, or education. Indeed, all options for improving mental health should be pursued to bring treatment to individuals. Some ways of delivering interventions, noted in later chapters, can circumvent many of the usual barriers and do not need to assume that batting down illiteracy or stigma is a precondition to getting people into treatment.

Other Factors

I have designated a third broad category of barriers that are not easily placed elsewhere, barriers that greatly influence whether care is and can be provided to all those in need of services. They are highlighted here but raise critical issues to which we return later in the book.

Case Identification

Mental health literacy usually concerns people in the community and the extent to which they are able to identify clinical problems and resources for treatment. This might be referred to as self-identification given the focus on clients, potential clients, and communities of clients (e.g., by cultural or ethnic groups). Consider case identification as a separate barrier to providing services with a shift in focus from potential clients to systems of care.

Case identification refers to the ability to identify cases (individuals who might be in need of care) as a function of various systems within society, such as the schools, the workplace, and the community. That is, we know individuals with problems exist in large numbers. To what extent can they be identified by systems within the community and directed to potential treatment or other interventions? The difficulty in identifying cases in need of attention is a barrier to providing services. We might call this *system mental health literacy*, the ability of systems to identify clinical problems and direct individuals to the services that would help them.[4]

Case identification can be explained using, as an example, shootings in public places (schools, movie theaters, churches, shopping malls, and so on). In these shootings, multiple people have been killed and wounded. In many such cases, news articles report that the shooter had some form of mental illness, undiagnosed or poorly treated, or otherwise not detected. The implication is that something could have and should have been done differently to prevent the crime.[5] Using a case identification approach, we ask what might be done to identify such individuals. Invariably following such violent incidents there are numerous calls and perhaps even some allocation of funds for increases in mental health services (e.g., Mueller, 2014). But even if implemented, the effect of such action is likely to be very small to nonexistent. This is because more services will not help in identifying people who need those services nor in bringing those people to the services that exist. More broadly, adding more funds to a system that is not very effective in providing services is of uncertain value, at best.

Case identification is a barrier to care because we have no systematic way of identifying cases in a proactive fashion. Because we know that most psychiatric disorders begin in childhood and in adolescence, those periods of life would be one place to begin to focus on case identification. Systems and settings in which many or most children are seen would be a logical place to implement systematic means to identify cases that might warrant attention. For example, elementary schools could conduct routine monthly evaluations of each child that focus on age-related functioning in social spheres (e.g., friends, interacting with others, victims or bullies or both), academic spheres (e.g., not so much achievement oriented but overall doing alright in role requirements), and other domains. Measures could be brief, and the resulting huge data sets could be used by researchers to refine items and their utility in predicting later problems and to address variations in region, ethnicity, and culture. All the measures would alert screeners to children who might be in need of supports (and not necessarily just from a mental health professional—this could mean volunteers, Big Brothers and Sisters, and the like).

Not all sources of dysfunction emerge in childhood and adolescence. We should have means of identifying people in need of services over the course of life through the school system, the workplace, and public service (such as the military). We need not begin with the daunting task of identifying all psychological disorders (>400 in contemporary diagnosis) and revamping multiple systems (elementary, middle, and high school; workplaces). Currently, we do not have procedures in place that are convenient, user-friendly, and brief and that could be used on a large-scale basis for even one or two disorders. Consequently, systematic efforts to identify cases in any setting and on almost any scale (e.g., school district) would be a good start.

Currently, when someone with undiagnosed or untreated psychological impairment commits a crime or completes suicide, we are led to wonder how the individual could have slipped through the cracks. There are no cracks—there are huge gorges. We do not look for individuals who are on the path toward needing care. In addition to increasing mental health literacy so that clients and their relatives can better identify who might be in need of treatment and what to do, we also need to have in place complementary, systemic procedures to identify such individuals as early in life as possible. Also, we want to identify dysfunction (subclinical) early in its progression because the longer the dysfunction goes untreated the more likely it will become a more serious disorder (or disorders). Thus some case identification is likely to be appropriate at multiple points early in life (e.g., pediatric visits, schools), but it has to be done quite systematically and in an ongoing way. I mentioned that there are obstacles in identifying dysfunction in childhood because of variation and the transient nature of many "symptoms." Yet these need not be a deterrent to case identification as we collect data systematically, looking for possible outliers or "profiles" that increase the risk for clinical dysfunction. Assessment is arguably as important as developing interventions.

Model of Intervention Delivery

An enormous but often overlooked barrier in reducing the burdens of mental illness is how we routinely deliver psychological treatment. Consider as a key distinction the difference between interventions and how they are delivered. We have evidence-based psychosocial interventions (EBPIs), which are the *interventions*; how they are provided to individuals is the *model of intervention delivery*. The vast majority of psychosocial interventions in various forms of cognitive behavioral, traditional, and other therapies are delivered in a common way (or model of delivery) that dominants mental health. That dominant model has three interrelated characteristics:

1. Treatment sessions are provided in person and one-to-one with a client (individual, couple, family);

2. Treatment is administered by a highly trained (e.g., master's or doctoral level) mental health professional; and
3. Sessions are held at a clinic, private office, or health care facility.

This model is so pervasive that it is usually seen as *the* way of administering treatment when in fact it is only *one way* (with many options as will be elaborated in later chapters). I mention here that the dominant model is a barrier because it is available to so few people in the United States and in other developed and developing countries. If we are interested in reducing the burdens of mental illness, this model can play *a* role, but it should be very different from the one in current use. Later I will engage in a more extended discussion of the model, why and how it limits access to mental health care for people in need, and how to surmount that (see Chapter 6). Here, it is important to mention the dominant model as a professional-system barrier: "professional" because the model is dictated by the professions that provide mental health services and "system" because this barrier is not inherent in the attitudes or perceptions of clients. Therapy almost always means individual psychotherapy of one sort or another. That is fine if you are fortunate enough to have access, but it is not viable as a means of helping a large number of people in need.

ADDRESSING AND SURMOUNTING BARRIERS TO TREATMENT

These barriers must be addressed if we are to provide mental health services on a large scale and reach the vast majority of individuals in need of services. There are two broad strategies for addressing these barriers. First, one can combat individual barriers directly. For example, to address financial considerations and cost as a barrier, we can make affordable insurance available for a larger number of people and also simplify the process of charging insurance for mental health services (though no small task, that). Providing reimbursement for treatment sessions is a step in the right direction for reducing cost as a barrier. In the United States, insurance programs are still not the same as providing free as-needed care, enabling clients to walk into a clinic or health care facility and not worry about payment, coverage, or an interrogation about one's insurance. In many other countries (e.g., some within the European Union), treatment is free, although of course it is paid for by taxes. In any case, better insurance coverage is an attempt to address cost as a barrier and obviously constitutes a direct assault on an important barrier.

Another example relates to mental health literacy. This barrier is addressed by ongoing efforts to distribute information and educational materials about disorders and their treatment. For example, in the United States, the Centers for Disease Control and Prevention (2016a) play a pivotal role in providing updated information on physical and mental health issues. Information and educational materials are provided in multiple languages. Moreover, there is a major effort to ensure that information about health care is presented in plain language (free from jargon) to improve health care literacy.[6]

Despite having provided two examples of direct efforts to reduce or eliminate barriers, it must be acknowledged that there will be no single way to overcome any individual barrier, and hence multiple efforts at multiple levels (federal, state, local) are important to continue and expand. In the vast majority of efforts, education is seen as the path to reducing barriers. If people knew more, they would behave differently, goes the thinking (this of course has so many counter-instances in research and everyday life, such as our diet and exercise behaviors). Nevertheless, the impact of an effort to reduce barriers is an empirical question. We need more trials to test different strategies to determine whether (1) a given barrier in fact was reduced; (2) the reduction led to more people being treated or taking care of themselves; and, arguably most important, (3) one could see palpable improvements in health as a result. Also, education and better understanding may be essential as part of a larger package that includes multiple ways of directly combatting the barriers.

A second and complementary strategy is to sidestep barriers entirely rather than addressing them directly and individually. By sidestepping, I mean making the barrier less relevant or irrelevant rather than trying to surmount it. For example, a barrier in physical health care has been getting people to treatment settings (clinics and hospitals). A breakthrough here was making the setting less relevant; many treatments can now be brought to patients by setting up clinics to do limited work in shopping malls, drug stores, and other settings (these include vaccinations, screens for cardiovascular disease, and much more). Referrals can be made from these settings when serious medical conditions are evident. Reducing the need to travel to clinics (with obstacles being transportation, parking, and scheduling appointments) increases the likelihood of receiving services. A related effort has been to set up small urgent-care centers. These are walk-in services often in fairly unassuming and nonmedicalized store fronts. The centers bring medical care closer to patients' lives and also alleviate the ordeal of going to a doctor or to a hospital. They help get people to treatment by getting treatment centers closer to people.

Mobile mammography has served as a model for bringing care to individuals. Busses equipped with diagnostic tests, materials, and information visit communities where people live and can provide services in the neighborhood. The model has been adopted to address all sorts of health issues (general health, cardiovascular health, oral health, and others; I do not provide citations here because most of these are commercial enterprises and can be found on the Web). In any case, bringing treatment and diagnostic services to people to some extent sidesteps the barrier of accessibility. Similarly, in mental health care there are ways to sidestep some of the barriers. This model of delivering treatment (through technology, social policy changes) provides several opportunities that I will take up later in the book.

Much of contemporary psychosocial research has focused on identifying EBPIs, a topic addressed in Chapter 4. Having treatments that are effective and with firm science behind them is pivotal. With piles of effective interventions in hand, now one looks to the other hand with a pile of barriers. Can we get all of these effective treatments to people in need? Devising effective treatments is only a part of what is needed if all of the barriers discussed here remain in place. That is why any discussion of reducing the burden of mental disorders requires at least a two-pronged approach: not only the development of treatments but also efforts to ensure that they can be delivered on a large scale.

SUMMARY AND CONCLUSIONS

We have learned that the vast majority of individuals in need of care actually receive nothing at all. And the proportion that does receive care gets a wide range of "interventions" that can involve any contact or even just one contact with a variety of individuals (counselors, healers, health but not mental health professionals), few of whom are directly trained in mental health care.

In this chapter I also discussed barriers to receiving care and highlighted several impediments. System factors were discussed, which refer to barriers outside of the individual that can impede receiving treatment. The financial cost of treatment in the United States is clearly a deterrent. When a person has insurance coverage, it is not always so clear what will be reimbursed. Policy and legal regulations were also noted as a systems barrier, and these reflect a panoply of influences dictating whether service facilities are available and whether various groups and clinical problems will be treated based on budgetary constraints. Also, trained mental health professionals are too few in number and are concentrated in places that limit their reach among the many who need services. Other limits (too few professionals to reflect the ethnicity and culture of the population, and too few trained to address problems where need is great, such as with children and older adults) provide further barriers.

Attitudinal barriers are considered to have an even greater impact in keeping individuals from treatment. I began with discussing stigma associated with symptoms of mental illness, including self-stigma or views individuals have about themselves and acknowledging symptoms as such. Mental health literacy was discussed and shown to relate to delays in identifying whether one has a mental disorder and is in need of treatment, as well as delays in action to obtain treatment. The lack of information and ability to recognize a disorder alone prevents individuals from seeking appropriate care, leaving aside barriers such as stigma.

Case identification and model of intervention delivery were two barriers rarely discussed that greatly limit providing services. The dominant model of treatment delivery has been and continues to be some form of individual psychotherapy, delivered in person, by a mental health professional and in a clinic or private practice setting. Evidence-based and non–evidence-based therapies are of this model. The dominant model of providing treatment and viable alternatives will be taken up in later chapters.

PART II

Current Status and Advances in Psychosocial Interventions

4

Evidence-Based Psychosocial Interventions

Advances and Challenges

Prior chapters have noted that the need for services for individuals with psychiatric impairment is enormous, that the majority of individuals in need of care receive absolutely nothing in the way of systematic or professional care, and that there are multiple barriers related to providing and receiving care. A critical "missing" piece concerns what we as mental health professionals have to offer in the way of psychosocial interventions. That is, if we *could* get interventions to individuals and individuals to interventions, would what we have to offer make any difference? In this chapter I will review the enormous progress we have made in developing evidence-based psychosocial interventions (EBPIs), the status of these interventions, and key questions and challenges in getting them to those in need.

My focus is on psychosocial or psychological interventions. The goals of these interventions are to reduce the full range of psychological sources of dysfunction related to affect, cognition, and behavior and psychiatric disorders that can impair everyday functioning. They employ a variety of psychological and interpersonal processes as methods of change, including psychoeducation, talk, feedback, modeling of new behaviors, altering decision making, altering cognitions, coping, emotion regulation, problem-solving strategies, practice and rehearsal, and engaging in specific activities outside of sessions.

HEALING AND PSYCHOLOGICAL INTERVENTIONS: HISTORICAL OVERVIEW

Psychosocial interventions and psychotherapy as a subcategory of those are relatively recent terms, yet many of the elements of psychological interventions have been used since the beginning of documented history in the context of healing, both for physical and mental health (Norcross, VandenBos, & Freedheim, 2011). Perhaps the most prominent example comes from religious and spiritual practices that span historical epochs, continents, and cultures. Religious and nonreligious (secular) traditions draw on a variety of practices, ceremonies, and rituals, as well as potions, herbs, plants, and other substances. Many of these are intended to alter, relieve, and cure mental, physical, and spiritual ailments. Religious and spiritual leaders, shamans, healers, and others with analogous cultural functions have been placed in helping and healing roles.

At various points in history, the causes of mental illness were thought to be religious or spiritual in nature. For example, possession by Satan was at one time considered to be the source of psychological problems, and many treatments (e.g., exorcism) were directed to redress the problem (e.g., Scull, 2015). Even today, exorcism as a treatment of physical, mental, and spiritual maladies continues to be used. With sources explaining how mental and physical health symptoms emerge, how one can determine whether exorcism is needed, and how to carry out the procedures (Michael, 2014; Nguyen, 2014; Sabry & Vohra, 2013)?

Without the benefit of research and careful documentation, we cannot know the outcomes and effectiveness of the many psychosocial procedures practiced through the ages. Yet I believe it is reasonable to assume that many of them often had good outcomes, that is, led to improvements. Two reasons support the reasonableness of this. First, in fact many symptoms of clinical dysfunction (both mental and physical) improve over time with or without treatment. Some sources of significant impairment (e.g., recurrent depression) are episodic, which means they come and go over the course of one's life. During some periods there is genuine improvement, and that can occur without treatment. If some treatment is provided, it would be natural to attribute the change to the treatment, even if the treatment itself did not lead to the change. The equivalent would be having special beverages, foods, or potions or engaging in various rituals or chants while one has a cold. Many of these might lead to relief, but the cold is likely to remit with or without any of these.

Second, we know that beliefs and expectations on the part of the patient can lead to very marked and dramatic changes both in mental and physical disorders. Treatments, even if they are "fake" (not based on procedures that would be likely to help given properties of the actual intervention), lead to improvements if they generate expectations for improvement on the part of patients. In fact, the more a given psychological procedure generates expectancies for improvement, the greater the therapeutic change (see Baskin et al., 2003; Boot et al., 2013; Grissom, 1996). Historically (and currently) interventions that generate strong expectancies for change were likely to have an impact.

The role of belief and expectations in relation to improvements in both mental and physical disorders is nicely illustrated in the work of Franz Anton Mesmer (1734–1815). He was Austrian physician who began a clinical practice in which he healed individuals of a variety of physical and mental sources of impairment. Mesmer's procedures included quite specific actions and rituals such as touching the body and having patients listen to music, at some points soft and at other points loud and intense. He had a theory of *animal magnetism* in which therapeutic change was achieved by realigning fluids and physical forces in the body. The practices and rituals within treatment served as the means of changing these forces and fluids and when successful would lead to cure.

Mesmer's treatment was apparently quite effective. He had a long string of successes in changing all sorts of mental and physical maladies (e.g., anxiety, blindness, congestion, convulsions, coughing, dizziness, fits of rage, hallucinations, headaches, hemorrhoids, pain, paralysis, spasms, stomachache, temporary blindness, toothache, vomiting, and more!) (Crabtree, 1993). Many of the changes were dramatic and evident in the daily functioning of the individual (e.g., walking without a limp, cessation of all coughing, restoring vision).

Formal evaluation of Mesmer's procedures was carried out by a group of scientists headed by Benjamin Franklin, who was in France at the time as America's first ambassador. The charge of the Franklin Commission, as it later came to be called, was *not* to determine whether Mesmer's treatments worked but rather to see if Mesmer discovered a new physical fluid and whether there was any basis for the claims Mesmer made regarding how this treatment worked. The commission carried out several observations and experimental tests that made it very clear that if people believed objects to which they were exposed had been magnetized (given the forces from Mesmer), they improved. In fact, it did not make much difference if the objects had been magnetized (imbued with special features); people improved if they believed the objects had been. The commission concluded that the benefits of Mesmer's procedures could be traced to imagination (expectations, placebo effects) on the part of the patients. In relation to the commission's charge, there was no evidence for special fluids or animal magnetism as the basis of the effects of the treatment. There was no real challenge to the fact that Mesmer changed people's mental and physical health. Indeed, the commission directly observed improvements in patients undergoing Mesmer's procedures. Yet Mesmer's explanation of these changes was rejected. I mention Mesmer in a little detail to illustrate my point about the likelihood that many procedures intended to help people probably often did. All sorts of procedures that might evoke expectations for improvement both on the part of the person who delivers the intervention and on the recipient are likely to have an impact. When "imagination" or "suggestion" or placebo effects are invoked to explain change, they tend to be used in a dismissive and pejorative fashion. In fact, they are reliable influences and indeed may play a key role in much of the effects of contemporary therapies for physical and mental health (e.g., Kam-Hansen et al., 2014). In any case, all of the many undocumented procedures by healers over thousands of years—and many continuing into the present—cannot be dismissed out of hand as ineffective. We now know that procedures (what is actually done in treatment) do make a difference but also that expectations about what those procedures will do can as well.

Psychosocial interventions constitute a major area of scientific research and have moved well beyond the unsystematic reports of the effects of treatment. The scientific study of variations of psychotherapy in particular and interest in treatment effectiveness can be traced to mesmerism, the development of hypnotism after that, and then psychoanalysis, although invariably one can pluck examples from ancient history that approximate many scientifically based treatments. Psychoanalysis brought a theory of the human mind into sharp focus and influenced our understanding, evaluation, and treatment of psychological disorders. The dominant views throughout history were that mental disorders were caused either by evil spirits or physical health problems (e.g., imbalance of fluids from Greek medicine, and even bad air). Mesmer unwittingly advanced the view that psychological factors were key, and this stemmed from conclusions about the importance of imagination as the basis of the changes his methods produced. Mesmer's work is an excellent example of formalization of psychotherapy and the role of expectations and belief in therapeutic change.

In terms of the development of therapy, leaving aside the matter of beliefs and expectations, the greatest impact and visibility are deserved by psychoanalysis, developed by Sigmund Freud (1856–1939). Psychoanalysis made a huge conceptual leap by advancing a view about how psychological problems came about and what processes in therapy are needed to eliminate the problems. This was not considered a very scientific view—no real evidence, anecdotal cases, and a theory that seemed slippery because it could not be well tested (e.g., Grünbaum, 1985). None of that detracted from Freud's putting psychotherapy on the map and prominent in the minds of health care professionals, artists of all types (e.g., authors, musical composers, painters, playwrights, sculptors), and the culture more generally. Although psychoanalysis is well beyond the scope of the present book, it is important to credit its treatment and conceptual view as the "big bang" of psychotherapies. Indeed, many theories of therapy and innovators of new treatments (e.g., nondirective psychotherapy, cognitive therapy, rational emotive behavior therapy, behavior therapy) used psychoanalysis and its limitations as a base for new lines of work that in fact generated sound scientific research. Creative inventors and proponents of these new treatments often included in their papers direct criticism of psychoanalysis as a point of departure and rationale for "new and improved" conceptual views and interventions and as important evidence (e.g., Ayllon & Michael, 1959; Ellis, 1957; Lazarus, 1961; Rogers & Dymond, 1954; Salter, 1952).

The inspiration for much of the psychosocial intervention research that has been conducted today can be traced to early evaluations of what was once a rather weak and skimpy empirical literature on psychotherapy. In 1952, Hans Eysenck (1916–1997), a prominent British psychological researcher, evaluated the sparse research literature on psychotherapy that was available at the time. The conclusion he reached from reviewing the research was that treatment was effective (i.e., was associated with therapeutic change) for approximately two-thirds of the patients who received treatment. This initial conclusion seemed promising—more than that—great news. But, somewhat disconcertingly, it was also found that among patients who did not receive any treatment, approximately two-thirds improved. With or without treatment, it seemed, improvements were about the same. The conclusions were challenged, and the evidence to support the finding was not all that clear (there were no truly randomized controlled comparisons of the type that are routine today) (e.g., see commentaries in Eysenck, 1966).

Interestingly, Eysenck was not alone in the general claim that the evidence, such as it was, did not support the view that psychotherapy surpasses the changes that occur over time without treatment (e.g., Levitt, 1957, 1963). Updating of the reviews by including more research did not change the conclusion very much but continued to generate vibrant discussion, controversy, and rebuttals (Bergin & Garfield, 1994; Eysenck, 1966; 1995). In the years following these critical reviews, psychotherapy research flourished. Conferences centered on psychotherapy research, special book volumes to consolidate the latest science, and research on treatment processes and outcome increased dramatically (e.g., Meltzoff & Kornreich, 1970; Rubenstein & Parloff, 1962; Shlien, 1968).

We now know that psychotherapy does lead to change. Seminal reviews of research in the mid-1970s and early 1980s identified hundreds of controlled studies and concluded that in fact psychotherapy in general was effective (Smith & Glass, 1977; Smith, Miller, & Glass, 1980). The evidence keeps pouring in, with increasing focus on the specific types of treatment as applied to various disorders. Psychotherapy research has continued to advance remarkably along many fronts, as evident by increases in the quantity and improvements in the quality of research, expansion in the conceptualization of treatment (e.g., to include concepts and techniques from Eastern traditions), development of treatments that span multiple disorders, integration of technology and social media, use of cognitive, social, and clinical neuroscience and computational models to better understand therapeutic change, and increased attention to critical ethnic and cultural issues (see Gelo & Pritz, 2015; Lambert, 2013).

CONTEMPORARY EVIDENCE-BASED PSYCHOSOCIAL INTERVENTIONS

Background and Delineation

A key advance has been the development of EBPIs. Perhaps this does not seem like an advance—was there a time when evidence was not important or relevant? With the development of scientific psychology, one must say that evidence is always relevant, but its importance has become more salient as natural, biological, and social sciences have progressed more generally. A scientific approach with emphasis on theory, empirical tests, and measurement, among many other tenets and practices, has profoundly influenced psychotherapy. In the early development of psychotherapeutic practices (e.g., mesmerism, hypnosis, psychoanalysis), the effectiveness of treatment was "documented" with anecdotal case studies rather than with the carefully controlled trials that are routine in contemporary research. Much of the documentation in medicine was of the same type, lacking standard practices evaluated carefully in empirical research.

In the 1960s and 1970s research in psychotherapy began to advance visibly, as reflected in the work on nondirective (also called *client-centered*) psychotherapy by the prominent psychologist Carl Rogers (1902–1987). Another, larger advance began in behavior therapy, which encompassed research drawing on conceptual models and practices from laboratory research on psychology of learning (see Kazdin, 1978b). Many different behaviorally based treatments were evaluated empirically and increasingly in well-controlled studies and with replications. The well-controlled studies were randomized controlled trials (RCTs) in which participants are assigned randomly to conditions. RCTs are commonly regarded as the "gold standard" in intervention research (in psychology, medicine, education, and so on) and have special status as a result. Research indicated that there was considerable evidence for the effectiveness of many different interventions (e.g., Bandura, 1969; Kazdin & Wilson, 1978). Through all of this, many hundreds of psychotherapy techniques continued to be in use (as they are still today), most having not been evaluated empirically (then and now).

In the mid-1990s, a committee comprising well-respected researchers and clinicians completed a very influential report to identify and designate treatments with supportive research (American Psychological Association [APA] Task Force, 1995). The report proposed criteria that might be used to establish whether a given treatment would be regarded as *empirically validated treatment*, a term soon replaced with *empirically supported treatment*. Revisions continued to refine the criteria and to provide an updated list of treatments. In a second revision, for example, the criteria and set of treatments were updated, as provided in Box 4.1. From the criteria, one can see that classifying a treatment as supported or not supported is not so straightforward. To rectify this, a more graded system was used by noting the level of support (well established, probably efficacious). In addition, the authors readily acknowledged, there are factors not covered by these criteria, including the quality of the study (whether the test was strong in terms of how it was conducted, sample size, and so on) and outcomes that might be important but that were omitted.

Enumerating criteria and designating treatments as having suitable support to be well established or probably efficacious was enormously important, but the process was not without controversy, which mobilized many researchers and clinicians (e.g., Chambless, Baker et al., 1998; Chambless & Ollendick, 2001). The sources of controversy included challenges to the criteria, what constitutes "evidence," the degree to which the evidence was applicable to circumstances in which treatments are used in clinical practice, the neglect of key influences in therapy (such as the therapeutic relationship), and claims of a potential bias favoring behavioral and cognitive behavioral treatments (see Eliott, 1998; Norcross, 1999; Tanenbaum, 2005). Perhaps the greatest achievement of this task force was making explicit the goal of clarifying the evidence base of treatment and acknowledging what many already knew: that most treatments in use are not supported by evidence and that many treatments are supported that are not widespread use.

Box 4.1

CRITERIA FOR "EMPIRICALLY VALIDATED TREATMENTS"

Well-Established Treatments

I. At least two good between-groups design experiments demonstrating efficacy in one or more of the following ways:
   A. Superior (statistically significant) to pill or psychological placebo or to another treatment
   B. Equivalent to an already established treatment in experiments with adequate sample sizes

   Or:

II. A large series of single-case design experiments ($N > 9$) demonstrating efficacy. These experiments must have:
   A. Used good experimental designs, *and*
   B. Compared the intervention to another treatment, as in IA.

Further Criteria for Both I and II:

III. Experiments must be conducted with treatment manuals.
IV. Characteristics of the client samples must be clearly specified.
V. Effects must have been demonstrated by at least two different investigators or investigating teams.

Probably Efficacious Treatments

I. Two experiments showing the treatment is superior (statistically significant) to a wait-list control group; *or*
II. One or more experiments meeting the Well-Established Treatment Criteria IA or IB, III, and IV, but not V; *or*
III. A small series of single-case design experiments ($N > 3$) otherwise meeting Well-Established Treatment Criteria

Note: Since the committee's early work and this report, the term *empirically validated* was changed to *empirically supported.* More generally, the term *evidence-based* is used, as noted in the text.

Source: Chambless, D. L., Baker, M. J., Baucom, D. H., Beutler, L. E., Calhoun, K. S., Crits-Christoph, P., . . . Woody, S. B. (1998). Update on empirically validated therapies, II. *Clinical Psychologist, 51*(1), 3–6. Reprinted with permission from the Society of Clinical Psychology, Division 12 of APA.

Since the original report, both the terminology used to refer to well-supported treatments and the criteria for their designation have evolved. To begin, various levels of support continue to be delineated, so treatments can vary depending on the strength of the evidence (e.g., Nathan & Gorman, 2015; Silverman & Hinshaw, 2008). That is, levels or amount of support (number and type of studies) are used to give gradations. As is evident in Box 4.1 with early iterations of the criteria, one can see that treatment evidence is viewed as more compelling when a treatment is compared with stronger control groups (other treatments or placebo conditions) than with weaker control conditions (e.g., no treatment).

A critical point is worth making here: The strength of the *studies* (or of the *evidence*) is not necessarily related to the strength of the *treatment* (i.e., the magnitude of the changes, the proportion of patients who improved). This is an important distinction that is occasionally lost; more studies do not mean a better (more effective) therapy, but rather that one can be more confident in the findings because they have been replicated. Indeed, the criteria for "evidence-based" do not require that the intervention really helps people in palpable ways, a topic to which I return later in the chapter.

Different terms are used to describe support and can vary significantly in their meaning. For example, *empirically supported* or *evidence-based treatment* refers to the interventions or psychotherapeutic techniques (such as cognitive therapy for depression, exposure therapy for anxiety) that have been carefully evaluated in controlled research trials. *Evidence-based practice* is a broader term and refers to clinical practice that is informed by evidence about interventions but in addition relies on clinical expertise and the clinicians' views of patient needs, values, and preferences and their integration into decision making for individual cases (e.g., APA, 2006; Goodheart, Kazdin, & Sternberg, 2006; Westen & Bradley, 2005). In short, the evidence is based on the interventions; adapting and adopting them in clinical practice as filtered by clinical judgment may or may not produce effects demonstrated in research. Thus evidence-based treatment is what has been supported in research. Evidence-based practice is not supported by research in the same way. After one takes the treatments from research and mixes them with several other components, including clinician discretion, we do not know if we have a treatment that is effective.

Empirically supported treatments as a term is still in use for the full range of psychotherapeutic interventions that have evidence. Yet "evidence-based" has been adopted, as in evidence-based psychotherapies or more broadly evidence-based psychosocial interventions—EBPIs. Among the reasons is that "evidence-based" is commonly used as a modifier in many disciplines (e.g., evidence-based: agriculture, chiropractic, dentistry, economics, law, medicine, nursing, ophthalmology, political science, public health, social policy, social work). Among the reasons to use "interventions" rather than "therapies" or "treatment," especially for the purposes of my discussion here, is that many influences can be used to improve mental health and psychiatric disorders (e.g., taxes that decrease addictive behavior, exercise that can improve depression)—but they are not at all "therapies" or "treatments" in the usual sense (although they can be therapeutic).

There is no universal set of criteria for designating treatments as EBPIs. Members of the original Task Force made refinements, and others have added to those (e.g., Chambless & Hollon, 1998; Chambless & Ollendick, 2001; Charman & Barkham, 2005), and further suggestions continue (e.g., Tolin et al., 2015). Moreover, the criteria used to designate treatment as evidence based vary among multiple disciplines (e.g., psychology, psychiatry, social work), diverse professional organizations within and among countries (e.g., in the Americas, European Union), and private and public agencies within a given country. Many insurance and health care agencies (as well as countries) are involved in defining the criteria in part to decide what treatment services will be reimbursed. All of that said, the criteria usually invoked are those listed in Box 4.2. In most designations, a treatment is considered to be evidence based if all or most of these criteria are met.

The minimal requirement is usually two well-controlled studies with replications by independent teams of researchers. However, outcome studies continue to pour—actually gush—from many well-established journals that routinely include multiple RCTs in their issues (e.g., *Journal of Consulting and Clinical Psychology, Behavior Therapy, Behaviour Research and Therapy*). Rather than looking to a couple of studies, more commonly conclusions about the effects of treatment are reached on the basis of reviews (meta-analyses) that bring multiple trials together for a quantitative review. The bar for meta-analyses of course is much higher than the minimal requirements of a few studies. By the time a meta-analysis is completed, a large set of studies is usually available and reviewed.

Meta-analyses of psychosocial interventions are now so readily common and available that they themselves often serve as the bases of reviews, sometimes referred to as a *meta-meta analyses* or *metasynthesis* (Johnson et al., 2010; Kazrin,

---

Box 4.2

Criteria to Delineate Psychosocial Treatments as Evidence Based

- Comparison of treatment with a no-treatment or other comparison control condition;
- Random assignment of participants to intervention and comparison or control conditions;
- Careful specification of the patient population (e.g., the disorder or problem and how the clinical problem is measured);
- Use of treatment manuals that specify in detail what the therapeutic procedures are;
- Multiple measures of therapeutic change, including measurement of the problem or disorder targeted in treatment;
- Statistically significant differences at the end of the intervention period between treatment and control or comparison conditions; and
- Replication of outcome effects, ideally by an independent investigator or research team that can reproduce the findings obtained in the original study.

Note: These are commonly used criteria culled from many different statements and recommendations. Variations of the criteria differ slightly across many interested parties involved in delineating evidence-based psychosocial interventions.

Durac, & Agteros, 1979).[1] Rather than individual outcome studies, the individual meta-analyses that encompass these studies are reviewed (e.g., Butler et al., 2006; Fabiano et al., 2015; Hofmann et al., 2012; Lambert & Ogles, 2013). With so many outcome studies and meta-analyses, we can now consider the impact of a broad range of treatments beyond the more familiar and more frequently reviewed cognitive behavioral interventions that have dominated the empirical literature.

How Many Evidence-Based Psychosocial Interventions Are There and What Are They?

Many interventions have been delineated as evidence based, and these can treat a wide range of psychiatric disorders and sources of impairment in psychological functioning among children, adolescents, and adults (e.g., Nathan & Gorman, 2015; Weisz & Kazdin, 2017). Making a list of or placing a number on available EBPIs must be done with caution for at least three reasons: (1) there is no single set of criteria that are in use universally, (2) some lists distinguish treatments by levels of support rather than whether they are evidence based or not, and (3) the list of treatments continues to grow. Even so, it is useful to provide illustrations to convey the treatments and the numbers involved.

At the time of this writing, a group within the APA has identified 80 EBPIs for mental disorders; these are provided in Box 4.3 (Society of Clinical Psychology, 2013). A few characteristics of the list are noteworthy. First, it is dominated by cognitive and behavioral treatments, which are the most well studied (e.g., Hofmann et al., 2012; Ougrin, 2011). The preponderance of cognitive behavioral techniques in this list does not imply that these treatments are more effective than non–cognitively based treatments in any given application; it is simply that the evaluation of non–cognitively based techniques has not caught up in terms of number of rigorous evaluations and grant-funded projects to investigate their effectiveness.

Second, the list is instructive, showing that there are not 80 different *techniques*. Some techniques are listed multiple times. For example, cognitive behavior therapy is in the box 17 times based on the problem to which the treatment has been applied and for which there is supportive evidence. So, it is important to be explicit about the multiple listing of individual techniques. Indeed, we know from experience in physical health care that a treatment (say, surgery or medication) is not effective in a general case or in the abstract but rather in relation to specific applications (for instance, surgery for appendicitis or lung transplantation, antibiotics for certain types of bacterial infections). With psychosocial interventions as well, a given technique might be effective with multiple problems. Yet the combination introduces a complexity in counting how many techniques there are and for what problems.

Other agencies, states, and professional organizations also provide lists of treatments with an evidence base. Perhaps the most prominent in the United States has been identified by a federal agency, which at the time of this writing has recognized more than 450 psychosocial interventions as evidence based; that number

Box 4.3

Sample List of Evidence-Based Psychosocial Interventions

1. Acceptance and Commitment Therapy for Chronic Pain;
2. Acceptance and Commitment Therapy for Depression;
3. Acceptance and Commitment Therapy for Mixed Anxiety;
4. Acceptance and Commitment Therapy for Obsessive-Compulsive Disorder;
5. Acceptance and Commitment Therapy for Psychosis;
6. Applied Relaxation for Panic Disorder;
7. Assertive Community Treatment for Schizophrenia;
8. Behavior Therapy/Behavioral Activation for Depression;
9. Behavioral Couples Therapy for Alcohol Use Disorders;
10. Behavioral Couples Therapy for Depression;
11. Behavioral and Cognitive Behavioral Therapy for Chronic Low Back Pain;
12. Behavioral Weight Loss Treatment for Obesity and Pediatric Overweight;
13. Biofeedback-Based Treatments for Insomnia;
14. Cognitive Adaptation Training for Schizophrenia;
15. Cognitive Behavioral Analysis System of Psychotherapy for Depression;
16. Cognitive Behavioral Therapy for Attention Deficit Hyperactivity Disorder (Adults);
17. Cognitive Behavioral Therapy for Insomnia;
18. Cognitive Behavioral Therapy for Anorexia Nervosa;
19. Cognitive Behavioral Therapy for Binge Eating Disorder;
20. Cognitive Behavioral Therapy for Bulimia Nervosa;
21. Cognitive and Behavioral Therapies for Generalized Anxiety Disorder;
22. Cognitive Behavioral Therapy for Obsessive-Compulsive Disorder;
23. Cognitive and Behavioral Therapies for Social Phobia/Public Speaking Anxiety;
24. Cognitive Behavioral Therapy for Chronic Headache;
25. Cognitive Behavioral Therapy for Panic Disorder;
26. Cognitive Behavioral Therapy for Schizophrenia;
27. Cognitive Processing Therapy for Post-Traumatic Stress Disorder;
28. Cognitive Remediation for Schizophrenia;
29. Cognitive Therapy for Bipolar Disorder;
30. Cognitive Therapy for Depression;
31. Dialectical Behavior Therapy for Borderline Personality Disorder;
32. Emotion-Focused Therapy for Depression;
33. Exposure and Response Prevention for Obsessive-Compulsive Disorder;
34. Exposure Therapies for Specific Phobias;
35. Eye Movement Desensitization and Reprocessing for Post-Traumatic Stress Disorder;
36. Family-Based Treatment for Anorexia Nervosa;
37. Family-Based Treatment for Bulimia Nervosa;
38. Family Focused Therapy for Bipolar Disorder;

39. Family Psychoeducation for Schizophrenia;
40. Friends Care for Mixed Substance Abuse/Dependence;
41. Guided Self-Change for Mixed Substance Abuse/Dependence;
42. Healthy-Weight Program for Bulimia Nervosa;
43. Interpersonal Therapy for Depression;
44. Illness Management and Recovery for Schizophrenia;
45. Interpersonal Psychotherapy for Binge Eating Disorder;
46. Interpersonal Psychotherapy for Bulimia Nervosa;
47. Interpersonal and Social Rhythm Therapy for Bipolar Disorder;
48. Mentalization-Based Treatment for Borderline Personality Disorder;
49. Moderate Drinking for Alcohol Use Disorders;
50. Motivational Interviewing and Motivational Enhancement Therapy for Substance and Alcohol Abuse/Dependence;
51. Multi-Component Cognitive Behavioral Therapy for Fibromyalgia;
52. Multi-Component Cognitive Behavioral Therapy for Rheumatologic Pain;
53. Paradoxical Intention for Insomnia;
54. Present-Centered Therapy for Post-Traumatic Stress Disorder;
55. Prize-Based Contingency Management for Alcohol Use Disorders;
56. Prize-Based Contingency Management for Cocaine Dependence;
57. Prize-Based Contingency Management for Mixed Substance Use/Dependence;
58. Problem-Solving Therapy for Depression;
59. Prolonged Exposure for Post-Traumatic Stress Disorder;
60. Psychoanalytic Therapy for Panic Disorder;
61. Psychoeducation for Bipolar Disorder;
62. Psychological Debriefing for Post-Traumatic Stress Disorder;
63. Rational Emotive Behavior Therapy for Depression;
64. Relaxation Training for Insomnia;
65. Reminiscence/Life Review Therapy for Depression;
66. Schema-Focused Therapy for Borderline Personality Disorder;
67. Seeking Safety for PTSD with Substance Use Disorder;
68. Seeking Safety for Mixed Substance Abuse/Dependence;
69. Self-Management/Self-Control Therapy for Depression;
70. Self-System Therapy for Depression;
71. Smoking Cessation with Weight Gain Prevention;
72. Short-Term Psychodynamic Therapy for Depression;
73. Sleep Restriction Therapy for Insomnia;
74. Social Learning/Token Economy Programs for Schizophrenia;
75. Social Skills Training for Schizophrenia;
76. Stimulus Control Therapy for Insomnia;
77. Stress Inoculation Training for Post-Traumatic Stress Disorder;
78. Supported Employment for Schizophrenia;
79. Systematic Care for Bipolar Disorder; and
80. Transference-Focused Therapy for Borderline Personality Disorder.

Source: Society of Clinical Psychology of the American Psychological Association. March 2016. Retrieved from http://www.div12.org/psychological-treatments/treatments/). Reprinted with permission from the Society of Clinical Psychology, Division 12 of the American Psychological Association.

continues to grow (Substance Abuse and Mental Health Services Administration [SAMHSA], October 2017b). Of course, the treatments are too many to list here (see http://nrepp.samhsa.gov/AllPrograms.aspx), and the list is constantly revised, with more techniques being added.

The list includes many interventions that might be familiar to mental health professionals engaged in clinical research or practice (e.g., cognitive behavioral techniques, exposure therapy, multisystemic therapy, relapse prevention therapy). Many others may be unfamiliar and are not routinely included in most books or journal articles that review EBPIs (for instance, accelerated resolution therapy, critical time intervention, peaceful alternative to tough situations, network therapy). I suspect these and many others listed are not taught in most mental health training programs either. Many of the interventions extend beyond direct treatment of psychiatric dysfunction and include, for example, community support and care for patients with schizophrenia, or interventions with elementary school children to prevent drug use.

These two separate lists of EBPIs (and there are others I have not explored here) should only be considered approximate guides for a variety of reasons. Many interventions appear on one list but not on the other. Many treatments that could arguably be considered evidence based are on neither list (more on this later). Occasionally, similar treatments (procedures) have different names, different treatments have similar names, and varying gradations and permutations of these make it difficult to discern whether there are two variations of the same treatment or whether the two treatments ought to be delineated (see Kazdin, 2000). In short, though we are certain that there are now quite a few such interventions, it is difficult to say with confidence how many, and in fact it may be wise to avoid such a number because "technique by disorder" should be our unit of measure (see Box 4.3), rather than just "technique." The better question to ask is whether there is an evidence-based intervention for this or that disorder or domain of functioning.

Expanded Range of Evidence-Based Psychosocial Interventions: The Midas Touch

As the EBPI research has evolved, two changes are noteworthy. First, we have gone well beyond the criterion of a couple of very carefully controlled trials to determine whether a treatment is evidence based. More often than not, scores of studies can be brought to bear, and hence reviews of multiple treatment studies are used to identify EBPIs. Second, we have moved well beyond the cognitive behavioral variations of psychotherapy (as in Box 4.3) that long dominated EBPIs. Many that are "traditional" forms of therapy and that antedated the move to cognitive behavioral treatments are now identified as evidence based. Let us look at these two shifts in more detail.

Meta-analytic reviews of the evidence, involving scores of studies, are commonly used to evaluate a given treatment, harnessing the strength of combinations of many studies and evaluating study features (such as clinical problem focus, quality of the study, types of outcome measures) that may influence their conclusions. Interestingly, as more and more treatments go through meta-analyses, we see something of a King Midas effect. As the reader will recall from Greek mythology, everything Midas touched turned to gold (www.mythweb.com/encyc/entries/midas.html). This included food and beverages as he tried to feast. As the myth continues, as Midas took his daughter by her hand to go to dinner, she immediately turned into a gold statue. Through more intricacies of the myth, this all was reversed, but Midas came to loath wealth and lived a more modest life. (The story of exactly how and why he started a franchise of shops to replace mufflers remains a matter of heated scholarly debate.) In relation to the present discussion, the Midas touch seems to be evident when many, if not most, psychotherapy techniques undergo meta-analysis. Table 4.1 lists several interventions

Table 4.1 SAMPLE OF MORE TRADITIONAL (NON–COGNITIVE BEHAVIORAL) EVIDENCE-BASED INTERVENTIONS

Technique	**Sample Reviews**
Animal-assisted therapy	Virués-Ortega et al. (2012)
Grief therapy	Allumbaugh & Hoyt (1999)
Humanistic therapies	Elliott (2002)
Hypnosis	Rotaru & Rusu (2016) Shih, Yang, & Koo (2009)
Marital and couples therapies	Snyder & Halford (2012)
Mindfulness	Creswell (2017)
Motivational interviewing	Lundahl et al. (2010)
Music therapy	Standley (2002)
Nondirective supportive psychotherapy	Cuijpers et al. (2012)
Paradoxical interventions	Shoham-Salomon & Rosenthal (1987)
Play therapy	Leblanc & Ritchie (2001)
Psychodrama	Kipper & Ritchie (2003)
Religious and spiritual adaptations of psychotherapy	Smith, Bartz, & Richards (2007)
Self-help therapies	Scott, Webb, & Rowse (2015)
Sensory integration therapy	Vargas & Camilli (1999)
Short-term psychoanalytic and psychodynamic Longer-term versions of these therapies	Leichsenring, Rabung, & Leibing (2004) Smit et al. (2012)
Wilderness/adventure therapy	Bettmann et al. (2016) Bowen & Neill (2013)

NOTE: I have selected one or two key references (for less frequently discussed treatments) to support the claim that these are evidence-based as concluded from a meta-analysis. For many of the techniques, multiple reviews are available. Also, I have referred to these treatments as non–cognitive behavioral treatments. Yet as cognitive behavioral therapies have evolved, they have drawn on and integrated some of the therapies in the table (e.g., mindfulness, motivational interviewing, many of the self-help treatments).

that might now be considered evidence based. They have meta-analytic reviews, have surpassed the criterion of a couple of controlled trials, and now are designated as evidence based.

Decades ago, when therapies were first actively investigated, behavioral and then cognitive behavioral treatments (such as systematic desensitization, exposure therapy, cognitive therapy for depression) were emerging, with many outcome studies sometimes replicated ad nauseam. At that time, the assumption was that these new therapies would replace traditional, unevaluated Brand X interventions that were probably not worth doing anyway. "Traditional" included interventions based on approaches that emphasized psychoanalytic, psychodynamically oriented, and insight-based treatments focusing on talk as the basic medium of change. The focus was on the inner workings of the mind, psychological processes, and facets of personality (like self-esteem) that were considered to underlie clinical dysfunction (e.g., London, 1986). Fast-forward to today, and many of these same very traditional therapies, omitted from early designations of EBPIs, now have evidence in their behalf. Many of these treatments are listed in Table 4.1 and draw on studies with RCTs. My point is that now many interventions are evidence based beyond the cognitive behavioral treatments that once dominated.

A few important caveats and qualifiers are in order. First, not all meta-analyses are of equal quality, nor are they the same in the scope of studies available to review. Some analyses, for example, draw on fewer than 10 studies, and others on a few hundred. Second, not all reviews have shown that the treatment in question is effective; some treatments that do not appear in the table have been reviewed, with findings of insufficient or nonexistent evidence to support their use (these include psychological debriefing for trauma, equine-facilitated psychotherapy for childhood disorders, and others) (e.g., Anestis et al., 2014; Litz et al., 2002). Third, many other treatments (like relational therapy, sand therapy, horticulture therapy, and smudge therapy [play therapy with paints]) have their own literatures (e.g., Loewenthal & Samuels, 2014; Predny & Relf, 2004), but insufficient information is available to draw any conclusions because of the paucity or complete lack of controlled rigorous scientific studies. Finally, although the list of EBPIs is long, it is still the case that hundreds of treatments are in use in the real world, and most of these have not been studied (for one list, see Kazdin, 2000). Add to this the fact that in clinical practice, interventions are often combined, and these combinations are rarely documented or evaluated in research.

Routine Care, Too, Can Be Called Evidence Based

The scores of EBPIs include a large set of cognitive behavioral interventions and many traditional therapies as well (see Box 4.3 and Table 4.1, respectively). An assumption with the development of EBPIs is that they can and probably ought to replace what is ordinarily done in clinical practice. Whether or not the extent to which EBPIs surpass the effectiveness of treatments usually provided in clinical care is obviously a critical question. There is now a reasonably well-developed research base that evaluates treatments as usually practiced in settings in which psychotherapy is provided.

Treatment as usual (TAU), also referred to as usual or routine care in a given setting, has included diverse forms of individual, group, or family therapy and an assortment of community services (see Kazdin, 2015). Some form of psychotherapy is the most commonly used type of TAU. Initially, TAUs were used primarily as control or comparison conditions for studies of other ("the real") treatments. As control conditions, TAUs have several benefits (e.g., clients in the primary treatment being studied and those in the control [as usual] conditions both receive some form of treatment; many of the common factors of therapy, such as meeting with a therapist, developing an alliance, and hearing a credible rationale are controlled in varying degrees). Yet the impact of TAUs is of considerable interest in its own right, well beyond its use as a mere control condition. Understandably, this is the case because most therapists are practicing TAUs, and the interventions cannot be dismissed out of hand without clear evidence that in fact they are inferior in their effects to the putative "new and improved" EBPIs.

The efficacy of TAUs has been examined in multiple meta-analyses. Two types of meta-analytic reviews speak to the effectiveness of TAUs (see Kazdin, 2015). In the first type of review, studies are accumulated that make direct comparisons between an EBPI and a TAU. In this type of review, RCTs form the main basis of comparison for the individual studies. Across all such studies, the difference in effect size (magnitude of effect) is computed to determine how or whether one class of treatments (EBPIs) is better than another class of treatments (TAUs) (e.g., Spielmans et al., 2010; Wampold et al., 2011; Weisz, Kuppens, et al., 2013). Overall, the conclusion from this type of review is that EBPIs tend to show greater therapeutic changes (effect size) compared with TAUs, but the difference is rather small ($\sim d = .2$ to .3) and not always statistically significant.[2]

Conclusions about the effectiveness of TAUs vary as a function of dose (amount) of treatment and whether the TAU was some form of psychotherapy or a community service that may or may not have been actually received by clients. For example, in the studies, often the EBPI was longer (more sessions, more time in therapy) than the TAU. When this or other differences are controlled, the difference in effectiveness between EBPIs and TAUs is not always statistically significant, and small differences (from uncontrolled comparisons) become even smaller. Based on this first type of review, it would be difficult to argue that one class of treatment is more effective than another.

The second type of review is based accumulated outcome data from TAUs in clinical settings and where the data are not from RCTs (e.g., Cahill et al., 2010; Hunsley & Lee, 2007; McEvoy & Nathan, 2007; Merrill, Tolbert, & Wade, 2003; Minami et al., 2008). The evaluations are based on computing effect sizes from assessments completed in clinic settings where various TAUs have been provided. The effectiveness of TAUs is based on *benchmarking*, that is, comparing the magnitude of the effect (effect sizes) of TAUs in clinical work, with the magnitude of effects of EBPIs in controlled clinical trials (see Delgadillo et al., 2014). The many reviews of TAUs based on benchmarking encompass multiple clinics, thousands of clients, and diverse outcome measures. The general finding from such reviews has been that that TAUs and EBPIs are comparable, that is, within the same range and not statistically different in the magnitude of effects. Also, both classes of treatment surpass the changes that occur with no treatment at all (the natural history or course of the disorder), as attested to in the reviews cited previously.

Both types of reviews raise doubts about the routine superiority of EBPIs over what is done in many clinical practice settings. Yet we ought to be careful in leaping to the conclusion that TAUs are equal to EBPIs, or even in implying that all TAUs (or EBPIs) are equal to each other within their respective treatment classes. There are huge ambiguities related to what TAUs even are; they are not usually described at all, and one cannot assume they are even consistent within a given clinic (as practiced by two different therapists) and of course across different clinics (see Kazdin, 2015). What this means is that TAUs cannot really be replicated across other settings. TAU is very much like a *soup du jour*—ordering soup of the day at the same restaurant on different days or at different restaurants on the same day may sound the same, but it is unlikely that the soup is the same, and no one could replicate the soup without details about the ingredients.

Overall, the evidence now suggests that TAUs, as a broad class of treatments, in principle can be as effective as EBPIs, as another broad class. Yet this is of little conceptual or practical use because we do not know which among the scores and scores of TAUs are effective and for what problems. Even so, we now have evidence-based "doubt" that calls for caution in assuming the EBPIs invariably are more effective than TAUs (for further discussion, see Kazdin, 2015). This is not a trivial matter because there are huge ongoing efforts to disseminate EBPIs to clinical practice settings. Given this investment, it is important to be confident that any new treatments put into place in a given clinic will surpass effects of TAUs already in place in these settings.

General Comments

There is now a long list of interventions that can legitimately be called evidence based (see Box 4.3 and Table 4.1), leaving aside the unspecifiable routine treatments (TAUs) practiced in clinical settings. Are all these treatments effective or equally effective? Evaluations of psychotherapy decades ago occasionally invoked the Dodo bird verdict from *Alice in Wonderland* (Carroll, 1865), namely, that "*Everybody* has won, and all must have prizes" (Chapter 3, www.alice-in-wonderland.net/books/1chpt3.html). This notion, initially applied to techniques of psychotherapy more than 80 years ago (Rosenzweig, 1936), was exhumed and made prominent again more than 40 years ago by an influential review of psychotherapy outcome research (Luborsky, Singer, & Luborsky, 1975) and continues to be used (McAleavey & Castonguay, 2015; Palpacuer et al., 2017). All techniques are not likely to be equally effective, of course, yet rarely are comparisons made to evaluate whether treatments differ in the outcomes they produce.[3]

So how are we to select from among the many options to recommend what treatments ought to be used in clinical practice and for what disorders? This is enormously important for patient care, for informing decisions as to what treatments ought to be disseminated to clinical practice and what treatments will be reimbursed by private and public agencies. Clearly, the selection is not just an academic exercise or a matter of scholarly debate. Various government agencies and organizations have taken on the task, including SAMHSA, a federal agency in the United States (SAMHSA, October 2017b). That agency's list of EBPIs, exceeding 450 interventions and growing, includes a variety of foci, including community supports for patients and prevention programs in the schools. Many state and insurance agencies also identify the treatments to classify not just best practices but also what will be reimbursed. In other countries, organizations evaluate the evidence and make recommendations. A prominent example is the National Institute for Health and Care Excellence (NICE, https://www.nice.org.uk/), an agency in the United Kingdom that reviews, selects, and recommends interventions based on the evidence for mental and physical health. Reviews of treatments are provided by clinical problem and by population (such as children, older adults). We will return to NICE recommendations in Chapter 5 in the discussion of dissemination of treatment. Suffice it to say that the evidence has filtered from reviews of research to recommendations to guide clinical practice.

EVIDENCE-BASED PSYCHOSOCIAL INTERVENTIONS IN PERSPECTIVE

Although lists of EBPIs continue to expand, fundamental questions remain concerning what the evidence means, how and why the treatments achieve therapeutic change, and how, whether, and the extent to which the findings from controlled research apply to clinical practice. There are extensive discussions and programs of research on these issues. I sample these here to place EBPIs in perspective.

Effectiveness of Treatment: What Can We Say?

Treatment Outcome Measures and Their Interpretation

Several measurement issues directly influence any conclusions we make about EBPIs and their impact. Consider the individual RCT as a starting point. In any given study that evaluates an EBPI, usually several measures are included to evaluate domains of patient functioning. The goal is to assess changes in the symptoms or disorders that initially brought the client to treatment. There are many such measures, and often these are completed by the clients themselves (like self-report measures of depression) or others (such as professional interviewers, relatives, therapists) who might have a perspective on functioning. A fundamental concern is whether the measures and summaries of the evidence reflect actual changes in patient functioning in everyday life.

Another way to frame this issue is to ask: What does it mean to say that a treatment is evidence based? That the treatment is effective in improving the lives of the clients who receive it? Not necessarily, given the following:

- Different measures (e.g., self- versus other-report; self-report versus direct observations) do not correspond very well and can lead to different conclusions about whether treatment is effective and about the strength of the effects (e.g., De Los Reyes, Aldao, & Augenstein, 2017);
- Psychological measures (standardized self- or other-report measures, tasks within the laboratory) do not necessarily "map on to" or reflect how the client is doing in everyday life (Blanton & Jaccard, 2006); and
- When authors complete an investigation of an EBPI, they often are selective in drawing only on certain measures out of all that were used in the study—specifically those measures that support the expected conclusions about the treatment. Measures that did not support expectations often are neglected (see De Los Reyes & Kazdin, 2006).

Psychotherapy studies are likely to focus on measures (e.g., self-report and interviews of depression), and these are less well established as directly related to real-life referents. That is, we do not know, as one illustration, the extent to which scores on a valid measure of depression (e.g., Beck Depression Inventory or Hamilton Rating Scale for Depression) relate to exactly how people are experiencing depression in everyday life (e.g., when they get out of bed in the morning, when they consider going to work, whether they eat, sleep, and engage socially with others). Self-report checkmarks and clinician ratings presumably are correlated with these other indices, but that is still indirect as a sample of experience. The point here is not about any single measure. In virtually all treatments, multiple measures may be relevant. Add to that, self-report is very important in its own right (e.g., happiness, quality of life). Yet interpretation of treatment effects could be greatly enhanced by direct measures that sample functioning in everyday life (e.g., proportion of days of going to work, reduced emergency department visits, and suicide attempts, or samples of mood both through self-report and physiological correlates in real-time by use of technology, as discussed later). These comments do not invalidate the measures but merely mean that further assessments are needed if we want to know about actual functioning in everyday life.

In short, the status of treatments as evidence based requires a cautionary note or qualification. Discussions of EBPIs usually skip over what individual studies actually show and what changes on the measures used in that study actually mean, whether all of the measures were considered, and so on. These points do not discount the excellent research, but rather temper conclusions about what the effects are.

Effect Size

Beyond the individual studies, consider multiple studies in meta-analytic reviews that are used to determine whether an intervention is evidence based.

Meta-analyses use effect size as a way to summarize how effective treatment is. Effect size and related indices are valuable in scientific research in general, beyond our discussion, because they provide a measure of strength of an effect in statistical terms and complement statistical significance testing.[4] Effect size is the difference in means between groups (e.g., treatment and comparison groups) as expressed in standard deviation units. This is a statistical concept. Nevertheless, the statistic (e.g., strong effect size) is often confused with the importance or the practical or clinical value of the treatment (e.g., Rutledge & Loh, 2004; Sun et al., 2010). Yet there is no necessary relation at all.

The limits of effect size as an index of practical significance are easily illustrated. For example, consider a hypothetical treatment for obesity in which the meaning of the outcome measure is more easily illustrated (Kazdin, 2013). We might recruit individuals who are at least 100 pounds (~45 kg) overweight and twice or more their ideal weight (criteria sometimes used to define "morbid obesity") and assign them randomly to treatment or no-treatment conditions. We follow cases for one year after treatment ends. Assume that everyone in the intervention group loses 2 pounds (.91 kilograms) and everyone in the control group gains 2 pounds. Yet at the end of the study all participants may still be very obese. Effect size for this result might be very large given how the statistic is computed, but this does not convey whether weight and health status have actually improved for anyone. Did treatment help anyone in palpable ways—that is, was there benefit in terms of weight that makes a clinically important or useful difference? We do not know from the effect size, but we know from understanding the measure on which it is based that a 2-pound loss is not very likely to qualify because the risk for serious health outcomes (e.g., diabetes, osteoarthritis, heart disease, or cancer) is unlikely to be affected by such a small change in weight. In other words, a large effect size has no necessary connection to clinical impact or practical significance for individuals or the group. This is easy to see in this example because weight and its connection to objective outcomes beyond that direct measure (e.g., morbidity, mortality) are readily apparent.

The example was one in which effect size was large, but practical significance or clinical impact arguably was trivial. The reverse scenario reveals the problem, too—a small strength of relation (correlation) can reflect an important practical effect. For example, individuals who experience clinical depression after a heart attack are at higher risk for dying in the following six months than are those without depression (see Rutledge & Loh, 2004). In fact, after a heart attack, individuals with depression are more than four times more likely to die than those without depression! Yet the strength of the relation, using correlation, between depression and dying is small ($r = .22$), with a small amount of shared variance ($r^2 = .048$, or 4.8 percent). Similarly, the utility of aspirin in preventing a second heart attack has an important practical effect. Indeed, one clinical trial comparing aspirin and placebo was stopped early because the results were so clear in favor of aspirin. Yet the strength of the relation was small ($r = .03$; see Rutledge & Loh, 2004).

For research purposes it is quite reasonable to draw conclusions about what is more effective based on effect size. Moreover, we want to know in this context whether some treatments are consistently more effective (have stronger effect sizes). But there is no implication that "more effective" by this index has any bearing on practical changes or differences in patient functioning and translates to influence functioning or symptoms in daily life. This may seem paradoxical but is simply what effect size means.

In short, when we say that EBPIs are effective, the meaning is well known to researchers but might be narrower than implied. Changes on standardized outcome measures reflect the impact of treatment. When multiple studies are combined, usually many measures are also combined, converted to a standard unit (effect size), and summarized. As a general rule, usually we do not know from these individual studies that treatment made genuine changes in the lives of individuals. There are exceptions. Occasionally, treatment eliminates a problem (from several to zero panic attacks), or the measures (e.g., blood levels to indicate success in changing diabetes or consumption of illicit substances) are known to capture real-life behavior. So, interpretation of impact can depend heavily on the measures and what they are known to reflect.

Use of Other Indices

Changes on the usual standardized measures in a treatment study are recognized for their limits; that is, they may not reflect a change that is very important to the client. The changes or effects of an intervention may be statistically significant, the main criterion used in scientific research in general. But for intervention research, whether for the treatment of depression, anxiety, cancer, or heart disease, we want to know more and specifically about practical changes that make a difference clinically.

Clinical significance refers to the practical value or importance of the effect of an intervention, that is, whether it makes any "real" difference to clients or to others in their functioning and everyday life. Some studies look at the amount of change people have experienced on various treatment outcome measures. The goal is to determine whether one can look beyond statistical effects and whether the changes people make are "clinically significant." Four of the more commonly used measures are:

- Whether the symptom levels that were present at the beginning of treatment fall within "normal" levels as experienced by the general public, or by a community sample that is not experiencing such problems. For example, clients coming to treatment for depression or anxiety by the end of treatment might show levels of these characteristics that are evident in populations who are doing fine (Kazdin, 1977; Kendall & Grove, 1988);
- Whether marked or especially large changes are made over the course of treatment for individual patients. Large or clinically significant changes are usually measured in standard deviation units. If an individual changes (improves) from pretreatment to posttreatment by two standard deviations, that would be regarded as clinically significant (Jacobson & Truax, 1991). The rationale is that the amount of change moves a person

outside the range of the dysfunctional population to which they may have belonged before treatment;

- Whether individuals who began treatment with a formal psychiatric diagnosis (e.g., major depression according to the *International Statistical Classification of Diseases and Related Health Problems* [ICD-10] or the *Diagnostic and Statistical Manual of Mental Disorders* [DSM-5]) no longer meet criteria for the disorder once treatment is completed; and
- Whether clients or others in contact with them subjectively evaluate the change they have made as important and meaningful and as having had a palpable impact on their lives (Kazdin, 1977; Wolf, 1978). The question addressed by this method of evaluation is whether changes have led to differences in how clients and other people see the change. The views of others may be especially relevant in some circumstances (e.g., with children or older adults) because people we interact with every day (parents, teachers, adult children) often have a critical role in identifying, defining, and responding to what they regard as dysfunctional or deviant. Subjective evaluations permit assessment of the extent to which the effects of an intervention are apparent to clients or to others.

Each of these measures reflects an improvement on merely looking at whether a result is statistically significant or whether the magnitude of effect in statistical terms (effect size) reaches a particular criterion. Yet each of the measures has its own strengths and liabilities and qualifications that makes interpretation not so straightforward (see Kazdin, 2017b). As one example, subjective evaluation may seem "loose" and perhaps limited in part because how clients evaluate their therapists, therapy, or improvements does not relate very much to actual improvements in symptoms. That is, one could "love" one's treatment and therapist but not be doing any better with the presenting problems. And yet subjective well-being and happiness have been well studied outside of the context of treatment (e.g., Diener & Chan, 2011; Lucas & Diener, 2009). Happiness is associated with many other indices of mental and physical health, socialization, and work productivity that are not subjective. Consequently, whether one genuinely feels better about one's life subjectively is important in its own right. Many of us (though not you the reader, nor I the writer) have personal characteristics and attributes that we might wish we did not. Whether or not any of these can change, life still would be so much better if we simply felt differently about them. Subjectivity is important.

The measures of clinical significance I have highlighted have been in use for decades. Concerns remain about what they reflect and specifically whether they relate to how individuals actually are doing in their daily lives (Kazdin, 1999, 2017b). Many other measures have been suggested but are not routinely in use, including:

- Conducting qualitative evaluation of patient change by intense, in-depth evaluation of the person's functioning after treatment (e.g., Hill et al., 2013);

- Using measures that focus on quality of life rather than just symptom change (e.g., Awad & Voruganti, 2012); and
- Measuring multiple domains that define "recovery," including how well one is functioning in such areas as having a purpose in life, socializing with others, being involved in meaningful relationships, being optimistic about the future, and so on (e.g., Leamy et al., 2011; SAMHSA, 2012).

In Chapter 2 I mentioned that epidemiological research has provided estimates of how mental illness impairs individuals in their daily lives. Reference was made to disability-adjusted life year (DALY; one year of healthy life that is lost due to some form of impairment, years lived with disability (YLD), and years of life lost to premature mortality (YLL). These measures are rarely used in psychosocial intervention studies, with notable exceptions (e.g., Nadkarni et al., 2016; Patel et al., 2016). These latter measures would not only address the applied impact of treatment but also connect intervention research more closely with research on the scope and impact of mental illness as a problem. Ultimately, we want multiple indices of therapeutic change but with increased attention to those that reflect impact in everyday functioning.

The metrics used in research are important, but we do not know in the vast majority of cases how these metrics translate to patient functioning. That is why new and different measures (such as qualitative measures) continue to be proposed. In selecting a treatment, it is prudent to elect one with strong effect sizes, but we must be cautious as to what that means. We want to select the treatments based on the best metrics currently in use. We also want to improve the metrics to be sure we are capturing changes that occur in everyday life. I will take up the topic of assessment again later and mention the use of technologies that have changed our ability to sample functioning of individuals in real time (for instance, by measuring stress, blood pressure, and intrusive cognitions).

Common Factors and Their Role in Therapeutic Change

There several hundred therapy techniques, encompassing EBPIs as well as the much larger number of treatments not in use and not yet rigorously evaluated. It is hard to believe by key tenets of science (parsimony and plausibility) that they all "work" for different reasons. A very long-standing and enduring discussion on this topic rests on the view that commonalities among the many different treatments are the reason that they work (e.g., Frank, 1961; Lick & Bootzin & 1975; Palpacuer et al., 2017). These commonalities are referred to as *common factors* (and on occasion also as *nonspecific treatment factors*) and include attending treatment sessions, having personal contact and a relationship with a therapist, hearing a logical rationale that describes the putative origins of one's problem, undergoing a plausible procedure directed toward ameliorating the problem, having hope mobilized by starting treatment, and expecting improvements. As one can readily see, these factors easily transcend individual treatments and encompass those in which there is direct, in-person, one-to-one contact with a therapist. These factors can generate their own therapeutic effects (e.g., Duncan et al., 2010; Frank & Frank, 1991; Lambert & Ogles, 2013).

Myth, Rituals, and Mobilization of Hope

At the dawn of psychotherapy research, a prominent researcher provided an explanation as to why therapy might work and what its common factors might be (Frank, 1961). The explanation cited two components of therapy: myth and ritual. The *myth* refers to the "story," or the therapist's theory and views about why and how the problem (anxiety, an eating disorder) came about (because of something in early child development, perhaps, or low self-esteem) and what is needed to correct that. The *ritual* refers to the activities (e.g., talk, use of imagery), or what is going to be done with, too, or for the client in light of the story that was provided. The therapist conveys to the client the idea that, "because this is your 'real' problem, or the 'real' cause of the problem, we must do this to correct or rectify it." A myth and a ritual are common factors, even though the specific myths (stories) and rituals (activities) may change among the varied therapy techniques. The myth and ritual are therapeutic in part because they mobilize hope, and that itself has therapeutic benefits (views, experience, daily activities). This view remains a very reasonable interpretation of why common factors lead to change.

When clients participate in treatment, they are likely to believe in the procedures and have faith that some therapeutic change will result (Lambert & Ogles, 2013). We have learned from many years of medical research on placebos that the belief and expectations that treatment will help are themselves important and therapeutic. In medicine, a placebo is a substance that has no active pharmacological properties that would be expected to produce change for the problem to which it is applied. A placebo might consist of a pill or capsule that is mostly sugar (rather than, for example, antidepressant medication) or an injection of saline solution (salt water) rather than some active medication for the problem of interest. Placebos given under the guise of treatment can alter a variety of disorders ranging in severity from the common cold to cancer (e.g., Benedetti, 2009; Finniss et al., 2010). Even more than that, we know that some placebos (e.g., active placebos that have side effects similar to medication) and some ways of administering placebos (e.g., larger pills versus smaller ones; injections rather than pills) even increase or strengthen placebo effects. Placebo effects, by definition, result from factors other than active ingredients in the substance itself. Hence the belief of the patient in treatment and perhaps the belief in the physician who administers treatment, and similar factors, appear to be responsible for change.

Two additional points might be especially interesting to note here. First, placebos can be very effective, even when clients are not deceived about them. That is, telling people they are receiving a placebo does not detract from the favorable impact on clinical dysfunction (e.g., irritable bowel syndrome, migraine headache, pain) (Carvalho et al., 2016; Kam-Hansen et al., 2014; Kaptchuk et al., 2010). Second, surveys of physicians indicate that in fact placebos are used in everyday clinical practice. The rates vary across countries but indicate between 17 and

80 percent of doctors have prescribed placebos in their routine clinical practice (see Howick et al., 2013). Overall, there is very extensive evidence in research on the effectiveness of placebos as well as evidence that they are used in clinical practice. All sorts of legal and ethical issues are raised by this, but they are well beyond our present scope.

Effects analogous to placebo reactions influence individuals who receive to psychotherapy, too. I mentioned the example of Mesmer in some detail previously. The effectiveness of Mesmer's procedures was not in question, but the effects ultimately were shown to be attributed to belief, suggestion, and expectations of the people he has treated. Mesmer's work is merely one example in a long chain of medical, therapeutic, and religious procedures that have been used and with reported effectiveness and with likely effects due to suggestion (Shapiro & Morris, 1978; Wampold et al., 2005). Hypnosis, for instance, is a treatment heavily reliant on suggestion and has evidence of effectiveness for psychiatric disorders (see Box 4.3).

I discussed earlier the research showing that the greater the expectations generated by a treatment or control condition in the context of psychotherapy, the greater the therapeutic changes. A very credible treatment or control condition that is purported to be a "real" treatment leads to greater therapeutic change than less credible conditions. The evidence does not warrant stating that expectations explain all changes in treatment or are the singular the reason that so many EBPIs lead to change. I believe it is fair to say that common factors, especially expectations that are generated by treatments, are rarely adequately controlled for or evaluated and cannot be ruled out as an explanation for treatment effects (e.g., Dew & Bickman, 2005; Kazdin & Wilcoxon, 1976; Kirsch, 1985; Locher, Hasler, & Gaab, 2016; Palpacuer et al., 2017). Because expectations often are viewed as artifacts or something to "control" experimentally, there have been very few efforts to optimize them to enhance the effects of treatment. The net effects are both conceptual (we do not have a clear understanding about the therapeutic change process) and practical (what should we do to maximize client change in relation to both specific and common treatment factors?).

Client-Therapist Relationship

A common factor that has been the subject of thousands of studies is the client-therapist relationship and warrants separate comment (Norcross et al., 2011). Among the many facets of the relationship, the *therapeutic alliance* is most frequently studied (Castonguay et al., 2011). Alliance refers to the quality and nature of the client–therapist relationship, the collaborative interaction, and the bond or personal attachment that emerges during treatment. A high-quality therapeutic alliance is associated with higher rates of treatment completion, greater compliance with treatment demands, and greater therapeutic change (e.g., Norcross et al., 2011; Orlinsky, Rønnestad, & Willutzki, 2004).

Because that relationship is common to many different treatments, it is a common factor. Yet the alliance is not "just" a common factor. Many traditional forms of therapy (e.g., psychoanalysis, psychodynamically oriented therapy, client-centered psychotherapy) viewed the relationship and alliance as the means for working through a clinical problem. That is, the "myth" or theory provided to the client emphasized early relationships in early child development as the putative causes of individuals' current problems, and therefore the relationship in treatment was the place to work through those causes (i.e., the ritual). Mothers were often viewed as the culprit in leading to psychological and even worse problems in the child (including autism, schizophrenia, and sudden infant death syndrome). Early relationships and especially blaming of mothers have gone by the wayside as playing a causal role in clinical dysfunction. Yet the role of the therapeutic relationship continues to be studied and viewed as pivotal in the context of psychotherapy.

The quality of the alliance predicts therapeutic change, a finding now supported by thousands of studies (e.g., Horvath & Bedi, 2002). Another now well-established finding is that the stronger the therapeutic alliance, the greater the therapeutic change (Crits-Christoph et al., 2013), although the magnitude of the relation actually is rather small ($r = .275$, or 7.6 percent of the shared variance between alliance and therapeutic change) (Horvath et al., 2011). Additional evaluations, including four meta-analyses in the context of child and family therapy, also found the alliance outcome correlations to be small (r ranging from .14 to .24) (Green et al., 2013). Symptom improvements early in therapy are associated with improved alliance, and improved alliance is associated with symptom change, that is, a bidirectional or reciprocal relation (Lutz et al., 2009; Marker et al., 2013). In any case, it is clear that for many treatments the alliance may play a role in change that transcends any treatment. However, evidence is not available that alliance is a cause of the change or how alliance would even lead to symptom changes.

Going forward, it is important that we try to better understand the role of common factors in EBPIs, how much they contribute, and whether they can be optimized or otherwise altered in some way to improve therapeutic change. For example, if expectations generated by the treatment are causally related to improvements, perhaps these ought to be enhanced as a routine part of treatment. If the therapeutic alliance plays a role, there ought to be ways of optimizing it with specific strategies and techniques that are part of treatment. On the other hand, we know now that many treatments can be quite effective without a therapist (e.g., self-help and on-line treatments; some "apps") and of course without that alliance (e.g., Harwood & L'Abate, 2010).

The advantage of common factors is that they bring parsimony to the morass of different evidence and non–evidence-based treatments that are in use. For the majority of treatments still in use clinically, the question of whether they are effective has yet to be answered. Assuming that they do, for the moment at least, then we would want to know how and why. Parsimony brings unity to the therapy literature by providing one explanation for the impact of many very different treatments. Moreover, parsimony brings in much of medicine where all sorts of placebos (e.g., pills, sham injections, sham operations) have demonstrated effectiveness based on expectancies and beliefs.

Mechanisms of Action: How and Why Treatments Work

The role of common factors, though I treated it separately in light of the attention in clinical research over the years, is part of a larger challenge: We do not really know how change occurs. But let me be more concrete. Let us say a patient comes to treatment for major depression and has a variety of symptoms (sadness, loss of interest in activities, hopelessness, diminished appetite, and poor sleep). The patient begins a regimen of cognitive therapy for depression, which stated simply focuses on changing maladaptive cognitions and engaging in activities outside of sessions that support that goal in everyday life. Depressive mood (sadness) and other presenting symptoms improve as well. This is great, and in keeping with massive evidence (e.g., Butler et al., 2006; Hollon & Beck, 2004). But precisely how did this change happen? I do not ask, notice, what caused the change—in the case of well-controlled research (RCTs), we usually can say the "cause" is the treatment. We can usually say that because of random assignment of clients to different conditions showing that one condition (treatment) was superior in its effects in relation to another (perhaps a control condition). Thus we know that cognitive therapy changes depression and is the cause. Rather, we are looking for something finer grained: What are the precise reasons, mechanisms, and steps through which the change occurred (Kazdin, 2014)? What are the treatment's "active ingredients"?

The difference between the cause and the process through which it occurs may be more easily conveyed in a different context. We have known for decades that cigarette smoking is a cause of lung cancer. Cross-sectional and longitudinal studies have linked smoking to lung cancer; experimental research with nonhuman animals has established a causal role. However, this leaves unexplained the mechanisms (i.e., the processes through which lung cancer comes about). There are many studies that provide a fine-grained analysis of what happens at the cellular level, with genes that control mutations leading to cancer. As one early example, a chemical (benzo[a]pyrene) found in cigarette smoke was shown to induce genetic mutation at specific regions of the gene's DNA that is identical to the damage evident in lung cancer cells (Denissenko et al., 1996). This finding suggests precisely how cigarette smoking leads to cancer at the molecular level. So, we have gone beyond cause to understanding better how one influence (smoking) unfolds in a step-by-step process leading to the consequence (cancer).

Back to psychosocial interventions. We do not have knowledge about precisely how change comes about in a step-by-step or basic process fashion. We know from a variety of actions and interactions with the client, through talk, rehearsal, practice, problem solving, self-statements, or other components of a given treatment, that change occurs in a domain of symptoms (e.g., lifting of mood, increase in activities, return of appetite, normalization of sleep). How does this happen? What changes in the brain influencing these latter symptoms are attributable to the actions of the therapist and his or her interactions with the client?

There are all sorts of theories and models, but these are a bit abstract. For example, stating that cognitive therapy works by changing cognitions is fine at a general level, but precisely how does that happen? Are there structures, functions, or other changes in the brain that act on symptoms and make them go away, or changes in psychological processes related to perception, learning, or memory that change and in turn act on symptoms? A critical research priority is to understand why and how therapy works, and this is not just an academic exercise. If we know what the underlying processes are that explain therapeutic change, perhaps we can focus on them in a more concentrated way and increase the effectiveness of treatment.

Two concepts are studied to better understand the basis for change: mediator and mechanism. *Mediator* is a construct that shows a statistical relation between an intervention and outcome. This is an intervening construct that suggests processes about why change occurs or on which change depends. Mediation is evident when several conditions are met: (1) the intervention leads to change in outcome measures, (2) the intervention alters the proposed mediator, (3) the mediator is related to outcome, and (4) outcome effects are not evident or significantly (statistically) less evident if the mediator did not change. These relations convey that change was mediated (e.g., correlated with, depended on) by some construct. However, even when these conditions are met, ambiguity can remain as to the precise role of the mediator (Bullock, Green, & Ha, 2010). The mediator may not explain precisely how the change comes about. For example, we know that expectations for improvement that are generated by treatment can lead to therapeutic change and that the more believable the treatment or control condition, the greater the therapeutic changes, as noted earlier. Expectancies are a reasonable explanation and mediator but does not tell us precisely how the change came about, what happens when expectancies are mobilized in the client, and how they actually reduce stress, anxiety, depression, or other symptoms that served as the basis for seeking treatment.

Mechanism refers to a greater level of explanatory specificity than mediator and reflects the steps or processes through which therapy (or some independent variable) actually unfolds and produces the change. Mechanism explains how the intervention translates into events that lead to the outcome or precisely what was altered that led to symptom change. To move more closely to mechanisms, psychotherapy research has benefitted from advances in cognitive, affective, and social neuroscience, as well as the development of noninvasive neuroimaging and other biological assays. The goal has been to examine the structure, function, and activity of the brain that are associated with clinical dysfunction (especially anxiety and depression) or changes over the course of psychotherapy among adults (e.g., Frewen, Dozois, & Lanius, 2008; Porto et al., 2009; Quidé et al., 2012; Roffman et al., 2005). Much of this work, but certainly not all, is correlational when characterizing disorders or change processes. Yet the strength of the research stems from moving closer to understanding the underpinnings of a particular disorder (e.g., anxiety) and change in those characteristics associated with treatment. For example, from the reviews mentioned previously, research has:

- Identified neurological characteristics associated with specific disorders and subtypes;
- Evaluated change in neural processes in "regions of interest" in light of characteristics associated with specific disorders;
- Experimentally induced or provoked symptoms (e.g., sadness manipulations in healthy samples, trauma stimuli in patients with posttraumatic stress disorder) to demonstrate experimentally brain areas implicated in dysfunction;
- Demonstrated "normalization" of neurological structures, function, and activity after therapy is completed;
- Elucidated similarities and differences in specific brain processes altered by different interventions (e.g., medication, psychotherapy) for a given disorder (e.g., major depression); and
- Documented some similarities in what brain processes are altered by the same intervention (e.g., cognitive behavior therapy) as applied to different disorders (e.g., obsessive compulsive disorders, depression).

I have sampled lines of work to convey what I mean by more fine-grained analyses. I highlighted research with humans and neuroimaging. Neuroimaging is moving rapidly to increasingly molecular levels of analysis, analyses of brain circuits, and analyses in real time, so what I have listed previously will be "primitive" very soon.

Nonhuman animal research also can elaborate processes that underlie therapeutic change. Brain receptors, intracellular signaling, and target genes that reflect analogues of human dysfunction and change have been studied using animal models. As one example, medications can alleviate depression. These antidepressant effects of medication relate to the expression of a protein in the brain synapses (brain-derived neurotrophic factor [BDNF]) that stimulates growth and differentiation of new neurons and synapses.[5] We know from several studies with humans that major depression is characterized by low BDNF levels and that these levels increase after successful antidepressant treatment (Sen, Duman, & Sanacora, 2008). In nonhuman animal studies, antidepressant effects can be manipulated experimentally to isolate the mechanism underlying these changes (e.g., infusing BDNF into the hippocampus directly, gene-knockout studies, blocking studies negating the operation of the *BDNF* gene, manipulating exercise that attains a therapeutic-like antidepressant effect and alters BDNF) (e.g., Duman et al., 2008; Shirayama et al., 2002). These studies move us toward identifying precisely what is involved in successful intervention and symptom change.

Understanding processes and the unfolding of therapeutic change is an increasingly active area of research in light of advances in the study of brain functions and processes and at increasingly finer levels of resolution. Biological and psychological processes increasingly are studied together (e.g., cognitive, social, and cultural neuroscience) to elaborate the connections, reciprocal relations, and conversions of experience and brain processes. Basic research on memory and cognitive processes outside of the context of therapy is likely to be quite relevant in explaining how therapy leads to change (Harvey et al., 2014). At this point in time, we have treatments that can lead to change without a very complete empirical understanding of precisely how these changes happen.

Generality of Findings From Research to Practice

The issue of the generality of findings from research to application applies to many areas in science where basic and highly controlled research demonstrates the impact of a variable or intervention (e.g., medicine, agriculture, engineering, computer science). In each case, the conditions of research emphasize experimental control over all sorts of variables and conditions, so the impact of a particular variable can be studied and well tested. Indeed, at the extreme, key phenomena and their processes are studied in animal models or petri dishes, with researchers knowing full well that application awaits better understanding.

The concern about whether findings from controlled psychotherapy research can be extended to practice has been discussed for decades (e.g., Borkovec & Rachman, 1979; Hoagwood et al., 1995; Kazdin, 1978a). These enduring concerns have to do with the many ways in which the conditions of research depart from the conditions of clinical practice. In Table 4.2 I have summarized some of the key ways in which treatment as studied in research differs from how it is applied in clinical practice.

We know that what is shown in research trials may not apply to clinical practice. To start, consider the clients seen in research versus those seen in clinical practice. In research, clients are usually recruited who have a very specific set of problems. Inclusion and exclusion criteria enable researchers to select a homogeneous set of clients with few complications (such as disorders other than those of interest in the study, or suicidal risk). Also, these clients must formally agree (informed consent) to be randomly assigned to various conditions, and these may include no treatment or a wait-list condition. If clients are chosen to receive treatment, they are likely to receive a fairly fixed regimen of therapy, after which treatment is ended. Merely agreeing to be randomly assigned to one of a number of possible conditions may make the samples seen in treatment quite different from those seen in clinical practice. In clinical practice, clients seek treatment for a problem that is having a real impact on their lives. All sorts of case complexities (comorbid disorders, other stresses of living related to relationships and work, and so on) are likely to be present—complexities that often disqualify participants from research studies. In clinical practice, usually all comers are taken (if treatment can be paid for in some way).

In research, the focus of the treatment is fairly well set. Indeed, clients are included and actively recruited because their psychological problems are suited to the treatment. In clinical practice, not only are there multiple problems, but also priorities may change over the course of treatment. We have known for decades that the problem that ends up being the main focus of treatment is often different from the one the client presented with at the beginning of treatment (e.g.,

Table 4.2 Sources of Difference in Treatment Research and Clinical Practice

Foci of the Concern	**In Research Trials**	**In Clinical Practice**
Sample or Participants	• Often recruited for treatment • Screened to have "pure" problems (inclusion and exclusion criteria) • Clients are randomly assigned (and accept that) to various treatment or control conditions, including no-treatment or wait-list controls • Clients may be able to wait (no urgency), so there is no crisis if treatment is delayed (wait list)	• Individuals seek treatment • Included even if multiple and complex problems or comorbid disorders • Select the treatment by virtue of coming to a particular setting and do not have to be part of random assignment • Clients in need of treatment—may be in crisis
Treatment	• Often rigid (e.g., session-by-session focus, number of sessions) and controlled by a fixed manual with some but not unlimited flexibility • Neat and very circumscribed with a narrow focus and not applicable to real cases • Treatment is usually brief and ends no matter how well or poorly the clients are doing	• Individualized and changing during the course in response to changing problem or perceived needs of the patient • Many different procedures may be used and combined • Treatment may be ongoing and of varying durations among patients, depending on progress
Therapists	• Often graduate students in training with much less experience in clinical work • Closely supervised treatment to be sure therapists stay on track with regard to the manual	• Trained practitioners usually with extensive experience • No supervision to monitor what is done, how well it is done, and how it is modified
Focus of Treatment	• Often on the presenting problem for which individuals have been screened • Rely on psychiatric diagnosis for selection and treatment focusing on disorders and neglecting personality characteristics and disorders that can influence treatment effects and outcomes • Treatment focus and measures aimed primarily at this one focus, unlike demands of clinical work where focus and criteria for improvement can change over time • Goals of treatment in clinical work are not always or only changing symptoms	• Presenting problems may be diffuse and include specific problem areas (e.g., depression), but many environmental and contextual conditions that influence content of treatment sessions (e.g., stress from living conditions, relatives, child issues) • Often the process is as or more important than the outcome, i.e., providing clients with an opportunity to air issues in a safe environment, have acceptance of the problem before moving on to any solutions

NOTE: Elaboration of these and other objections and concerns can be found in several sources (e.g., Borkovec & Rachman, 1979; Bruce & Sanderson, 2005; Chambless & Ollendick, 2001; De Los Reyes & Kazdin, 2006; Herbert, 2003; Kazdin, 1978a; Nelson & Steele, 2006; Wampold & Imel, 2015; Westen, Novotny, & Thompson-Brenner, 2004).

Sorenson, Gorsuch, & Mintz, 1985). In clinical practice, maximal flexibility is needed to respond to patient presenting problems, changes in the problems, and emergent issues in everyday life (e.g., relationship problems, work stress).

In short, whether treatment studied in research generalizes to clinical practice is a reasonable concern. As it turns out, some treatments (such as cognitive therapy for depression, exposure-based treatments for anxiety, multisystemic psychotherapy for violent children and adolescents, parent management training for children with conduct problems) have been well tested in scores of studies with quite different patient samples (Nathan & Gorman, 2015; Weisz & Kazdin, 2017). The samples have included very severe cases (the hospitalized and incarcerated, suicidal individuals). Hence one can be reassured that the findings are not restricted to narrowly defined and circumscribed samples. But the point remains: Favorable results obtained in well-controlled studies in research settings are very promising. The extent to which the intervention is effective in applied settings requires additional study.

SUMMARY AND CONCLUSIONS

Earlier chapters lamented the high prevalence of mental disorders and the fact that most people with these disorders, or who are otherwise in need of services, receive no intervention aimed at their psychological impairment. The EBPIs discussed in this chapter are examples of available treatments with scientific support, even though they come with significant caveats. Yet we can say that, in principle, if we *could* get treatment to people, we could make a difference. This assumes that treatment would be delivered as intended and developed in research.

As I mentioned, there is no single count of EBPIs, and this is influenced by the fact that there is also no single set of criteria universally invoked to define EPBIs. For many problems in adults, adolescents, and children there are now multiple treatment options that can be said to be evidence based. Actually, the range of treatments now with an evidence base is vast and includes large categories of cognitive and behavioral treatments and a variety of traditional therapies (e.g., play, therapy, psychoanalysis). Interestingly, the highly variable class of interventions referred to as "treatment as usual" also has evidence in its behalf, but that is very difficult to interpret for reasons I noted. Yet the overall conclusion is that we have interventions that can change many clinical problems.

Despite great enthusiasm about the emergence of EBPIs, there remain core ambiguities about what that status means. For example, measures from individual studies, effect sizes from meta-analyses, and selective use of measures by investigators reporting on their results all introduce ambiguity as to what can be said about a given treatment and its impact on client functioning. Common factors are also a complication because it remains to be seen to what extent hundreds of different treatments achieve outcomes because of some factor that is common to them all. The expectations for improvements that treatments generate in the clients is one common factor that contributes to, if not accounts for, change. Apart from the now large literature on expectations in psychotherapy, there is now an older sister literature on placebo effects, which are likely to operate through similar means. There is great power in belief, and its role in therapy remains to be elaborated and perhaps eventually better harnessed. Mechanisms of change are also an issue because we want to know precisely how treatment leads to change—what psychological and biological processes are altered. Neuroscience that looks at changes in biological and psychological processes (such as how environmental events change the brain and how those changes result in symptom change) is beginning to describe the change process in fine detail. Finally, an enduring question concerns the extent to which the effects of treatment, when studied under highly controlled settings, with specially selected samples of clients (and therapists), and with treatment monitored and closely supervised, will lead to results that cannot be applied or easily transferred to clinical settings. Efforts are ongoing now to extend treatment research to clinical practice, including alterations of the treatments themselves to simplify the process. These are topics for Chapter 5.

5

Current Trends in Treatment Research and Practice

The development of evidence-based psychosocial interventions (EBPIs) represents a major advance and provides multiple treatment options for many different mental disorders and sources of impairment. Psychosocial intervention research is extremely active on several fronts and extends well beyond outcome studies. In this chapter I discuss four extremely active areas of research and clinical practice. The areas include efforts to:

- Disseminate and implement EBPIs into clinical practice;
- Integrate physical and mental health care in providing services;
- Develop EBPIs that can be applied broadly across clinical problems; and
- Use technology and social media to provide treatment.

I highlight these areas because they relate to the overall goals of at once improving intervention services and reducing the burdens of mental illness. At the same time, some of the seeming obvious trends and movements may not actually do much to chip away at those burdens.

DISSEMINATION OF TREATMENT: ADDRESSING THE RESEARCH–PRACTICE GAP

Research has now identified scores of interventions with a strong evidence base. Perhaps the initial priority of research would be to ensure that the treatments with the best evidence are those that are used in clinical practice. Indeed, a major priority and challenge in current research is to disseminate EBPIs so they are being carried out in clinical practice (Barlow et al., 2013; Weisz, Ugueto et al., 2013).

The *research–practice gap* is the term used to refer to the fact that what has been shown to work well in research is not what is being carried out in practice. The gap in integrating findings from research to clinical practice is evident both in physical and mental health care (Institute of Medicine [IOM], 2001). Recognition of the availability of EBPIs for the treatment of psychological dysfunctions has led many government agencies and professional organizations to recommend adoption and use of these techniques (e.g., American Psychological Association, American Medical Association, National Institutes of Health, US Department of Defense). In the United States, the President's New Freedom Commission on Mental Health (2003) lamented the lack of availability of evidence-based treatments and the inconsistent and uneven quality of the use of the treatments when they are available. Concerns over the lack of disseminating evidence-based mental health care and recommendations convey interest in and broad attention to the issue of the research–practice gap. Unfortunately, neither of these translates very quickly, if at all, to actual changes in clinical practice. Much more is needed both in conceptualizing the task of moving treatments from the laboratory (controlled trials, often in university settings) to clinical settings (hospitals, clinics, private practice office), evaluating the effectiveness of different strategies to do that, and even developing treatments in ways that may facilitate their dissemination.

Overview of the Task

To begin, dissemination of treatment is a multistep process. In broad strokes, the major steps include:

1. Involving agencies, administrators, and clinicians in the importance, utility, and value of providing treatments that depart from what might be going on routinely already (i.e., treatment as usual);
2. Providing training experiences that will develop the requisite skills of the therapists;
3. Implementing procedures to ensure that the skills and interventions are carried out as intended;
4. Including a means within the clinical service to sustain the quality of the interventions and to ensure that the interventions are administered with fidelity over time; and
5. Evaluating therapeutic changes among the clients who receive the treatment and assessing whether the changes in clinical practice resemble those that had been achieved in the well-controlled clinical trials that established the evidence base of the treatments.

Each step has its own set of decisions, tasks, practices, and hurdles. Consider just a few of the steps in more detail. To begin, involving agencies, administrators, and clinicians to disseminate treatments is a huge challenge. It is unlikely that any one is "against" EBPIs, but adopting them is another matter. There may be little incentive to adopt new interventions. One might say that agencies are incentivized or forced to use new techniques in order to receive reimbursement from insurance. However, receiving reimbursement is a matter of *reporting* what was done in therapy, and that may differ from what was *actually* done, a topic to which I return in a moment.

Ponder the initial challenge and disincentives that may operate against dissemination. To use EBPIs, agencies would have to pay trainers to come in and train and supervise clinicians in the new treatments. Also, clinician time spent in training means time not spent in sessions with clients, earning money for themselves and the agencies. Related, administrators and those who set policy for a given clinical service may not automatically embrace the view that the new treatments will improve on the care that is routinely provided. That is, there may be little perceived need for new treatments. Patients are not clamoring for something different, and clinicians tend to be pleased with what they are doing. In any case, step one of the dissemination process is not minor.

Second, and related, training of therapists requires development of skills. Training usually begins with didactic experiences (e.g., webinars, workshops, seminars, use of instructional materials), but this by itself is not likely be effective in developing actual techniques and strategies that therapists will use in sessions with clients. Knowledge, information, and instruction all are likely to be necessary, but unlikely to be insufficient for developing the relevant skills (e.g., those needed to administer cognitive therapy for depression). In this context, administering psychotherapy is like learning a musical instrument, learning to fly an airplane, or mastering a sport. In each case, there is a lot to know, but knowing is not the same as practice at doing, and practice and supervision are needed so that the doing achieves some level of competence. In developing the use of EBPIs, skill training, practice, and direct supervision of clinical cases are needed to reach an adequate level of competency. In addition, after the skills are trained, some form of supervision is needed so that the skills are sustained over time.

Even with my brief comments on a couple of the steps, one can see that there are challenges in disseminating treatment. Another related matter that circumvents the steps is a default position. Clinical services and clinicians often provide or attend a workshop or two on an EBPI, return to their services, and integrate what they learned into their treatment as usual. The service or clinicians may now state (e.g., Web page, Facebook, business cards) that they provide a particular form of treatment, but there is no quality control over such claims. So, if I say I do cognitive behavior therapy for depression, this could mean my own adopted and adapted version as woven into my "regular" therapy. There is no check on whether I am doing "real," high-quality, evidence-based cognitive behavior therapy. This is pernicious because most lay people would have no idea that not all claims of delivering an EBPI are the same. And from the standpoint of disseminating an EBPI, administrators or clinicians might well claim to already be providing the treatment, or integrating parts of it into their service. Rarely are data available to address these issues, such as whether diluted versions in use produce worse outcomes than the high-fidelity version and whether the EBPI in diluted or full form produces improvements that really make a difference in patient improvement, as reflected in indices of mental or physical health, impaired functioning, or quality of life.

The steps I have noted are challenging but not insurmountable. In fact, adoption of EBPIs often is highly recommended or mandated in ways that help move dissemination forward. Perhaps the marked influence is when an agency (government or nongovernment, insurance, third-party payers) goes beyond "recommending" treatment and notes that treatment will not be reimbursed if it is not one of the interventions that has been approved in advance. Reimbursement will require a statement to the effect that the treatment was one from a list of EBPIs. Yet clinicians often integrate components of multiple treatments and may well be able to say legitimately that they used a particular technique. Whether the treatment was implemented well or in a way that it was studied in research is unknown. So, there is no assurance of exactly what was done in treatment.

Examples

Dissemination is a very active area of research with many efforts to extend EBPIs on different scales (e.g., individual clinics and hospitals, national programs throughout a country). Those dissemination programs that are most prominent and visible are large-scale efforts that have financial and institutional support from governments. Completing the steps I listed is greatly facilitated by the ability to set policy within an organization, policy that may encompass priorities, guidelines, and requirements for a given service. In addition, the means of providing financial support to enact those priorities are critical. For example, the training of practitioners to competence and sustaining their skills are staff intensive and costly. Ability to provide financial support is also very important. Guidance from the top (by those who enact laws and regulations and set policies) does not negate the need to work with and persuade local administrators in the value of implementing EBPIs. Yet initial authorization, funding, and expectation set the stage and help to scale dissemination efforts to reach many practitioners and services where treatment is provided. Consider two illustrations of well-developed and large-scale dissemination programs.

Veterans Health Administration

In the United States, the Veterans Health Administration (VHA) operates the largest health care system in the country and provides services for the physical and mental health needs of veterans. Dissemination of EBPIs began with identifying EBPIs that would be relevant to the most common problems seen in the population (veterans) and that would be feasible to train. Table 5.1 lists the treatments that were selected as a point of departure (Karlin & Cross, 2014). When identified,

Table 5.1 Evidence-Based Psychotherapies Being Disseminated in the Veterans Health Administration

Evidence-Based Psychotherapy	**Condition**
Cognitive processing therapy	Posttraumatic stress disorder
Prolonged exposure therapy	
Cognitive behavioral therapy for depression	Depression
Acceptance and commitment therapy for depression	
Interpersonal psychotherapy	
Behavioral family therapy	Serious mental illness
Multiple family group therapy	
Social skills training	
Integrated behavioral couples therapy	Relationship distress
Cognitive behavioral therapy for insomnia	Insomnia
Cognitive behavioral therapy for chronic pain	Chronic pain
Motivational interviewing	Motivation and adherence
Motivational enhancement therapy	Substance use disorders
Contingency management	
Behavioral couples therapy	
Cognitive behavioral therapy for substance use disorders	

SOURCE: Karlin, B. E., & Cross, G. (2014). From the laboratory to the therapy room: National dissemination and implementation of evidence-based psychotherapies in the US Department of Veterans Affairs Health Care System. *American Psychologist, 69*(1), 19–33.

there was a multilevel focus to develop implementation of these EBPIs in clinical services. These levels included:

1. *Policy level:* developing specific policies to guide practice about what treatments are provided to veterans and to recruit and obtain more staff as needed to administer the services;
2. *Provider level:* providing details about the training programs to develop competence, including materials to be used to train therapists and evaluate their competence;
3. *Local systems level:* devising methods and identifying and training staff at the level of individual services to coordinate, support, and facilitate a culture change as well as adoption and implementation;
4. *Patient level:* ensuring that veterans are informed of treatment choices and EBPIs, enhancing processes that can augment treatment such as fostering motivation, socialization to the treatment process, and the relationship with the therapist; and
5. *Accountability:* measuring several facets of implementation, including documentation of competence of delivery and evaluation of therapist and patient outcomes.

My comments merely highlight key components, but each has extensive documentation, training, and means of implementation.

There have been many reports of the implementation of EBPIs in the VHA. As an illustration, as of 2012, more than 6,400 staff were trained to administer an EBPI for posttraumatic stress disorder (PTSD)—a high-priority treatment among veterans. All the facilities provide cognitive therapy or exposure therapy for PTSD, the most common mental health diagnosis in the VHA system. One of these treatments was required in the dissemination effort, but almost all facilities provided both. Several evaluations have been reported on multiple facets of the program (e.g., therapist competence and completion of training, treatment rate of patients, patient alliance with the therapist) (see Karlin & Cross, 2014). Importantly, evaluation of patient outcomes showed that patients improved with the treatment and with the same degree of change evident in controlled research trials of those treatments (e.g., Eftekhari et al., 2013). Quality of life improved as well.

The program has continued to develop, expand, and document the successful implementation of strategies to disseminate treatment. I have provided an example in which the focus was on disseminating treatment for PTSD using cognitive behavior therapy and exposure. Other treatment interventions (as noted previously in Table 5.1) have been included as well, and the focus has greatly expanded to other problems experienced by veterans (e.g., depression, insomnia, substance use disorders, chronic pain, and dementia-related behaviors) (e.g., Drapkin et al., 2016; Karlin et al., 2013; Stewart et al., 2015; Trockel et al., 2015). With successes in hand, still much work needs to be done, including decreasing the variability in quality of implementation across the many sites, decentralizing the process so that local facilities have means to train and monitor treatment, hiring more staff to increase the scale of implementation, ensuring that implementation quality is sustained, and providing treatment through telehealth to extend the reach are some of the foci. The main lesson is that ensuring high-quality treatment is not a matter of training therapists alone but rather of changing systems of care at many levels and ensuring that the advances can be sustained. All of this is in the context of evaluating quality and fidelity implementation and impact on treatment outcomes for patients.

Improving Access to Psychological Therapies

In England, a large-scale program has been in place to greatly increase the availability of effective psychological treatment for depression and anxiety (Clark, 2011, 2012). This is a government-based program within the English National Health Service. Both clinical and policy developments served as the background. On the clinical side, the National Institute for Health and Care Excellence (NICE) is a national resource that provides guidance to improve health and social care. NICE is a resource to review the best available evidence for the full range of mental and physical disorders (see www.nice.org.uk/).

NICE reviews of treatment identified cognitive behavior therapy as an effective intervention for depression and anxiety disorders.[1] From these, specific guidelines for treatment were also provided. Add to this further work that was completed on the likely economic benefits of effectively treating depression and anxiety. The collaboration of a clinical researcher (David Clark) and economist (Richard Layard) completed analyses to show that the effective treatment of depression and anxiety on a large scale would pay for itself by reducing the costs of these disorders if untreated (e.g., in welfare benefits and medical costs and the loss of revenue from taxes and productivity). The case was made in academic articles and other resources (e.g., pamphlets and reports, some of which were sponsored by various mental health organizations and charities) that went to politicians, administrators, clinicians, the public, and the media (published in the Sunday edition of the national newspaper, *The Observer*) (e.g., Layard et al., 2006, 2007; Layard & Clark, 2014).

As a result of the convergence of the broad communication efforts, the central government of the United Kingdom the made a commitment to implement two pilot programs to recruit and train therapists. The programs were successful in training therapists, in treating a large number of patients (>3,500 in the first year), and in demonstrating improvements in patient outcomes as reflected in reductions in depression and anxiety. Following this, the government provided funds for the extension of the program nationally to train therapists. After 3 years, 95 percent of the services that provided care were participating in the program. More than 3,600 new therapists had been recruited. Services saw approximately 310,000 and 399,000 patients by the end of years 1 and 2, respectively, per year, with the goal of scaling up to 900,000 per year. Improvements in clinical outcomes were documented. Moreover, data were collected to show that thousands of patients (>13,000) were no longer receiving sick pay or state benefits in light of their recoveries. As mentioned previously, one of the arguments for this large-scale implementation was that the program would reduce costs in other areas of social services. Consequently, these latter data were relevant outcomes. Indeed, the projected cost savings by providing effective treatment surpassed original estimates. That is, treatment paid for itself (and more) in terms of government savings.

The program continues with further government funding (to 2020), improvements and extensions in training, and planned extensions in the clinical problems treated. Part of these planned extensions is development of treatments for children and adolescents, as well as extensions to individuals 65 years and older, who tended not to be well represented in the initial extensions. Also, the program will include further treatments (e.g., mindfulness) and make treatment available on the Internet (Clark, 2016).

Several facets of the program, including recruitment of therapists, implementation of assessments, and monitoring and supervision of treatment, are part of the success. The program is one of few dissemination efforts showing large-scale extension of treatment not only to training therapists in place already but also in recruiting new therapists and services to extend the reach of treatment. Ordinarily, dissemination of treatments consists of training the existing cadre of therapists. The Improving Access to Psychological Therapies (IPAT) program is unique in greatly adding the staff to provide the services.

General Comments

The VHA and IPAT represent large-scale efforts to disseminate, and they have special characteristics, including multilevel intervention and centralized support at policy and financial levels. There are scores of other dissemination programs that do not operate at that level but rather within a state or province in the United States or Canada (e.g., for hospital and third-party payer systems) (e.g., Hoagwood et al., 2017; McHugh & Barlow, 2010; Novins et al., 2013).

Although there are many different settings and systems of care, it is likely that key features or steps I mentioned previously will continue to be relevant, including prioritizing delivery of EBPIs at the administrative level and then at the clinical level, developing the means of competency-based training including direct supervision of treatment, programming the means of sustaining treatment quality, and monitoring process and outcomes of the dissemination efforts. Yet, for small clinical services, whether funded by local or state government, or private business, the model is not easily applied. The lack of funds to support trainings and ongoing supervision means core elements of dissemination are not available. Commonly, these smaller, less-resourced services have clinicians participate in webinars or attend a workshop or two. Missing are an evaluation of whether the training in fact developed the requisite skills, whether the skills were carried out faithfully in the clinical services in which the clinicians work, and whether patients improved or made greater changes after the new procedures were in place.

Challenges and Critical Questions

Conceptual Model of How to Disseminate Treatment

There are a number of challenges for disseminating treatment into routine clinical practice (Addis, 2002; Waller & Turner, 2016; Weisz, Ng, & Bearman, 2014). They begin with the concern and some evidence that when treatment is disseminated, the effectiveness drops off. This is not inevitable and may be more a measure of the effectiveness of the dissemination and implementation model (Brownson, Colditz, & Proctor, 2012; Fixsen et al., 2005; Schoenwald & Hoagwood, 2001). Even so, large-scale application can be expected to have variable results, with some clinicians and services more than others having success in implementation and better outcomes for their patients as a result. Part of the infrastructure of dissemination is likely to require ongoing methods of training, sustaining gains, and intervening to help improve implementation when evidence suggests this may be an obstacle. And if there is no strong support at the level of policy, administration, and finance, it is difficult to envision how dissemination will take place. This not a pessimistic statement. Rather, I consider this stance to come from aspects of treatment we take for granted, such as how we administer treatment (mostly in-person individual therapy), how we develop treatment in research (mostly without considering how the technique will translate to clinical practice), and what those treatments are (often complex and requiring commensurate levels of training). Yet all of these can change and, as I argue, ought to.

The usual way we develop treatments may be a detriment to extending their use in clinical practice. Typically, as we develop treatments, we begin with a focus on a clinical disorder, a model or theory of how that disorder may come about, how treatment can address key components of the disorder, and what we might draw from the human and nonhuman animal research (e.g., extinction, fear conditioning) in the way of principles or techniques. We then begin tests of treatment under well-controlled conditions. These steps sound reasonable and exemplify many of the virtues of good science (e.g., developing a conceptual model, testing under carefully controlled conditions so that all sorts of biases and artifacts that interfere with drawing conclusions are minimized or eliminated). The difficultly emerges when one wishes to generalize the finding to applied settings, in this case clinical practice. As I noted in Chapter 4 (see Table 4.2) the conditions in treatments as carried out in clinical practice are likely to depart from the conditions in which treatment is developed and conducted in research settings. Understandably and as previously noted, the applicability of findings from research is a concern that has come up repeatedly over the course of psychotherapy research. What is different now is that we have a set of evidence-based treatments and increased accountability from agencies (federal and private) to justify procedures that are in use and what will be reimbursed. Clinical services and clinicians are under pressure (if they want to be reimbursed for services) to use approved EBPIs. Dissemination is not just an academic topic or a luxury. For services and perhaps at some point clients, the focus will be on providing the most well-supported treatments. Thus there are ethical and moral considerations here as part of our accountability: Are we providing the best available treatments, and if not, how can that be justified?

The contrast of conditions from therapy as studied in research and as applied in clinical practice is not an unavoidable constraint. Our model or conceptual view of how to move treatments from the laboratory to the clinic could be the greatest limitation toward effective dissemination. What is our model of moving from evidence to application? An implicit one might be termed the "build-it-and-they-will-come" model. This expression, paraphrased from a popular movie (*Field of Dreams*, 1989) has lingered in contemporary US culture well beyond the original context (e.g., Adams, 2010). In relation to dissemination, this "build-it" model is based on the optimistic hope that after everyone sees our wonderful evidence, they will swarm our labs, seize our manuals, and rush back to their clinics where they will implement our interventions with abandon. That is, everyone who sees our remarkable effects will want to benefit. We have abandoned that model. As discussed, there is little incentive for services and clinicians to learn the techniques as they are intended to be administered; it is not always so clear that research-based treatments will be more effective or even useful given the complexity of clinical work. Also, the scientists who do the clinical trials research are mostly talking to themselves (in journals, grant review panels, and convention symposia), rather than to clinicians or consumers of treatment.

Obviously, another model is needed that narrows, if not eliminates, the gap between research and practice and between generating and applying treatment. One suggestion is that we develop treatments in the settings in which they are ultimately to be used, or at least be attentive to those conditions from the beginning (e.g., Fixsen et al., 2009; Lyon & Koerner, 2016; Weisz et al., 2015). For example, in one model, several dimensions are proposed to be considered from the very outset at the stage of developing the treatment (Lyon & Koerner, 2016). The dimensions include:

- *Learnability:* providing clinicians with opportunities to quickly learn to use the treatments;
- *Efficiency:* attending to the time, effort, and cost of using the treatment;
- *Memorability:* ensuring that critical elements of treatment can be remembered and successfully applied without added supports;
- *Error avoidance and recovery:* facilitating recovery from errors or misapplications of treatment;
- *Acceptability/satisfaction:* ensuring the interventions are viewed as acceptable to clinicians;
- *Low cognitive load:* keeping the interventions simple; and
- *Exploit natural constraints:* making sure the interventions will fit the contexts in which they will be used.

While the model points us in a needed direction, it is too early to know precisely how the challenge will be operationalized. That is, if I am ready to develop a treatment, where do I begin, and how do I ensure that multiple dimensions of the model in fact are addressed? There is the added task. We have now devised a few hundred EBPIs that have not taken into account these dimensions. No doubt some treatments already but unwittingly include features of these components. Perhaps the challenge is to retrofit current treatments in ways that make them more readily adaptable for clinic use. In any case, the model provides a finer-grained evaluation of the task of disseminating treatment and the dimensions to which we ought to attend early in the development of interventions.

Evaluating Treatment Outcomes

Efforts to disseminate treatment ought to include means of evaluating outcomes to ensure that patient functioning is altered. We are going to great lengths to replace treatments in place at a given clinic with those that are evidence-based and putatively "new and improved." Yet evidence is still essential to ensure that dissemination makes a difference in client outcomes.

The large-scale programs I mentioned as illustrations (the VHA and IPAT) included client outcome assessment. Yet many efforts to disseminate treatment do not (see McHugh & Barlow, 2010). Collecting data on the impact of clinical practice would be desirable in its own right apart from any efforts to disseminate treatment. That is, we do not usually know from the way most clinics operate whether patients improve with the treatments they receive. Systematic assessments before, during, or after treatment (with validated scales) to evaluate symptoms, impairment, or daily functioning are routinely *omitted* in clinical practice. Yet, when disseminating a treatment designed to provide "new and improved" patient care, we would want to be sure that the outcomes produced are favorable and ideally resemble those evident from research. Perhaps most pertinent, do the new treatments surpass the effects obtained with routine treatments provided? As

I discussed in Chapter 4, routine treatments (treatments as usual), when evaluated, are often just as effective as EBPIs. In general, we want to evaluate patient outcomes to be sure treatments are helping, and this assessment alone can improve treatment outcomes (Poston & Hanson, 2010). The importance may be even greater with ambiguity about where and when an EBPI improves on treatment as usual. The IPAT program I mentioned in England evaluated patient changes as well as cost savings associated with the dissemination of EBPIs. Among the findings were that the EBPIs in clinical practice obtained equivalent effects to those obtained in research studies.

Diverse Treatment Venues and Mental Health Professionals

A challenge for disseminating treatment is reaching practitioners in quite diverse settings, including individual private practice office, small practice settings with multiple therapists, health care settings, hospitals, and in some cases, large systems of care (e.g., national agencies) with thousands of professionals who deliver treatment. And clinics and practitioners can vary widely in whom they see (e.g., children, adolescents, and adults) and where they are (e.g., urban, rural). How to reach the different therapists is not obvious. Yet we do not have many venues for carrying out training at the level of individual therapists, leaving aside scaling training up to reach thousands of mental health professionals and across the main disciplines that provide treatment (psychology, psychiatry, social work).

In addition, the task of learning a new treatment is part of the challenge. Learning an EBPI is not a matter of reading a book, participating in a webinar or two, or attending a workshop. As I mentioned previously, many of the treatments require mastery of procedures that have to be done in a particular way. There might be some academic instruction, but hands-on instruction and supervision are also likely to be essential. Clinicians usually cannot take the time away from their practices to learn a treatment in any formal way. Also, graduate training programs in mental health still do not routinely include EBPIs as part of their curricula. And it would be difficult to exert control or influence among diverse disciplines that have their own traditions and views about what treatments are appropriate.

Public Treatment Literacy

Disseminating treatment also involves educating the public. It would be helpful if lay people knew more about what EBPIs are and asked for them when they seek services. Consumer-based marketing of treatment (also referred to as direct-to-consumer advertising) is common in the context of medication, where media blitzes tell the public about a new drug to treat this or that physical or mental health problem (Gallo, Comer, & Barlow, 2013). Moreover, the pharmaceutical industry goes well beyond direct advertising to the public. Extensive, multifaceted, and sophisticated marketing efforts include a large workforce and budget devoted to promotion of drugs. Individuals referred to as detailers, who work for pharmaceutical companies, meet directly with physicians, but also with those in positions to make decisions (e.g., for approved medications used in hospitals) about new drugs (e.g., Larkin et al., 2014; Manchanda & Honka, 2005). Direct-to-consumer advertising and direct-to-physician marketing (detailing) consume billions of dollars in the United States to promote the interest in, desire for, and use of prescription medications.

Psychological treatments are not promoted to the public and professionals in a way that even comes close to the promotional machine of pharmaceutical companies, although such efforts have been encouraged (Gallo et al., 2013). There is no profit to be made in the way that is the case for medications. That is, EBPIs are not the product of a for-profit industry, and therefore no budget is available for systematic and large-scale advertising or promotion. Individual investigators occasionally franchise their technique and more often receive money for providing workshops for their programs, but this is a practice promoted by a few individuals for a few therapies, and not the same as national and international promotion.

Educating the public about the availability of EBPIs would likely require many venues for disseminating information (e.g., media, Web). This is a major challenge. Information is readily available to the public on all sorts of interventions for mental health problems (e.g., online treatments, applications ["apps"], self-help treatments). There is no easy way to tell which among these is evidence based. Moreover, we ought not to assume that "evidence based" is a criterion that the public would accord great weight without education about what that is. Already we know from the discussion of mental health literacy in Chapter 3 that the public often sees psychosocial interventions as not very effective, and many prefer doing nothing rather than seeking treatment. In addition, there is a huge reliance on complementary and alternative medicine and practices, that is, interventions that are not conventional and mainstream for a given clinical problem (e.g., the use of herbs, special diets, acupuncture, probiotics). Educating the public about standardized and complementary treatments and those with and without a strong evidence base is a major challenge. Providing more information, though always valuable, by itself may not be very effective or persuasive (e.g., as evident with healthful diets, the importance of vaccinations, the importance of breastfeeding).

Several factors have converged to heighten the significance of and attention to dissemination, including as I mentioned the emergence of EBPIs as well as increased accountability as two examples. But there are broader influences that extend well beyond psychosocial interventions and affect health care more generally. First is the development and expansion of implementation science (e.g., Birken et al., 2017; Proctor et al., 2009). The overall focus is the scientific study of methods to promote the uptake and use of research findings into applied settings, organizations, and policy. Second is the attention to translational research. This area has as its goal moving research from the laboratory (basic wet laboratory or "bench" science), to clinical application (bench to bedside), and to community levels (bedside to community) (e.g., Bardo & Pentz, 2012; Woolf, 2008). Both implementation science and translational research are united in aims to recognize, and make significant efforts to surmount, the delays in moving breakthroughs in research to application so that they might help people in everyday life. Both topics are beyond the present scope but place in context the heightened significance and attention to dissemination and implementation.

The dissemination of treatments addresses the research–practice gap (moving techniques studied in research to clinic settings). Addressing that gap could improve the treatments for the small proportion of those in need who actually receive treatment. Yet dissemination does not address the treatment gap, namely, reaching the many individuals in need of treatment who receive nothing. The dominant model of delivering treatment is in-person, one-to-one sessions with a mental health profession and in a special setting. That model limits the extent to which treatment can be scaled up to address people in need of services (Fairburn & Patel, 2014; Kazdin & Blase, 2011; Kazdin & Rabbitt, 2013). Stated another way, if all the therapists provided EBPIs (i.e., all therapists administered treatments with a strong evidence base), it would not have much, if any influence, on the burdens of mental illness. This is not an argument against dissemination; we want people to receive the best possible treatment. But because most people are completely missed by the current treatment model and do not even receive the non–evidence-based interventions, arming therapists with putatively better treatments will not really help those who are outside of the elite group that receives services. Chapters 7 and 8 underscore interventions and models of delivering them that can better reach those people in need of services.

INTEGRATED CARE: PRIMARY CARE AND BEHAVIORAL HEALTH

Traditionally, the care of physical health is handled in primary care facilities that are devoted exclusively to medical concerns. We are most familiar with these facilities as we go to our doctor to check on our health and to receive medical care for an acute or chronic medical problem. Needless to say, mental health and substance abuse problems are not usually treated in that setting. They might not even emerge as issues because there is not likely to be a formal screening or assessment process that would readily detect problems unrelated to the visit. Also, the professionals who are expert in mental disorders and substance use and abuse disorders are typically working in other settings, such as mental health or specialty facilities or (if at a large hospital) in other departments not connected to the setting in which physical disorders are treated. In short, separate "types" of clinical dysfunction are treated in separate settings and by separate sets of professionals who may be in little or no communication with each other.

This traditional care often is described as "fractionated" because services address only a segment or fraction of the needs of individuals. Integrated care is a model of bringing together multiple resources to address the range of physical, mental health, and substance use problems one may experience and in this sense is opposite from fractionated care (see Substance Abuse and Mental Health Services Administration [SAMHSA], 2017a).[2] In addition to the focus on physical health problems, integrated care focuses on lifestyle issues (e.g., diet, exercise, cigarette smoking) that directly relate to physical and mental health.

Background and Rationale

Interest in, calls for, and implementation of integrated services are not at all new (e.g., Starfield, 1992; World Health Organization [WHO], 2001b). Many government and nongovernment organizations in the United States and internationally have called for integration of physical and mental health care and have brought us to where we are now (see Collins et al., 2013; Crowley & Kirschner, 2015; Kazak et al., 2017). Although the concept of integration of services is not new, there is renewed attention to the importance of integration and accelerated efforts to facilitate the changes in health care delivery. These changes in the United States were augmented relatively recently by changes in laws that ensure parity of mental and physical health services and provide incentives for states to integrate services (Mental Health Parity and Addiction Equity Act in 2008; Patient Protection and Affordable Care Act in 2010).

The rationale for integration of services is based on four major considerations. First, mental and physical health problems go together (e.g., Lehman & Dixon, 2016; Scott et al., 2016); a mental health problem is likely to be associated with a physical health problem, and vice versa. For example, 68 percent of individuals with a mental disorder have one or more chronic physical conditions (SAMHSA, 2017a). Also, individuals with mental illness are much more likely to have high blood pressure, heart disease, diabetes, obesity, and asthma. Lifestyle characteristics also overlap with mental illness and physical illness. Individuals with mental disorder are more likely to smoke cigarettes, abuse substances, and eat high-fat diets and are less likely to exercise than the general population (e.g., Chwastiak, 2015). Perhaps understandably and tragically, individuals with mental illness are more likely to die at a much younger age than expected. I will return to the connections of mental and physical health and lifestyle because they have other implications for intervention beyond integrated care. For now, the rationale for integrating mental and physical health and substance use care is that they are quite related and that services that only treat one or the other make less sense in terms of sharing information, assessment, and intervention.

A second rationale is the fact that when individuals with mental disorders do go to treatment, they are likely to go to a primary care (e.g., internal medicine) service. In fact, a significant proportion of patients who are seen in primary care treatment are there for a mental disorder. Estimates vary worldwide and by type of disorder, but approximately 30 to 40 percent of visits to a primary care service relate to a mental health problem (e.g., Ansseau et al., 2004; Wittchen et al., 2003). The estimates are approximate because, across studies, different diagnoses and diagnostic systems are used, and the disorders (clinical and subclinical) themselves vary in the proportions seen in medical practices. Add to this the fact that a significant proportion of these disorders are not detected, diagnosed, assessed, or treated by the primary care physician. Thus one reason that mental disorder is not treated is that it is not diagnosed or recognized as such when individuals show up at their medical visits. Now add one more relevant fact, that in the United States people visit their doctors approximately once per year (e.g., Chen, Farwell, & Jha, 2009). That single visit in a primary care service might be the only opportunity to diagnose and treat mental disorder.

A third rationale stems from barriers to receiving mental health services, a topic I have discussed. Multiple barriers are involved here—as mentioned, the stigma of going to mental health services certainly is one worth noting. With integrated care, one can go to a primary care facility (as one would for physical condition) and have seamless care there that also addresses any mental health issues. Access to care, another barrier, would be improved as well if primary physical health facilities had on-site resources for treating mental illness and behavioral health issues. A related barrier is negotiating different health care needs and systems. If an individual has a mental and physical disorder, the obstacles of finding suitable treatment for each and following through are significant deterrents. Another barrier that served as the impetus for integrated care has been a simple lack of treatment services, especially in developing countries. When any service is available it would be better to ensure that multiple problems could be treated (WHO, 2001b).

Finally, the rationale for integrated care involves the critical role of behavioral health, that is, what people do to maintain their own health and address conditions that will improve both mental and physical health. Lifestyle practices include diet, exercise, cigarette smoking, managing stress, and social isolation, as examples, and relate both to the onset and course of mental and physical disorders and the effectiveness of many treatments (e.g., through adherence to treatment or serving as risk factors for a poor outcome). These lifestyle issues are not likely to be covered in traditional care, although advice might be given to engage in this or that practice (e.g., "you ought to stop smoking, drinking, and begin exercising). Integrated care provides a venue in which to address critical lifestyle issues that otherwise might be missed or treated superficially, and behavioral health care, when integrated into primary care, provides an array of strategies including EBPIs to address these lifestyle, health-related issues.

Key Characteristics

Integration of services is a model of care, actually several different models of care. These models vary as a function of the setting in which services are provided, the range of disciplines and services included, professionals as part of the team, and the population that is served. Amid the diversity, the model of care includes several common characteristics:

- *Comprehensive care:* among multiple disciplines to help with the range of medical and psychological services;

- *Patient-centered care:* emphasis on the whole person and partnering both with the individual and family and the integration of culture, values, and preferences of the patient;
- *Coordinated care:* linking, managing transitions between types of care and settings if needed;
- *Accessible services:* facilitating receipt of services with shorter wait times and easier access to contract of the team; and
- *Quality and safety:* commitment to using evidence-based practices, shared decision making with patients and families, measuring patient experiences (Agency for Healthcare Research and Quality [AHRQ], 2017).

There are many services that are integrated, some of which are large scale. I mentioned the VHA earlier as the largest fully integrated health care system in the United States and encompassing more than 1,700 sites of care. *The system* serves approximately 9 million veterans each year (www.va.gov/health/). This can serve as a model, but also has several unique features, such as central federal government oversight and control of budgets, practices, and other features that allow widespread extension of services. Yet recent changes in health care in the United States (Patient Protection and Affordable Care Act, signed into law in 2010) provide incentives and supports for states to integrate primary care and behavioral health care in their services. Further, there are enormous resources available to provide training, consultation, and resources to facilitate integration of services (AHRQ, 2017; SAMHSA, 2017a).

Benefits and Challenges

Integrated care allows treatment of several clinical problems that tend to go together. Consequently, the treatment and care of the patients are likely to be much better because disorders outside of one domain (e.g., medical) are more likely to be detected and treated, patients can visit a single setting (e.g., "regular doctor's office) with less or no stigma, and communication among professionals caring for different problems is likely to be better. Typically, professionals in different contexts do not have much contact with one another in relation to services provided. The lack of communication does not serve the patient very well—indeed patient protections preclude routine communication among professionals in different services unless special consent by the patient is sought and provided. Common records (e.g., electronic) in an integrated care setting, but also more informal collaboration among a treatment team, is likely to produce better outcomes. The better outcomes are likely because the disorders are often intertwined and one condition (e.g., depression) can greatly influence adherence to medical regiments for another condition (e.g., taking HIV, cardiac, and cancer medications). So, neglecting one component can detract from treatment outcomes of other conditions.

There may also be cost savings in integrated care in relation to both the direct and indirect costs I have covered previously (SAMHSA, 2017a). It is not only treating a given condition more efficiently (in one setting) but also treating conditions that otherwise might be overlooked. Those overlooked conditions (e.g., depression among patients, substance use) can influence the effectiveness of treatment of the "primary condition" (by better patient adherence) but also reduce the consequences of the otherwise untreated conditions (e.g., emergency department visits, disability-adjusted life years).

There are many challenges of integrated care. A set of challenges relate to critical decision points with no single, simple, or empirically based answers. These include deciding optimal ways to assess and screen individuals to decide the services they ought to receive, what among evidence-based treatments (medical and psychosocial) will be available for different types of physical and mental health problems and behavioral health foci, precisely how the services are integrated and funded, practical procedures such as billing, and training individuals in providing services in a collaborative way. For example, a recent set of case studies with eight individuals representing different health care organizations in different states in the United States identified barriers to integrated care (Buche et al., 2016). Five themes emerged:

1. Too few staff;
2. Disagreements about the roles of the different providers;
3. Limits on sharing information about the patients;
4. Policies from both state and federal government that hamper reimbursement for care; and
5. Management of the workflow and logistics (use of physical space in the patient flow).

These themes have emerged in qualitative and quantitative studies of integrated care (e.g., Scharf et al., 2013).

Diverse professions are involved (physicians, nurses, psychologists, social workers, licensed professional counselors, marriage and family therapists, and peer support personnel), and standardized training within any given profession, let alone between professions, is not at all worked out. Also, different professional organizations have models and recommendations about how to integrate services (e.g., American College of Physicians [Crowley & Kirschner], 2015; American Psychological Association [Cubic et al., 2012]). The diversity of models and organizations involved signal that integration is well underway, but many issues remain to be resolved and unified.

Evidence has supported the effectiveness of integrated care and treating mental disorders as part of the care for physical disorders (e.g., Asarnow et al., 2015; Coventry et al., 2015; Sharpe et al., 2014). Comparisons of integrated care versus primary care, the likelihood of detecting and treating various conditions, and the outcomes have promising data. Yet there are so many ways of integrating services and variations on what actual services are provided in a given setting.

Consequently, at this time it is difficult to identify one specific model or form of integration that has a strong evidence base for the treatment of mental and physical disorders and behavioral health issues to support well-being and health.

General Comments

Will integration have an impact on reducing the burdens of mental illness? Will more people be seen for their mental health problems (scalability), and will people be seen who otherwise do not receive services (e.g., ethnic minorities, children, older adults)? These are critical issues for our discussion. Integration provides greater opportunity to reach a segment of the population that seeks physical health care and in that process will also have access to mental health care. Of course, there are many who do not seek or obtain physical health care. And, in relation to mental health, too few professionals are available to treat the vast majority in need if we continue to insist on the usual degrees and credentials in the mental health professions. Perhaps it is too early to address the issues of scalability and reach to special populations in need. It is not clear at present that integration, as beneficial as that might well be, reaches the vast majority of those who receive no treatment. If it makes a little dent, that would be a significant contribution.

DEVELOPING BROADLY APPLICABLE TREATMENTS

The development of EBPIs has focused on matching treatments to specific psychiatric dysfunctions such as anxiety disorders, major depression, bipolar disorder, and a few hundred more, as specified in the dominant diagnostic systems (*International Classification of Diseases* [ICD-10], *Diagnostic and Statistical Manual of Mental Disorders*, [DSM 5]). The interest of treatments in relation to specific disorders can be seen in the sample list of EBPIs I provided in Chapter 4 (see Box 4.3), in which techniques are listed in relation to clinical problems. Focusing on specific psychiatric disorders has been a reasonable approach and has the appeal and precedent of the treatment of many physical disorders.

The entire matter of "specific psychiatric disorders" is now easily challenged. Many disorders go together (comorbidity). Among comorbid disorders most commonly discussed are depression and anxiety. This raises the question of whether the disorders are distinct at all or whether they ought to be defined differently to begin with. That is, maybe there is another way to diagnose that encompasses both depression and anxiety and some common underlying process, even though those processes can lead to slightly different symptom manifestations—and so on for other disorders that may go together.

The current diagnostic approach of describing and counting various symptoms (phenomenology) by itself may not be optimally helpful in reaching diagnoses and understanding the nature of various conditions. We know from everyday life in medicine, too, that there are many symptoms (e.g., headache, nausea, fatigue) that go across disorders, and merely noting that the patient has them is barely helpful until laboratory tests can rule out alternatives or provide data that are more specific to one or two problems. Currently, psychiatric diagnosis does not have the laboratory tests to determine what the underlying problem and disorder might be. That so many diagnoses may be comorbid raises the prospect that we might profit from different ways at looking at disorders.

As we have been developing specific treatments for specific disorders, we have been fully aware that the delineation of disorders is clear at the margins (e.g., pure, severe, and extreme schizophrenia or autism), though many disorders and symptoms blend into one another. Adding the challenge of developing disorder-specific treatments is the monumental task—more than 400 psychiatric disorders are recognized (ICD-10; WHO, 2010). Do we need to devise unique treatments for each of these? And, since the "one-size-fits-all" cliché noting that any one specific treatment does not work with everyone is true for virtually all interventions (psychological, medical, social, educational), one treatment for each disorder might not even be enough. Numerous influences have led to an alternative strategy to developing disorder-specific treatments, with two interrelated areas of work having emerged: transdiagnosis and transtreatment. These serve as models for understanding clinical dysfunction, underlying processes, and intervention.

Transdiagnosis

Transdiagnosis refers to the study of processes that span many different manifestations of clinical dysfunction (e.g., Eaton et al., 2015; Harvey et al., 2004; Kring & Sloan, 2009). Transdiagnosis focuses on the nature of the disorders (e.g., risk factors and etiology) rather than the pure phenomenology (description) of the presenting symptoms and seeks underlying commonalities among multiple disorders. Several factors have served as impetus for a transdiagnostic conceptualization of psychopathology, including the following findings:

1. There are high rates of comorbidity, as I mentioned, so that individuals (children or adults) who meet criteria for one disorder are likely to meet criteria for at least one other disorder as well (e.g., Kessler et al., 1994; Wichstrøm et al., 2012). I mentioned depression and anxiety that go together as one example; many other combinations are evident, too (e.g., multiple anxiety disorders with each other; schizophrenia and bipolar disorder; conduct disorder and attention-deficit/hyperactivity disorder);
2. Underlying processes that maintain "different disorders" often are quite similar (e.g., Fairburn, Cooper, & Shafran, 2003; Green et al., 2010; Hettema et al., 2005). For example, eating disorders (bulimia, anorexia) share many common factors, as do many anxiety disorders (generalized anxiety disorder, panic disorder, and agoraphobia);

3. Several disorders share common biological underpinnings, as reflected in brain structures, neurotransmitters, and genes (e.g., Kendler et al., 2003; Meyer-Lindenberg & Tost, 2012; Smoller et al., 2013);
4. Common viral and bacterial infections during pregnancy trigger immune responses that can affect the brain development of the offspring and underlie a variety of psychiatric disorders (e.g., Estes & McAllister, 2016; Knuesel et al., 2014);
5. Broad characteristics have been proposed and are beginning to be elaborated that might explain the onset or risk for a variety of disorders. Examples include a general psychopathology factor (a "p factor"), neuroticism, perfectionism, sleep disturbances, deficiencies in cognitive control, and tolerance of uncertainty (Barlow et al., 2014; Caspi et al., 2014; Egan, Wade, & Shafran, 2011; Goschke, 2014; Harvey et al., 2011; McEvoy & Mahoney, 2012). Each is proposed to underlie or mediate many different disorders; and
6. A number of EBPIs (e.g., cognitive behavior therapy, mindfulness) are effective across a range of disorders, suggesting some common mechanisms or core processes in the nature of these disorders (e.g., working memory, emotion regulation) (e.g., Harvey et al., 2014; Johnston et al., 2013).

It is still the case that many disorders look quite different from each other, even though in many cases common factors can be identified. How common underlying factors (e.g., genetic, environmental) are manifest in different symptom patterns is an important line of work actively under investigation. That is, do individuals share a very similar or common vulnerability, which later branches out over the course of development into different disorders, or are the different paths distinct at the outset? Continued advances in assessing and charting brain and genetic processes are core parts of addressing these and related questions. Overall, from a treatment standpoint, looking toward etiology and underlying processes rather than phenomenology (what the symptoms are and look like) may allow more generic treatments that can be effective without assuming that different presenting symptom patterns require different interventions.[3]

Transtreatments

Transdiagnostic conceptualizations support a focus on interventions that might well have broad applicability, beyond quite specific disorders. We saw this emerge already in the delineation of EBPIs, where a few treatments (cognitive behavioral treatment, interpersonal psychotherapy, and acceptance and commitment therapy) are effective with different disorders (see Chapter 4). The apparent applicability of a few treatments immediately challenges the dominant thinking that specific treatments are needed for each disorder. Investigators began to cull factors from treatments, especially cognitive behavioral treatment, which had the largest applicability across disorders.

From the broader view that multiple disorders might be addressed with a given treatment, we now have *transdiagnostic treatments*, that is, interventions that can be used for or span multiple disorders. Multiple terms are used for these as they have developed concurrently but separately. The terms include transdiagnostic treatment, transtherapeutic approach, transdiagnostic cognitive behavioral treatment, and unified treatment protocol (e.g., Greeson, Garland, & Black, 2014; McEvoy, Nathan, & Norton, 2009; Norton, 2012). They are not all identical but overlap greatly because they distill components from EBPIs that can be adapted and applied broadly.

For example, the unified treatment protocol is a transtreatment applicable to emotional disorders (e.g., anxiety, depression) (Barlow et al., 2011). The treatment draws heavily on cognitive behavior therapy, which has been well studied in the context of these disorders. The unified version distills core strategies that can be applied widely, including becoming mindfully aware of an emotional experience; reappraising emotion-laden attributions; identifying and preventing behavioral and emotional avoidance, and facilitating exposure to cues (both internal and situational) associated with emotional experiences. The unified treatment, as well as other cognitively based transtreatments, has supportive evidence and, in light of individual studies and their own meta-analyses, readily meets criteria for an EBPI (e.g., Newby et al., 2015). Primary applications have been with depression and anxiety.

Some of the transtreatments consist of multifaceted elements, components, or modules (terms used interchangeably here). Components are identified that can be culled from EBPIs, and these are applied as needed based on the symptoms and diagnoses of the clients. Using the components as needed is not the application of specific treatments to specific disorders per se; rather, a small number of components are selected, and these individual components have wide applicability.

One such treatment is referred to as the Common Elements Treatment Approach and draws on components of EBPIs (Murray & Dorsey, 2013; Murray et al., 2013). The focus of the treatment has been primarily with individuals exposed to trauma and experiencing symptom domains often associated with that including, depression, anxiety, and alcohol use. The approach is interesting from a transdiagnostic standpoint. By selecting individuals exposed to trauma, the implied view is that trauma is a common feature from which a range of diverse symptoms might emerge.

As an illustration, in one trial nine elements (or components) were part of treatment and were deployed based on presenting symptoms of the clients (Bolton et al., 2014). The clients were Burmese individuals who had experienced trauma and who had been displaced to Thailand (Bolton et al., 2014). Client symptoms included depression, anxiety, and many reactions associated with trauma. Counselors were trained to implement the different elements of treatment and to decide how and when the elements were to be applied. Some of the nine elements were presented to all clients (e.g., introduction to the program and orientation, cognitive coping and restructuring, graduated exposure [because all had trauma history]); other elements (e.g., behavioral activation, anxiety management, motivational interviewing) were based on whether symptoms were related to depression, anxiety, or alcohol abuse. In this study, the Common Elements treatment led to marked improvements in clinical dysfunction, as reflected in specific symptom domains and overall functional impairment compared with a wait-list control. The impact of treatment has been replicated in another country (Iraq) and with individuals who were survivors of trauma (Weiss et al., 2015).

There are several other noteworthy features of the Common Elements treatment model and its use, including simplified elements that could be easily trained, use of individual (counselors) with no mental health training to administer treatment, and cultural adaptation of treatment. These features will be quite relevant to novel ways of providing services more broadly to people in need and will be part of discussions in Chapter 6. In the discussion of dissemination of treatment earlier in this chapter, I mentioned a model of beginning treatment development with an eye to clinical applicability (e.g., simplified materials for training). The Common Elements model developed with many of the issues in mind that would facilitate dissemination and broad adoption.

Another modular approach has been used in the context of child therapy (e.g., Chorpita & Weisz, 2009; Ng & Weisz, 2017; Wood et al., 2015). Modules or components of treatment were selected that are likely to have wide applicability among youth referred clinically, and that can be taught to therapists and applied clinically. For example, in one demonstration, three modules (cognitive therapy for depression, cognitive therapy for anxiety, and behavioral parent training) were used and applied as needed to children referred for treatment in 10 outpatient services (Weisz et al., 2012). Depression, anxiety, and conduct problems constitute frequent bases for child referrals. Also, children may experience more than one of these, such as high rates of comorbidity. Therapists were trained in three modules and could then apply each module as needed. The primary presenting problem that served as the focus was identified at the outset of treatment and was re-evaluated throughout the course of treatment. Responsiveness to treatment influenced whether a different module was needed or whether one that has been applied would be repeated. A direct test showed that the modular approach produced much greater clinical benefits compared with treatment as usual (Weisz et al., 2012).

Transtreatments and modular treatments have several strengths. The most salient perhaps is an effort to simplify the vast number of EBPIs to some core of well-studied treatment components. This facilitates dissemination of effective treatments by requiring therapists in clinical practice to learn a few core modules rather than select from hundreds of techniques. In addition, the approach takes into account that individuals who come to treatment are likely to have more than one diagnosis or presenting problem. Therapists can be equipped to have a single treatment or a few core elements or modules that can address many different patients and referral problems.

Transtreatments, at least those I have mentioned, meet criteria for EBPI and could be added to our burgeoning list. I have not included them in prior lists (see Chapter 4) because most of the treatments or components (modules) fall within the broad rubric of cognitive behavioral interventions. Of course, drawing on cognitive behavioral interventions is not a necessary condition. That is, transtreatments in principle could be drawn from any set of therapies. For example, treatment referred to as mindfulness is applied widely to many different disorders (Germer, Siegel, & Fulton, 2013). Mindfulness involves attention to and awareness of the present moment (e.g., focusing on present thoughts, feelings, sensations) (see Germer, 2004). Acceptance is often part of that and entails willingness to experience diverse thoughts and emotions without being judgmental. The treatment fosters reduced anxiety, arousal, rumination, and depression and increased emotional regulation and acceptance of oneself or circumstances. Mindfulness can be considered as a transtreatment because it is applied quite widely across psychiatric disorders and with a strong evidence base spanning children, adolescents, and adults (e.g., Khoury et al., 2013; Perry-Parrish et al., 2016; Zoogman et al., 2015).

Many research questions remain for transtreatments. For example, the modular approach that takes core components of other EBPIs is relatively new, and some basic questions have yet to be answered. There are many commonalities among the transtreatments now (e.g., mostly variations of cognitive and exposure-based interventions). It would valuable if the field could settle a bit more on a transtreatment or set of components, or on the main ones that we ought to focus on in training of therapists. We do not want the proliferation of transtreatments with the new challenge of which one to select among that set. Also, research questions of interest might consider transtreatment as part of a *stepped-care approach*. Stepped care refers to beginning treatment with a general and relatively lower cost intervention before specialized care. For example, we know from many different studies that lay individuals (non–mental health workers) can effectively administer psychosocial interventions to individuals with psychiatric disorders (e.g., Nadkarni et al., 2016; Patel et al., 2011, 2016; Singla et al., 2017). Perhaps lay counselors could administer transtreatment as a first line of attack, and only when that proved to be ineffective would we resort to the costlier and specialized service. (We will return to the topics of stepped care and lay counselors in more detail in Chapter 9.)

A clear research priority is to integrate transdiagnosis and transtreatment. They have developed somewhat separately so that transtreatments are not so much based on better understanding of risk factors, etiology, and factors that are common to and differentiate disorders. Presumably at some future point, transtreatments will be based on a clearer understanding of how disorders unfold and when and where to intervene. The intervention might be a transtreatment or an intervention that at least is sufficient to treat a superordinate category or broad type of disorder (e.g., depression in its many forms, anxiety in its many forms).

For present purposes, the primary point to make is that there has been a change in treatment development. That change is a move from identifying a specific treatment for each specific disorder to treatments that can be applied to multiple disorders or a few components that can be deployed as needed based on variations of the symptoms clients present in treatment. Already there is an extensive research showing that transtreatments are effective. The approaches of transtreatment widely applied versus a disorder-specific treatment are not necessarily incompatible and might form part of a stepped-care approach.

USE OF TECHNOLOGY TO IMPROVE MENTAL HEALTH OUTCOMES

The use of technology to deliver psychological interventions is an extremely active area of research and clinical application. For the present purposes, I shall use the term broadly to include all the interventions that use the Internet; all media involving devices and their many platforms (e.g., virtual reality, smartphones, smartwatches, tablets, and much more); video, verbal, and text communication; and all sorts of exciting and emerging hardware and software. For purposes of noting this trend, I will group these together but in Chapter 8 will elaborate separate genres of interventions that are quite different in their delivery (e.g., use of social media, social robotics, television, and radio).

The use of technology in health care is not new. *Telemedicine* refers to the use of communication and information technology to extend the reach of medical practice and has changed how and where patients receive medical care (e.g., Roine, Ohinmaa, & Hailey, 2001; WHO, 2009). Telemedicine has been around for a long time in some form—at least 40 years (www.americantelemed.org/). Technological leaps in both hardware and software have extended the range of remote applications, as reflected by the development of diverse specialty areas (e.g., telepsychiatry, telesurgery, teleophthamology, teleaudiology, teleneurology) (e.g., Buck et al., 2016; Martini et al., 2013; Wooton, 2003). (As of this writing, there is no teleproctology, which of course is understandably "behind.") Each of the areas permits extending routine as well as highly specialized services to areas (e.g., rural areas, in any country) where the needed services are not usually available.

The revolution and evolution in the use of computers and use of the Internet and other media in everyday life have quickly filtered into health care in ways well beyond traditional telemedicine. *Telehealth* often is used as the broad term to encompass these many uses, but no one term can capture the range of interventions.[4] In everyday life, millions of people are actively involved with social media, or are connected to the Internet in one or more of many available ways. There are many indices of how pervasive the use of technology is. For example, for social networking, the number of users worldwide is estimated as 2.5 million people (very roughly one-third of the world population) (Statistics Portal, 2016). People are "connected" and beyond social interactions receive and provide all sorts of services (purchases, movies, video games, music). With each year, technology extends to further aspects of everyday life (e.g., self- or partially self-driving cars, gadgets to protect or clean one's home, clothing with sensors for use in relation to mental and physical health, an impersonal [rather than personal] trainer to help with exercise, and robotic toys for children as well as adults). In classrooms of young children through college students, assignments, discussion groups, and entire classes or undergraduate degrees are available on line. The age at which technology is integrated into life continues to fall, with younger and younger children increasingly at home with technology and social media. As an early entry point toddlers and young children often chat routinely with relatives through cell phones and video chat tools (e.g., Skype, FaceTime). Familiarity with and access to technology make it not all that surprising that at least one nine-month-old accidentally rented a car online (Kim, 2015). The overall point is clear. Technology is central to our everyday lives and awaits newborns as they enter the world. (Actually, there are many apps parents can use to monitor and bond with the fetus so that the fetus can begin exposure to technology without having to sit through the entire gestation period!) With each new birth cohort, a wider range of technology options are available, and these become the norm or at least pervasive rather than novel gadgets. In this context, mental health services that draw on technology may be a rather natural next step.

The use of technology to deliver mental and physical health care services includes many media, platforms, and venues, including primarily the Internet, apps, and short message services ("texting") through smartphones and other devices (e.g., tablets, smartwatches), as well as the use of virtual reality (Table 5.2). Developments in research continue to expand the interventions in how the techniques are used, new variations, and extensions to new uses in mental and physical health care. Applications through the Internet dominate, and there are tremendous variations in the options and ways through which this is done. For example, Internet-based interventions can vary along many dimensions and categories, such as whether and to what extent a trained mental health professional is actually involved in the delivery of treatment and whether treatment is delivered in specific sessions or available online at the discretion and schedule of the client.

Examples

Many technology-based treatments are available and encompass a broad range of psychiatric disorders and problems in everyday life. As with current trends in psychotherapy, cognitively based treatments for depression and anxiety may be the dominant foci, with many options available on line (e.g., Andrews et al., 2010; Arnberg et al., 2014; Spek et al., 2007). These programs often include the same core cognitive behavioral treatment sessions as used with in-person treatment (e.g., identifying and challenging cognitive distortions, engaging in positive activities) and are divided into sessions (with video clips describing key information and assigned homework) that patients can complete from virtually any location.

Online treatments can vary in the extent to which they are done completely by individuals on their own or use some assistance in varying degrees. For example, a well-known and long-established program for depression is referred to as

Table 5.2 Major Platforms, Formats, and Means of Technology-Based Psychosocial Interventions

Modality Delivery	Key Reviews or Discussion of Issues
Internet	Andersson et al. (2014)
	Barak et al. (2008)
Smartphones and eMobile devices	Donker et al. (2013)
	Gee, Griffiths, & Gulliver (2016)
Telephone (cell or landline)	Jackson et al. (2016)
	Lichtenstein et al. (1996)
SMS (texting)	Depp et al. (2010)
	Luxton et al. (2011)
Videoconferencing	Backhaus et al. (2012)
	Chakrabarti (2015)
Virtual reality	Opriş et al. (2012)
	Turner & Casey (2014)
Social robots	David, Matu, & David (2014)
	Rabbitt, Kazdin, & Scassellati (2015)

NOTE: The modalities have multiple variations. The variations, outcome evidence, and critical issue that each raises are beyond the purposes of this chapter. Key references are provided with reviews of the evidence and critical implementation and research challenges.

Beating the Blues (www.beatingtheblues.co.uk). The computerized treatment is interactive, multimedia, and computerized, and draws on cognitive behavioral treatments. Treatment is carried out without the need for a therapist and begins with a 15-minute introductory video; then eight weekly sessions are provided by computer. The sessions assign activities to do at home. Separate modules are presented (e.g., related to automatic thoughts, core beliefs, attributional style), and treatment can be individualized by additional modules that may also apply (e.g., graduated exposure if the patient has anxiety). Evidence supports the effectiveness of the program (e.g., Richards & Richardson, 2012).

Another program reported an online course for treatment of depression and included weekly therapist contact by phone or email (Titov et al., 2015). This was an uncontrolled large-scale study (>7,000 participants recruited) and yielded outcomes (effect size) on par with those obtained from (benchmarked against) face-to-face treatment using the same (cognitive behavioral) interventions. Although therapists were used in this program, the intervention could be administered to more people than usually would be the case because of their minimal contact (mean therapist time per case was 112 minutes). Thus each therapist had a case load of 20 to 50 patients.

Currently, there are scores of studies, often randomized controlled trials, showing that variations of online treatment with no or minimal contact with a lay counselor or trained mental health professional can produce treatment effects among clinic populations. It is still the case that very few of these demonstrations extend treatment on any scale that could have an impact on many in need of treatment. Exceptions are nicely illustrated in the context of cigarette smoking. One such telephone-based programs is referred to as "quitline" (see North American Quitline Consortium, 2016a, 2016b). Tobacco users call in and receive an evidence-based intervention that provides materials by mail, prerecorded messages, real-time phone counseling or a return phone call from a counselor, access to quitting medication, and taped calls to address possibilities of relapse (Graham et al., 2011; Lichtenstein, Zhu, & Tedeschi, 2010). Staff with bachelor's or master's degrees typically deliver the counseling services, although computers carry out much of the quitline counseling. In the United States, quitlines are offered in all 50 states and Guam, Puerto Rico, and Washington, DC; an estimated 1 percent of smokers in the United States use the services annually (see Cummins et al., 2007). Quitlines reach underserved populations; African American smokers are more likely than any other ethnic group to use these services, and Asian-immigrant smokers are as likely as European American smokers to use them (Maher et al., 2007; Zhu et al., 2010).

One large-scale application consisted of a Web-based intervention for smoking cessation (Muñoz et al., 2016). The program was available in two languages (Spanish and English) and was visited by more than 290,000 individuals from 168 countries. Data reported for more than 7,000 participants revealed smoking quit rates ranging from 39 to 50 percent at different points of assessment up to an 18-month follow-up. This program advanced the notion of massive open online interventions (MOOIs) to resemble the model of massive open online courses (MOOCs) in education. MOOIs would make available interventions that could reach individuals on a scale, as the demonstration in the context of cigarette smoking.

The Internet programs can include a variety of types of support with a continuum in the amount of support and the level of training of those who provide that support. Thus programs can include a continuum of external support, including complete independence, group support, and guidance by volunteer, semi-professional, or professional help from minimal to full-time aid (Harwood & L'Abate, 2010). Also, beyond the Internet, those interventions that a person can access and use on one's own are part of a larger genre of self-help interventions and can draw on various media (i.e., audio recordings, books, video, the Internet) to address numerous mental health concerns. In general, self-help interventions have an immense literature encompassing numerous approaches with various degrees of involvement by professionals. There are many effective interventions and many self-help resources available for a wide variety of conditions, including anxiety and mood difficulties, eating disorders, addictive behaviors, and personality disorders. Evidence suggests their effects are comparable to those obtained with individual in-person therapy (Bennett-Levy et al., 2010; Harwood & L'Abate, 2010). Yet they get lost in a sea of countless self-help books and websites that have no basis in theory or research. There is no easy way for laypeople to distinguish among fad, opinion, and research-based self-help techniques.

Apps for smartphones are being developed and applied to treat an array of mental health problems, including depression, anxiety, substance use, sleep disturbances, suicidal behavior, self-harm, psychotic disorders, eating disorders, stress, and gambling (Donker et al., 2013; Singh, 2014). Although there are many controlled studies, they are dispersed over many different programs and many clinical problem domains. Evidence at best is modest, and a reasonable conclusion would be that the vast majority of apps are not yet evidence based. The apps often have marketing hype and in that sense share a feature with the likes of fad diets, in which claims far outstrip evidence, and here, too, most people cannot readily discern what the evidence-based options are. The same might be said of texting, for which interventions including reminders and prompts to engage in therapeutic strategies to combat problems (e.g., depression, anxiety) are not sufficiently studied (Ben-Zeev et al., 2013). What is equally clear is that the evidence base for apps and other technology-based interventions is changing rapidly with an increased array of controlled studies with strong control groups (e.g., EBPIs delivered in the traditional way, treatments as usual in the clinic).

Benefits and Challenges

There several benefits associated with the use of technology-based treatments. Specific benefits and challenges vary by each by modality (e.g., apps, Internet, self-help, texting), but some broader issues can be identified. First, use of technology for administering psychological services or treatment involves an ever-increasing range of options in both hardware and software. These options are excellent in light of the focus of this book. Most people in need do not receive treatment, so we want multiple ways of reaching people with the hope that more will be served. Second, interventions can be extended to everyday life (rather than restricted to sessions in a therapy room or at a computer screen in one's home). The intervention through an app or link to a clinic can be provided in real time while people are going about their daily routines. If anxiety emerges, for example, coping statements and other interventions can be accessed or provided immediately. Third, technology can serve many roles, as reflected in providing the intervention or as a supplement to another form of intervention. Most forms of psychotherapy now involve "homework assignments," that is, therapeutically relevant behavioral tasks that will enhance treatment. Technology can provide these on a screen, prompt the activities, or be called up as needed. Fourth and related, in traditional forms of therapy, invariably there is a concern about what happens when treatment with a therapist ends. With apps or the Internet, therapy does not have to end in the usual way and can be drawn on as or when needed. This is critical because many forms of psychiatric dysfunction are episodic (come and go over time) or become more salient at times of stress or crisis. Technology affords the use of interventions as needed.

Finally, a unique advantage in relation to psychological intervention is the role of assessment of client functioning. Many of the apparatuses currently available (e.g., smartphones, watches, wrist monitoring bands) and apps associated with them can assess psychological and biological processes (e.g., stress, mood, heart rate, activity) in real time. This is often referred to as *experience sampling* and usually consists of prompting individuals to assess their state (e.g., mood, thoughts, or activities) through some device (e.g., smartwatch, smartphone) that the person carries or wears. The assessment can be directly connected to an intervention. When the patient signals that he or she is experiencing symptoms or some dysfunction, a preselected set of strategies (e.g., self-management, coping, stress management) can be delivered to a device for immediate use. All of this is readily automated and individualized to the problem, assessment domain, and programmed interventions.

To illustrate, biofeedback (as one intervention for stress) in years past required traveling to a facility (e.g., a laboratory) with the suitable equipment. One was "hooked up" to the equipment with an array of wires and monitors or some apparatus to help provide the feedback. Currently, many portable and affordable devices (for measuring heart rate, blood pressure, blood glucose levels) are available to the public and can provide the necessary feedback or periodic monitoring in everyday life (i.e., wherever the individual is at a given point in time) (e.g., Pallavicini et al., 2009; Zhang et al., 2010). Sensors that monitor heart or breathing rate and provide information immediately (e.g., in color or graphical display) can prompt the use of relaxation and other self-management techniques (e.g., RelaxLine, 2010; StressEraser, 2012). Apps for smartphones and tablets are constantly emerging and now allow assessment, feedback, and applications of interventions that can change mental health care. Smart clothing that tracks a variety of biological measures, used more commonly in relation to exercise and athletics, will no doubt find its way into assessment and treatment feedback loops. Better assessment can readily mean better treatment because the information can be used to make decisions about the intervention (e.g., more, less, different) and bring to bear better data about the impact on functioning in daily life.

In highlighting technology, I have emphasized delivery of treatment interventions. Yet the use of technology, including mobile apps, texting, and other applications, overcomes many of the barriers of participating in treatment (e.g., obtaining information about the available treatment options, avoiding stigma associated with seeking formal treatment at a clinic, assessing whether the treatment will be covered by insurance, and cost) (Price et al., 2014). Also, new resources are available to help track many of the available treatments (e.g., "apps") with client ratings of them (PatientView, 2016). Just tracking all the options is an enormous task and accomplishment.

Many challenges and issues remain to be resolved. First, there are many well-controlled treatment studies of various Internet, self-help, virtually reality, and other programs. However, the applications are not as well studied and established as in-person administered EBPIs. Reviews note that much of the evidence supports the effectiveness of technology-based interventions and that they are as effective as those administered in the traditional way (e.g., Andersson, 2014; Donker et al., 2013; Riper & Cuijpers, 2016). Many problem domains, especially depression and anxiety in adults, have the strongest evidence, but a surprising range of disorders (e.g., schizophrenia, bipolar disorder, conduct disorder, substance abuse, gambling) have been addressed and have evidence as well. In addition, treatments have been applied to children, adolescents, and adults. Dividing the studies by disorder and sample underscores the paucity of work for any given focus. In short, evidence will need to catch up to the enthusiasm for the use of technology.

Second, psychotherapy research has a long history of studying factors that can contribute to treatment outcome (see Gelo & Pritz, 2015; Lambert, 2013). Client, therapist, and relationship factors are among the leading categories. We do not yet have an idea if influences in the context of in-person therapy play a similar role in some of the technology-based treatments. For example, traditionally much attention is given to the therapeutic alliance, that is, the bond between the therapist and the client, and how that is important in treatment. In many of the technology-based treatments, alliance shows a similar relation with treatment outcome (e.g., Jasper et al., 2014; Preschl, Maercker, & Wagner, 2011). Yet alliance is not needed or relevant in many treatments (e.g., self-help Internet-based treatments), some of which include no therapist. Some technology-based treatments involve robots, and the therapeutic relationship presumably has a different meaning. In general, there could be decades of research exploring what factors influence the various technology-based interventions. That would be daunting.

Many ethical and legal issues are raised by the notion of technology providing services. To begin, protecting patient security is essential. Data available in computers or cyberspace (e.g., the cloud) require very special encryption, and individual practitioners and small clinical services are unlikely to have the resources to keep up on maintaining a secure server and hack-proof information. Larger organizations (e.g., major hospitals, universities, insurance providers) are more likely to have such resources, but they are hardly foolproof, and interest in hacking often is greater for larger organizations. Protection of data and privacy is a definite issue in the use of technology and is heightened because of the many formats, platforms, and types of equipment involved in storing data.

Second, professional and legal issues also come into play. Professionals who administer psychotherapeutic services are usually licensed on a state-by-state basis in the United States. Yet technology-based treatments often are provided well beyond state boundaries. Clients from anywhere in the country or the world with access to the Internet can call up an online treatment or work with a clinician located in one state. Strictly, the delivery of services in this way is not covered by most licenses, so is it all right to administer such treatments? Insurance and litigation for malpractice also are new territories when treatment can be practiced anywhere and a client feels inappropriately or unethically treated. Does the client have recourse if in another state or country? Professional, legal, and clinical issues can also emerge during the treatment if the client becomes worse or continues in the treatment without improving. Without a therapist to monitor the course of treatment, there may be untoward consequences in the clients' lives, including in the extreme: harm to themselves or others. Professional and legal responsibility and client resource are at best ambiguous areas with most technological applications and self-help versions of treatment. These points sample a range of issues that new technologies raise in delivering services. I will return to technology later in the context of innovative models of treatment delivery.

The directions that psychosocial therapeutic applications of technology will take are hard to predict but exciting to imagine. Technology development for medicine, space exploration, astronomy, business and industry, and military, among other domains, fuel continued advances. Artificial intelligence, voice recognition and conversation, and human–machine social interaction are making astounding advances that are relevant to health care. Psychosocial interventions will also profit from these advances.

Even with what we have now, intriguing as well as amusing therapeutic scenarios are easy to envision. For example, we have smartcars that drive themselves. Perhaps it will be only a little while before the public finds these acceptable. When they are, a psychologist and computer scientist no doubt will collaborate to develop a module for that car that provides psychotherapy of some kind (e.g., traditional talk therapy may be standard; cognitive behavior therapy or mindfulness may be options for a little extra cost; and at the luxury end there may be a special comorbidity package that includes all EBPIs and a couple of treatments as usual). The car will be able to detect cues from the passenger (e.g., electrical, physiological, or olfactory—now already quite possible with sensors in clothing). (Already driver alcohol consumption can be detected in one's car.)

Based on data derived from these sources, a warm and friendly computer voice (while the car is self-driving) begins. (As is the case with many car global positioning systems, in our scenario the passenger gets to select the language, dialect, accent, and gender of the voice.) The computer voice begins in a mellifluous and comforting tone, perhaps with a charming French accent, "Sidney [name of the passenger], I can tell you are tense. Are you still having problems with your (*computer voice presents options*: boss at work, relationship, golf swing, mom)? We have 12.37 minutes until we arrive at our destination; perhaps we could talk about it or at least cover one self-defeating cognition." Now the exchange between Sidney and the voice begins. Perhaps when the ride ends, the computer voice gives one concrete suggestion of a therapeutic assignment to try and complete within the next hour or two. Given the connectivity of things, it would be rather easy to have the computer in the car speak to Sydney's smartphone to follow through with prompts of the assignment.[5]

Already, virtual therapists can appear on a screen and respond therapeutically (e.g., Robinson, 2015). A client driving his or her own car could put on one of those helmet-mounted display systems that fighter pilots use and have the image of a virtual talking therapist right there! All the technology I note is available now. I mention this merely to convey possible qualitative changes that may be forthcoming. One can envision some of the research questions that follow, for example: Does treatment of stress of a male or female in their car on the way home from work improve the quality of interactions with their partner and children once they arrive at home?

In Chapters 7 and 8, novel models of presenting treatments will be discussed. Variations in how treatment is delivered will benefit from breaking down the conglomerate category of the use of technology in treatment. However, as a broad trend, a considerable amount of attention now is being placed on how to convert advances in hardware, software, and social media and the pervasive penetration of smartphones, smartwatches, tablets, and new platforms into improving physical and mental health.

SUMMARY AND CONCLUSIONS

I have highlighted four active areas in which intervention research and practice are changing. These included efforts to disseminate the EBPIs, to integrate physical and mental health care services, to develop treatments (transtreatments) that can be used to treat multiple disorders, and to exploit the range of new technologies available (e.g., Internet, apps) as a way of providing interventions. These areas of research are among those most relevant to the goals of this book, namely, providing interventions in ways that can reduce the burdens of mental illness.

The chapter did not review evidence that has emerged in the areas I have highlighted. Evaluation of the outcome literature was well beyond the goals of the chapter and would not be feasible in a single chapter. Indeed, technology-based interventions need to be reviewed exhaustively and separately by modality (e.g., Internet, virtual reality, texting, apps), or in some cases within modality by problem domain. More reviews of the literature continue to emerge, often in journals specializing in one or more of these technologies.

Perhaps the most significant lesson overall is that treatment is changing. Arguably, the most dramatic changes in the coming years will be those that emanate from technology. Within this context, the use of technology as a viable way to receive critical health care information and interventions or as a complement to traditional in-person services will become increasingly natural and maybe even the norm.

PART III

Expansion of Interventions and Models of Their Delivery

6

Need to Expand Interventions and Models of Intervention Delivery

Disseminating treatments to clinical practice, integrating care for mental and physical health, developing transtreatments that can be applied across multiple psychological problems, and exploiting the benefits of technology are four priorities that dominate intervention services and research, as elaborated in Chapter 5. Each of these is likely to improve and extend what patients receive. Providing the best available treatments in clinical practice is obviously critical, and nothing here challenges that, yet there are limitations in contemporary research on evidence-based psychosocial interventions (EBPIs) that the four priorities do not help very much, at least at present.

The purpose of this chapter is to convey a key implicit limitation of psychotherapy as delivered in clinical practice and investigated in research. That limitation is a major contributor to why most people do not (and without change will not) receive the interventions they would need to reduce mental illness. I will refer to the *dominant model of delivering treatment* (or interventions more generally) to describe that limitation and use that as a point of departure to propose characteristics of treatment delivery models that are needed to extend treatment. That is, we know that the dominant model cannot reach most people, but what characteristics or features of interventions or models of delivery are needed? Finally, the chapter conveys the promising options we currently have that include the critical characteristics to deliver treatment more widely. This chapter provides background to the next two chapters, in which novel models of intervention delivery are presented.

DOMINANT MODEL OF PSYCHOSOCIAL TREATMENT DELIVERY

Distinguishing Technique From How It Is Delivered

Most psychosocial interventions are provided as some form of psychotherapy. Whether the treatments are evidence based or not, and whether they come from one conceptual view rather than another, they usually share a common feature. That feature is how they are delivered or provided to people in need of services. I refer to how the intervention is delivered as the *model of intervention or treatment delivery*. Consider the distinction between an *intervention* or treatment technique and the *way that intervention is delivered*. The distinction is easily conveyed in multiple contexts, including our everyday lives.

For example, in our daily lives, our "to do" list (the intervention) notes the set of tasks we wish to accomplish and serves as a reminder to complete these tasks. That list can come to us in many ways, including smartphone alerts, calendar reminders, a physically printed copy of a list (how quaint), and verbal appeals from a loving partner. The list represents the intervention, and the many ways in which it can be presented to us are the models of delivery. Consider a very different context. In physical health care, some vaccines (the intervention) can be provided by injection, by nasal spray, orally, or through a needle-free patch (the models of delivery). In the context of mental health care, we also can distinguish the intervention (e.g., cognitive behavior therapy, some transdiagnostic treatment) from the model of delivery (e.g., by a live or virtual therapist, smartphone "app," or the Internet).

In relation to various forms of cognitive behavioral, traditional, and other therapies, one model has largely dominated how treatments are delivered. As I mentioned earlier and repeat here for convenience, that model has three interrelated characteristics:

1. Treatment sessions are provided in person and one to one with a client (individual, couple, family);
2. Treatment is administered by a highly trained (e.g., master's or doctoral level) mental health professional; and
3. Sessions are held at a clinic, private office, or health care facility.

To be sure, there are variations on this model, as in the use of technology, and I return to that later. Even so, in research and clinical practice, the model continues to rule. If you seek psychological services for yourself or a relative, it is almost certain that that service will involve the model with the three characteristics I have noted. And that is likely to be true in traditional settings (e.g., a clinic) or more forward-looking integrated care settings (e.g., clinics with multiple professionals and services).

This model of delivery with these characteristics has strong historical connections to medicine, and in that context the model is referred to as the *physician's practice model* (C. Christensen, Grossman, & Hwang, 2009). Indeed, many early psychological techniques (e.g., mesmerism, hypnosis, psychoanalysis) were provided by physicians (e.g., Franz Anton Mesmer [1734–1815], James Braid [1795–1860], and Sigmund Freud [1856–1939], respectively) and followed medical practice. These early psychosocial intervention techniques have played pivotal roles in the development of contemporary psychosocial therapies, which have followed the usual medical practice model of seeing the doctor for individual sessions.

Once in a while, the setting was not at a clinic, as in the famous case of Anna O, which is credited as the modern beginnings of "talk therapy."[1] The therapist (Josef Breuer) made house calls to conduct individual sessions with Anna (Breuer & Freud, 1957). And historically, sometimes treatment was administered to groups of clients as well as individually and in the home of the doctor (e.g., mesmerism). Yet these are exceptions. Currently in the United States, most psychosocial treatments are administered in the in-person, one-to-one therapy model, with a mental health professional, and at a setting to which the client must go. This model has been enduring, is in demand, and can deliver many EBPIs. It is so common that it is rarely perceived as a model or option, or as one of many alternatives. If treatment seekers are fish, the in-person, one-to-one therapy model is the proverbial water in which they swim.

Limitations of the Model in Reaching People

The dominant model limits the degree to which treatment can reach many individuals in need and in light of each of the characteristics of the model. Let us begin with the fact that the model relies on mental health professionals. I detailed in Chapter 3 that trained professionals represented a multipronged obstacle to providing services that reach most people in need. The obstacle includes too few trained mental health professionals in the United States, their heavy concentration in urban areas rather than being dispersed throughout the country in areas with few or no services, and limited training in many problems and populations for which there is great need (e.g., children, adolescents, and older adults). In addition, the ethnic and cultural diversity of mental health professionals does not come close to matching the diversity of the population in need of treatment.

For these reasons, expanding the workforce to deliver treatment with the usual, in-person, one-to-one model of care, a trained mental health professional, and in a special setting is not likely to have major impact on reaching the vast number of people in need of services. More of the same of what we have now will not much improve our ability to reach people in need.

Professional organizations and funding agencies provide support for trainees and incentivize professional development in areas of need (e.g., training in rural psychology, mental health services for special groups), but the scale of these is minute in relation to the need, and it is not clear they have had any impact. Of course, we would never want to turn down more resources to provide services. It is just that as a solution to the challenge of increasing the scale of interventions, more of what we are doing now in relation to the model of delivery will not suffice in closing the gap between the number of people who need services and the number of services that can be provided. In fact, the illusion that doing more of the usual or funding more of the usual is really helping may actually delay moving to solutions that make a real difference.

Another feature of the dominant model raises similar concerns in reaching individuals in need. Requiring clients to go to a special setting (e.g., clinic, private office) is also a constraint. Going to a setting raises at least three of its own interrelated obstacles. First, settings where services are provided are not readily available for many individuals. They are not nearby for large swaths of citizens, unless one lives in or near a city. Even inner cities are not likely to have nearby psychological service facilities. Second, "going" to a setting can raise practical issues such as transportation and child care. Too much effort is required. Finally, going to a "treatment" facility is likely to evoke concerns about stigma, including self-stigma. The effort to go to and schedule mental health services at a facility makes salient the notion that one has a problem, and that recognition may actually deter seeking help.

A current advance in health care is *integrated care*, which refers to providing services for general health as well as mental health and substance use and abuse in a single setting that coordinates services (Heath, Wise, & Reynolds, 2013; Vasan et al., 2014). This has several benefits in delivering a range of services and is perhaps especially important because a high proportion of individuals with physical health problems also have mental health problems, and vice versa. Having a setting where the patient can receive treatment rather than one facet of health makes great sense. Presumably there are fewer barriers (e.g., stigma) when one can go for a physical health problem and seamlessly be triaged into services for a mental health problem. Further, for present purposes, this does not alter the dominant model, that is, going to a place for mental health services. I will return to other facets of the dominant model, including many promising ways in which the limiting characteristics are being, and can be, addressed. I have already mentioned the use of technology, which is extremely promising as one avenue to alter the dominant model.

In-person, one-to-one therapy is referred to here as the dominant model because clinical practice, graduate school training, clinical program accreditation, predoctoral and postdoctoral internships, and research on psychosocial interventions draw heavily, and indeed almost exclusively, on this model. The dominant model has benefits that are already well known. To begin, it has served as the basis for identifying and developing EBPIs in research, and long before that for administering the treatments in clinical work. In addition, surveys show that adults who have received some form of psychotherapy generally are very satisfied and believe they have benefitted from the treatment (Consumers Union, 1995), although a small proportion (approximately 5 percent) report negative effects of treatment (Crawford et al., 2016). Yet, in light of the overall perceived benefits, the dominant model has proved itself to be viable. Nothing of my comments detracts from these remarkable gains. And for individuals who have access to that model, there may be little need to provide new ways of delivering treatment. My focus pertains to what would be needed to reach the largely underserved majority of individuals in need of mental health services. In that regard, the dominant model falls quite short.

The central point to convey here is that the vast majority of psychosocial treatments in the context of therapy are mostly delivered by the dominant model, which is just not feasible or practical for most people. Consequently, it is not so surprising that about 70 percent of people in need of services in the United States receive nothing, or that the 30 percent who do receive some service do not usually receive psychotherapy at all, but rather some contact with a health care provider, who might be their internal medicine practitioner, religious leader, or other service. Something more and different is needed to reduce the burdens of mental illness. That includes interventions that can effect change and at the same time reach the large number of individuals who are not yet served.

The need to move to additional models has been recognized for decades (e.g., A. Christensen, Miller, & Linds 1978; Collins et al., 2013; Ryder, 1988). The opportunity to move to novel models is new, as is our recognition that the need is enormous for better mental health care in developed and developing countries. Epidemiological data on a worldwide basis are better than ever before. Add to that, viable models for delivering interventions are clearer than ever, including, but well beyond, the use of technology. The models themselves will be elaborated in the next chapters.

DELIVERY MODELS TO REACH PEOPLE IN NEED OF SERVICES

Treatments and Models of Delivery

Typically, as we develop treatments, we begin with a focus on a clinical disorder, a conceptual model of how that disorder may come about, how treatment can address key components of the disorder, and what we might draw from the human and nonhuman animal research in the way of principles or techniques. We then begin tests of treatment. If one considers cognitive therapy for depression and prolonged or graduated exposure for anxiety, for example, many of these steps have been critical for developing these interventions. The viability of this model needs no more proof than the successes of these and many other EBPIs.

Conceptually, treatments have varied tremendously over the years. Pioneers of treatment techniques illustrate this nicely. Examples that occupy special places in the history of the development of psychosocial therapies include pioneers such as Carl Rogers (1902–1987; client-centered psychotherapy), Albert Ellis (1913–2007; rational emotive behavior therapy), Andrew Salter (1914–1996; conditioned reflex therapy), Joseph Wolpe (1915–1997; systematic desensitization), Aaron Beck (1921–; cognitive therapy for depression), and Arnold Lazarus (1932–2013; multimodal therapy). Each of these pioneers provided a new and different conceptual view of treatment and different procedures from what preceded them. Each of them also noted the conceptual (and empirical) limitations of psychoanalytic and psychodynamic therapies and how the new model that each proposed was more viable and connected to laboratory research or concepts derived from that research (see Kazdin, 1978b).

With remarkable conceptual creativity and connecting that to research, we in fact had changes in treatment, but what was not changed, challenged, or questioned was the dominant model of treatment delivery. Further research has provided a continued flow of creative interventions (e.g., dialectical behavior therapy, acceptance and commitment therapy, interpersonal psychotherapy, multisystemic therapy). Yet here, too, the model of delivery has continued (in-person, one-to-one sessions with a mental health professional in a special setting). That model of delivery is a barrier to reaching most people in need. The model need not be abandoned, but certainly must be supplemented by an array of other models.

Key Requirements and Characteristics of Scalable Models

Before presenting other models (in the next chapters), it is useful to step back a bit. What is the problem we are trying to address and indeed solve? That problem is to reach people in need of services with effective interventions; that is, our goal or target is to reach a large number of individuals who are unserved or underserved by current treatments. Before jumping to new treatments or models, it is useful to begin with the question: What are the key characteristics needed for the interventions and models of delivery required to achieve that goal? We know we do not want characteristics of the dominant model, but that does not tell us very much about what we do want. Table 6.1 summarizes several characteristics that should guide our development of interventions and focus our attention on delivery. The characteristics overlap but are not redundant.

Scalability is clearly a place to begin in pondering what characteristics models of delivery should include. With most people in need of treatment receiving nothing, scalability becomes critical from the outset. Will we be able to scale a particular form of treatment so that a large number of people can receive it? Scalability addresses the treatment gap, namely, the discrepancy between those who need treatment and those who actually receive an intervention. From the outset in considering the model of delivery, we ought to be concerned with making sure it can reach very large numbers of individuals in need. Remember, we are talking not necessarily about the intervention itself (e.g., cognitive behavior therapy), but

Table 6.1 Key Characteristics of Models of Treatment Delivery to Reach People in Need of Services

Characteristic	Definition
Scalability	The capacity of the intervention to be applied in a way that reaches a large number of people
Reach	The capacity to extend treatment to individuals who are not usually served or well served by the traditional dominant service delivery model
Affordability	Relatively low cost compared with the usual model that relies on individual treatment by highly trained (master's, doctoral degree) professionals
Expansion of the nonprofessional work force	Increase in the number of providers who can deliver interventions
Expansion of settings where interventions are provided	Bring interventions to locales and everyday settings where people in need are likely to participate or attend already
Feasibility	Ensure that the interventions can be implemented and adapted to varied local conditions to reach diverse groups in need
Flexibility	Ensure that there are options and choices because no one model of delivery is likely to have the reach needed
Acceptability of the model of delivery	Ensure that the intervention is acceptable to potential consumers of treatment and those who provide treatment. Acceptability refers to judgments by laypersons, clients, and others about whether the intervention procedures are appropriate, fair, and reasonable for the problem that is to be treated. The extension here is that the model of delivery must be acceptable and is separate from the acceptability of the intervention.

rather about whether it can be delivered in such a way to make it something other than a boutique intervention for the special few who have access.

Reach as a criterion overlaps with but is distinguishable from scalability. Many groups are especially excluded from treatment and for a variety of reasons. Ethnic and minority groups, individuals who are living in poverty or in rural areas, and other subgroups within our population (e.g., children, single-parent families, older adults, victims of violence) are much less likely to receive treatment than are individuals with none of these characteristics. Scaling treatments so that more people receive them does not necessarily handle disparities in treatment. We could be scaling up to reach more of the people (e.g., majority group members, living in urban areas); that would address one problem (making treatment available to more people) but perpetuate another problem (neglecting the same groups we are neglecting now). Reach extends the criterion of scalability to ensure that those groups at the greatest disadvantage for receiving care are specifically targeted by our models of delivery. This criterion addresses health care disparities.

Affordability is important because cost is a major and multifaceted barrier to receiving or providing care. On the receiving side, cost of individual sessions (without insurance and even with insurance) can stop people from seeking or remaining in a treatment that is otherwise available. Perceptions of affordability might be included here because most of us have little idea of what mental health services are covered and to what extent by any plan we have. In addition, enough insurance claims for mental health services are rejected as to induce anxiety and reticence in seeking treatment. (It is an interesting ploy, tactic, or consequence of insurance [whether for mental or physical health, one's car, or home] that there is a little fear that if one uses the insurance [actually files a claim], one will be punished in some way [e.g., higher rates, rejection of renewing the policy].) All of this means that many whose costs might be covered are kept from seeking an available treatment. This perception might overlap with the concept of mental health literacy.

Apart from affordability from the perspective of the client, there is the other side, namely, affordability from the standpoint of those who fund or actually deliver services. Federal and state governments in the United States, for example, routinely lament the costs of providing mental health services; that is, services are not sustainable because of costs. As I noted earlier, budget reductions include mental health services as one of the early places to cut spending. In any models of delivery, we have to be sensitive to cost both for the client and for the service provider. You may recall from Chapter 5 that the program (Improving Access for Psychological Therapy [IPAT]) in the United Kingdom promised, and then demonstrated, that providing treatment of depression on a large scale would in fact *save* money for the government. Scaling up the treatment, training many mental health professionals, monitoring quality of care and treatment outcome, and scores of other steps are all very expensive. Yet depression has measurable monetary costs, including welfare benefits and medical costs and the loss of revenue from taxes and productivity. Treatment in fact was cost-effective and saved more money than it cost to implement. Thus affordability may not mean that treatment delivery is inexpensive—even an expensive and seemingly nonaffordable treatment might well be affordable once cost savings are considered. In any case, when considering models of delivery, costs for providing and receiving services are essential to consider. Nonaffordability at either end would preclude large-scale extensions of treatment.

I mentioned earlier that the administration of treatment by trained mental health professionals as part of the dominant model of delivering treatment all by itself limits reaching many people in need. The number of professionals, where they are located (urban areas), the restricted range of what they treat in relation to need, and the paucity of a diverse ethnic and cultural diversity all are limits in relation to reaching people. The obvious question is: Who else but highly trained mental professionals can administer psychological treatments for significant mental health problems? We will say more about this later in the discussion of novel treatments that rely on laypeople. Sufficient to emphasize here, highly trained mental health professionals are not always and perhaps not even usually necessary to administer psychosocial interventions effectively. Evidence supports the notion that individuals without an advanced degree or training in psychology, psychiatry, or social work can effectively administer treatment and are no less effective in doing so (e.g., Nadkarni et al., 2016; Neuner et al., 2008; Patel et al., 2016; Poser, 1966; Stanley et al., 2014). In the mental health professions in the United States, the mental health service infrastructure includes regulation by the states and the professions in which people without a special license or training (e.g., in clinical psychology, psychiatry, social work) cannot provide "psychotherapy" nor advertise that they do. This is designed to protect the public from quackery and untrained service providers. But a more cynical spin is that it is also designed to protect practitioners from competition. Whatever the "spin," the trade-off or downside of the regulations is not allowing expansion of the workforce in ways we know now to be effective.

Laypeople can administer treatments and certainly could serve as the first line of treatment. Mental health professionals might well be reserved for cases in which their special talents are essential, in which the first line of defense by a person with less training has not been effective, or in which special privileges (such as prescribing medication) are needed. Needless to say, I do not advocate requiring no training or poor training of individuals who administer treatment. Rather, treatment can often be simplified, placed into trainable modules, and administered by individuals with little or no advanced training in the mental health professions—and still be effective and still produce favorable outcomes that are enduring (e.g., Barlow et al., 2011; Bolton et al., 2014; Patel et al., 2010, 2011). In any case, one characteristic we probably want of novel models of treatment delivery is that there are more people—thousands more—who can provide them.

Expansion of the settings where interventions are provided addresses another limitation of the dominant model of delivering therapy. Currently, most EBPIs require individuals to "go" to a clinic, hospital, or private practice office. That raises physical obstacles (e.g., transportation, location) and may heighten attitudinal obstacles (e.g., stigma). Those obstacles aside, the current physical settings would not be able to accommodate treatment that was scaled to reach large numbers and those in special areas (e.g., inner city, rural areas) where few facilities and services tend to be available. Of course, the use of technology (e.g., Internet, apps) moves treatment out of physical locales and brings treatment to people's homes. The integration of mental health services in settings where physical health care is provided (integrated care) might bring more people into mental health services. But other locations to which people have access could also be used to provide services (e.g., schools, shopping centers, urgent care centers), with examples to come in detail in the next chapter.

Feasibility has to do more with practical features of the delivery model. In fact, can the model be implemented given the circumstances of the local conditions? These conditions may include physical characteristics or infrastructure (e.g., access to computers or any health care facilities), but also to cultural and ethnic beliefs. That is, a very scalable treatment in principle might still not be scalable in practice because delivery is not likely to occur or be subscribed to in light of obstacles specific to the locale. Also, the intervention delivery (e.g., by nonlocal counselors or assumptions of the intervention) may be objectionable on grounds of beliefs or cultural practices. The intervention must be practical and likely to be subscribed to. Texting, for example, can be a highly feasible intervention in cultures where there are remote rural areas and no landlines, but cellular phones are very prevalent (e.g., Lester et al., 2010).

Flexibility is important in developing novel models of delivery. One of the problems with the dominant model that I did not emphasize is that for most therapists and clients, it is not just the dominant model; it is the only model. That is, if one wants psychotherapy, usually this is the model—take it or leave it. To reach people in need, it would be valuable to have multiple delivery models as options. By options, I mean that a given intervention (e.g., cognitive behavior therapy, graduated exposure) could be available or provided in multiple ways. Multiple models are needed not just to overcome the specific limits of the dominant model (in person, one-to-one sessions at a special setting) but also to have options that vary on accessibility and acceptability. Any given model will have its own limitations and obstacles. Multiple models are needed. Flexibility and choice of models may be the best way to meet the reach criterion of ensuring that groups with the greatest health care disparities receive services.

The final characteristic is referred to as *acceptability,* and that concerns consumer views of how appropriate, suitable, and reasonable the intervention is, that is, the means or procedures that are used to achieve change. The concept has been evaluated extensively in the context of the acceptability of various treatment options such as psychotherapy, medications, and behavior-change interventions (e.g., Carter, 2007; Kaltenthaler et al., 2008). From that literature, we know that acceptability can influence the likelihood that clients will continue in or drop out of the intervention, whether clients carry out the procedures prescribed during the intervention, and whether professionals (e.g., educators, therapists) actually use the procedure correctly (e.g., Allinder & Oats, 1997; Arndorfer, Allen, & Alijazireh, 1999; Kazdin, Holland, & Crowley, 1997). We know there are cultural and ethnic differences in seeking treatment, using clinical services, and treatment preferences (Boothe et al., 2005; Miranda et al., 2005). It is likely that acceptability influences each of these. Thus acceptability is not a property or characteristic of treatment per se, but rather is a characteristic in the context of ethnic and cultural perspectives in relation to that treatment.

For this discussion, we are focusing on a slightly different topic from acceptability of *treatment* or *an intervention,* namely, the acceptability of the *model of delivery*. Presumably, for many an intervention requiring one to visit a place labeled "clinic" and see a "therapist" is less acceptable than an intervention in which one can work using a video chat service (e.g., Skype or FaceTime, or the equivalent) from one's own home. Overall, we need interventions that not only are acceptable but also are acceptable models of delivery. Flexibility of the intervention is relevant here because multiple models are needed precisely because acceptability is likely to vary for different groups of individuals.

Some general points should be raised about the characteristics of models of delivery to be considered when developing interventions. First, the characteristics I mention might be considered as a guide rather than a comprehensive list. Second, the characteristics are not completely independent but they are different enough (e.g., scalability and reach) to make them worth distinguishing. Third, characteristics are each a matter of degree. Models of delivering treatment could vary on a continuum for each characteristic. Fourth, no one model is likely to address each or even most of the characteristics very well. The point is to have multiple models of delivery so that treatment can reach many people in need in different ways. A model with strengths even in only one or two characteristics in particular might still be extremely valuable. For example, a highly affordable intervention that people find acceptable could make a huge contribution. Across multiple models, all the characteristics need to be reasonably covered, which increases the options for models we can use.

More than the characteristics, it is useful to consider the overall goal we are trying to achieve. I have stated that goal as providing effective (evidence-based) interventions for the vast majority of individuals in need of services and to reduce the burdens of mental illness. Thus we begin with that goal and build interventions and models of delivery around it. This is in sharp contrast to the historical and current model of developing treatments (the dominant model) that begins with developing an effective intervention for a given clinical problem, without explicit attention to whether the treatment ever could be in widespread circulation among individuals in need. Neglect of the characteristic mentioned previously (see Table 6.1) means that our effective treatments from the outset might not be of much use to many people.

ENCOURAGING LEADS WITHIN THE MENTAL HEALTH PROFESSIONS

Within current psychotherapy research and clinical practice, the dominant model of delivery remains well ahead of any alternative model. Yet, within the mental health professions, there is movement toward other models that have some of the desired characteristics and that would help treatments to reach more people. In the prior chapter I mentioned that one trend in psychotherapy research is the use of technology to deliver treatment. The dominant model involves a client going to a clinic setting (whether traditional or integrated), whereas Internet and app versions of therapy can be accessed from home or elsewhere (e.g., public library, coffee shops—wherever there is computer and Internet access). Apps are also available 24/7 and do not require logging into a computer.

Technological applications are not merely novel models of delivery but also have changed critical aspects of the intervention. These include the assessment of client functioning (e.g., depression, anxiety, stress) while people live their lives. Experience sampling, mentioned in the previous chapter, refers to measurement of momentary samples of experience usually on multiple occasions throughout the day and over one's smartphone or other such device. The assessment can be connected with automatically delivered treatments or be used to prompt the client to invoke coping or other therapeutic strategies. These advantages extend beyond how to deliver a given treatment to encompass the integration of assessment with treatment in a seamless way.

Another change in treatment that technology has fostered is what happens at the "end of therapy." With the dominant model, therapy usually ends after a relatively small number of sessions (median is less than five sessions in the United States) when a client drops out (Gibbons et al., 2011; Hansen, Lambert, & Forman, 2002). Some of the technologies do not require ending treatment at all. The client can continue to be "in therapy" by using the intervention available from the Internet or apps. We know well from medicine that many disorders (e.g., diabetes, asthma) require ongoing care and treatments (e.g., kidney dialysis, immunosuppressant medication to prevent rejection after organ transplantation) are not expected to end, at least at this point in treatment development. Many psychiatric disorders also are chronic or episodic, and others might re-emerge or be exacerbated by environmental events (e.g., stressors). Having more treatments that are available lifelong is essential. Technology can readily facilitate this by providing continued treatment as needed. Thus, as a model of delivery, technology adds considerably to what we have beyond the dominant in-person model.

The use of diverse technologies to deliver treatment is relatively new, and there are, and will be, many new ways of administering interventions. Even so, to date many of the interventions continue to be extensions of the dominant model of delivering treatment. For example, many extensions that use the Internet are referred to as Web-based or on-line treatments and include one-to-one treatment with a therapist. The therapist is still involved but remotely. This is a huge advance from the dominant model nonetheless because clients do not have to "go" to a clinic to "see" a therapist there. The privacy of Internet treatment and ability of clients to have sessions in the comfort of their own homes may also reduce reticence and stigma in starting therapy.

Technology is advancing at a remarkable pace, which will change more facets of treatment in the coming years. While the formats and interventions are proliferating, there is an unexploited opportunity for creativity that goes beyond current application. Perhaps more can be done beyond finding improved ways of reaching people to developing entirely new interventions. A useful distinction has been noted in a discussion of the "physical Internet," which is an active area of work in industry, engineering, and manufacturing.[2] As one researcher noted in that context, "It's [the physical Internet] not about a better way of doing what you now do. It's about doing things you've never thought of doing before." (Gue, as quoted in Wible, Mervis, & Wigginton, 2014, p. 1106). The comment is instructive by keeping both facets in mind. We want to do things better (i.e., deliver therapy better, more broadly, with greater reach, and so on). We also want to rethink all facets of treatment and what technology offers that are not just novel ways of delivering what we have available now.

The distinction is not dichotomous but sensitizes us to consider options and foster truly novel ways of helping people that do not follow standard treatments (i.e., what we do now). For example, for both treatment and prevention, fully automated and individualized interventions can be designed to promote physical exercise (e.g., Hurling et al., 2007). Participants received solutions individually tailored to barriers they perceived, a scheduled weekly plan with mobile phone and email reminders, a message board to share their experiences with other participants, and feedback on their activity level on a wrist-worn device. This completely automated program increased exercise significantly. Also, for individuals with stress, psychological symptoms, and impairment, multiple Internet support programs are available and have evidence in their behalf (e.g., Bouma et al., 2015). Programs like these permit individualization but can still be provided on a large scale.

Let us be more ambitious in how such interventions are extended and take on a pervasive problem in both physical and mental health care, namely, treatment adherence (e.g., Dunbar-Jacob & Mortimer-Stephens, 2001; Howren & Gonzalez, 2016). Adherence is a problem for major (and minor) diseases and includes follow-through on treatment (e.g., taking medication as prescribed or at all, monitoring biological states through self-testing at home, getting follow-up checkups, filling and refilling medication prescriptions). Adherence is an issue with a direct impact on disability and mortality (e.g., cardiovascular disease, cancer, diabetes, HIV/AIDs). Moreover, psychological dysfunction (e.g., especially depression and anxiety) is a detriment to adherence in medical care that could be addressed by technology and have a broad impact on physical disease (e.g., DiMatteo, Lepper, & Croghan, 2000). Many psychosocial interventions (e.g., variations of cognitive behavior therapy and exposure therapy) have homework assignments, and carrying these out are challenges of adherence.

In short, attacking a problem like adherence with the use of psychological science and technology could have an enormous impact and affect millions of individuals and encompasses diverse health conditions. Many areas within psychological science (e.g., research on decision making, use of priming to promote behavior, social norming, message framing, feedback) could directly guide and form the basis for the interventions; technology could provide options of delivery to provide automated, disorder-specific, individually tailored, and large-scale application formats. This would be one example of going beyond doing what we are doing now. Technology-based interventions that address a pervasive limitation of many treatments for many diseases and dysfunctions could change what we do and also go well beyond diseases and dysfunction to address lifestyle changes that promote mental and physical health. We will return to technology and its use in treatment once more because it is part of a larger set of novel models of delivery.

SUMMARY AND CONCLUSIONS

Interventions (what actually is done to achieve therapeutic change) can and should be differentiated from how they are delivered (model of delivery). The dominant, in-person, one-on-one model of our past has proved to be quite valuable. After all, virtually all EBPIs have been developed, researched, and applied using exactly this model. But this model of delivery is not likely to be of help in treating individuals or reducing the burdens of mental illness on a large scale.

To say that one-to-one, individual therapy with a mental health professional cannot help on any large scale does not demean the value of that model of delivery. From this dominant model, research already has made enormous advances. And from that model we may well eventually understand what are the mechanisms of therapeutic change so that we can develop more effective treatments and deliver those on scale. Finally, a small minority of individuals with the means (their own funds, insurance) do seek and obtain treatment through the dominant model of delivery. So, we ought not to say that the dominant model should be abandoned. Rather, we need many other models of delivery that are not shackled by the limits of the dominant model now in use. In the next two chapters, I will discuss novel models that depart considerably from what the usual mental health professions use as a way of delivering psychosocial interventions.

7

Novel Models of Delivery 1

Expanding the Ways of Providing Available Interventions

The dominant model of administering psychosocial interventions serves a useful and important function even though it is available only to a small group of individuals in need of mental health services. Happily, there are many additional models that could be systematically brought to bear to make an enormous difference in mental health. These models can be evaluated in light of the characteristics noted in Chapter 6 (scalability, reach, affordability) that would be required to extend treatment beyond the confines of therapy administered with the dominant model. Several models are available, but for the most part, they are outside of the usual thinking and foci of the mental health disciplines.

In this chapter and in the next, I discuss many different models of delivering interventions. Because I have culled models from multiple disciplines and influences (e.g., physical health care, business, social policy), there is no easy classification to neatly group them along similar dimensions or categories. As an approximate grouping, I have delineated models that primarily deliver current treatments such as evidence-based psychosocial interventions (EBPIs) covered earlier. In these models, the treatments are not necessarily different from those we have been discussing (e.g., cognitive behavioral interventions), but they are provided differently. In the next chapter, more models are considered that can deliver many forms of treatment, though often the nature of the intervention itself is completely different from how we conceive of traditional treatment (e.g., use of television shows, taxes, and social policy).

This chapter covers three models: task shifting, disruptive innovations, and interventions in unconventional settings (Table 7.1 provides a summary of key characteristics for easy reference). I will elaborate on these, provide examples, and explain how they complement the dominant model of psychotherapy as a way of reaching people in need of services.

Table 7.1 Novel Models of Delivering Treatment

Model	Key Characteristic	Examples	Sample References With Illustrations
Task shifting (and sharing)	Expanding the workforce by using lay individuals to administer interventions that otherwise might be delivered by health professionals	Used worldwide for treatment and prevention of HIV/AIDS Recently extended to mental health service delivery	WHO (2008b) Fulton et al. (2011)
Disruptive innovations	A process in which services or products that are expensive, complicated, and difficult to deliver move in novel ways to alter these characteristics In health care, services are brought to people more than bringing people to the services	The delivery of health screening and treatment in shopping malls, drug stores, and grocery stores Use of smartphones, apps, and tablets to assess and deliver mental health interventions	C. M. Christensen et al. (2009) Rotheram-Boris et al. (2012)
Interventions in everyday (unconventional settings)	Expansion of health care beyond clinics and traditional settings to places that people normally attend for other reasons Overlaps with disruptive innovation but comes from different tradition and draws on different settings (e.g., schools, workplace, churches, hair salons, barbershops)	Delivery of health screening and education messages in hair salons	Linnan et al. (2014) Luque et al. (2014)

NOTE: Additional models are presented in Chapter 8.

TASK SHIFTING AND SHARING

Task shifting develops a workforce of lay individuals who usually are trained to implement and deliver health interventions that ordinarily might be provided by highly trained and credentialed professionals. The term *task shifting* helps convey how this operates, namely, by shifting tasks reserved for highly trained professionals to others, with the goal of greatly expanding the workforce. The model began in the context of providing physical health care services but applies to and has been extended to mental health care.

Definition and Background

Task shifting is a method of strengthening and expanding the health care workforce by redistributing the tasks of delivering services to a broad range of individuals with less training and fewer qualifications than traditional health care workers (e.g., doctors, nurses). This redistribution allows an increase in the total number of health workers (e.g., nonprofessionals, lay individuals) to scale up the scope of providing services. *Task sharing* is a related term that is sometimes used interchangeably with, but occasionally distinguished from, task shifting. *Sharing*, when distinguished, can mean that lay individuals work along with professionals, that is, share in the activities and tasks rather than completely taking over those activities (e.g., A. Walsh et al., 2010). However, the distinction is not consistently made. Moreover, they can easily represent a continuum only clear at the margins based on the extent to which professionals are involved in any of the treatment delivery tasks (direct care, supervision of lay counselors). For this chapter, I refer to task shifting to encompass both.

The concept and practice of task shifting in physical health care are not new. For years, the practice has been in place in many developed countries (e.g., Australia, England, United States), where nurses, nurse assistants, and pharmacologists provide services once reserved for doctors. Community health workers, a term defined long before task shifting was developed, have provided specific health services (e.g., birthing, neonatal care, immunization) in developing and developed countries and with demonstrated efficacy (e.g., Bang et al., 2005; Greenwood et al., 1989). These workers consisted of individuals trained outside of traditional medical training positions. Task shifting represents an extension of these applications in scope of health foci and scale.

Task shifting emerged from global health initiatives, particularly in developing countries. These initiatives focused on treating and preventing infectious (e.g., malaria, HIV/AIDS, tuberculosis) and noncommunicable disease (e.g., cardiovascular disease, diabetes, cancer, respiratory disease) and improving living conditions and education (e.g., Institute of Medicine, 2010, 2011; United Nations, 2000; World Health Organization [WHO], 1978, 2011a). These initiatives provide an important context for the present focus on delivering mental health care services. Delivering physical and mental health services typically contended with and shared key challenges of meeting health care needs in many cultures, under a variety of conditions (e.g., enormous resource constraints, geographical obstacles in reaching people), where people in need of services were not likely to receive them. Key strategies to address the problems included reorganizing and decentralizing health services to accommodate the limited traditional resources and infrastructure (e.g., medical personnel, hospitals).

Task shifting began in earnest with specific attention to the treatment of HIV/AIDS (WHO, 2008a). The epidemic and spread of HIV/AIDS heightened the need to increase quickly the delivery of services to unserved individuals and to reduce the burden of the epidemic. The need for services in many developing countries stood in sharp contrast to the medical infrastructure available to provide those services, at least using traditional medical care. For example, approximately 95 percent of individuals with HIV/AIDS reside in developing countries, and almost two-thirds of them in sub-Saharan Africa. Yet sub-Saharan Africa has only 3 percent of the world's health workers and provides less than 1 percent of the world's health expenditures (WHO, 2008a). Early estimates noted that an additional 2.4 million doctors, nurses, and midwives would be needed to meet national and international goals (WHO, 2006). The United Nations agreed to work toward making prevention, treatment, care, and support programs accessible by 2010. To that end, the range of workers recruited for health care expanded and included nurses, midwives, and community residents (some of whom were individuals living with HIV/AIDS) who could provide specific services, support of others, and help to overcome stigma and discrimination in their local communities. The majority of task-shifting applications have focused on physical health in developing countries (e.g., Ethiopia, Haiti, Malawi, Namibia), where shortages of human resources and the burden of illness (e.g., HIV/AIDS) have been especially acute.

An important feature to underscore is the research and evaluation associated with implementing of task shifting. Empirical evaluations showed that task shifting rapidly increased access to services in the context of HIV/AIDS, reached large numbers of individuals in need, and yielded good health outcomes and high levels of patient and counselor satisfaction (WHO, 2008a). The utility and effectiveness of the procedure were shown in high-income as well as resource-constrained countries. This evidence also controverted concerns that task shifting leads to low-quality care or that lay counselors would be less effective than professional workers in the outcomes they achieve. Task shifting continues to be in widespread use in physical health care and has evidence attesting to its effectiveness (e.g., Fulton et al., 2011; Maier & Aiken, 2016; Sokhom et al., 2015).

Applications to Mental Health

As physical health initiatives expanded globally, mental health received increased attention and became the source of its own set of international initiatives.[1] For example, in 2007 an international group of health researchers noted that expansion and scaling up of mental health services were "urgently needed" (Lancet Global Mental Health Group [LGMHG], 2007, p. 1242). The reasons were the burden of mental illness worldwide, the enormous proportion of individuals not receiving treatment, and the availability of effective interventions—points emphasized in prior chapters of this book.

A critical theme and topic that emerged and that is arguably even more present today is the interrelation between physical health and mental health (e.g., Boehm & Kubzansky, 2012; *Lancet Psychiatry*, 2015; LGMHG, 2007; Nordentoft et al., 2013; O'Donohue & Cucciare, 2005; Prince et al., 2007; Sharan et al., 2009). Indeed, a widespread view connecting these is reflected in the often-cited statement that there is "no health without mental health" (Prince et al., 2007, p. 859; WHO, 2005, p. 11).[2] As I have noted previously, physical and mental health problems more often than not go together and that was part of the rationale for integrated care.[3]

Task shifting was extended to mental health problems because it can be scaled up to provide services to individuals who otherwise did not have access to care and because of its adaptability to diverse countries, cultures, and local conditions. The extensions to mental health have not reached the scope of use of the approach achieved with physical health. Even so, there are many applications, and they continue to multiply (e.g., Hoeft et al., 2017; Singla et al., 2017).

An exemplary application of task shifting to mental health was a randomized trial of treatment of anxiety and depression in India (Patel, Weiss, et al., 2010). Twenty-four public and private facilities (serving more than 2,700 individuals with depression or anxiety) received a stepped-care intervention beginning with psychoeducation and then interpersonal psychotherapy, as needed and as administered by lay counselors. The lay counselors had no health background and underwent a structured two-month training course. Medication was available as part of the stepped-care as needed, as was specialist attention (health professional) for suicidal patients. At six and 12 months after treatment, the intervention group had higher rates of recovery than did a "treatment-as-usual" control group administered by a primary health care worker, as well as lower severity symptom scores, lower disability, fewer planned or attempted suicides, and fewer days of lost work (Patel, Weiss, et al., 2010, 2011). Overall, the study showed that lay counselors could be trained to administer interventions with fidelity and that their interventions reduced prevalence of disorder in a large sample.

This illustration conveys that task shifting, at least in developing countries, is beyond the stage of potential utility in delivering mental health services for individuals meeting criteria for psychiatric disorder. Since this evaluation, evidence from many other studies has revealed the effectiveness of task shifting as a model of delivery for the treatment of depression, anxiety, eating disorders, trauma, schizophrenia, and alcohol abuse (e.g., Balaji et al., 2012; Bolton et al., 2014; Kilpela et al., 2014; Nadkarni, et al., 2016; Patel et al., 2016; Rahman et al., 2008, 2016). These demonstrations not only establish the clinical utility of task shifting but also add to the evidence that lay counselors can deliver effective treatment and that outcome effects are not sacrificed in the process. Moreover, several of the studies have evaluated outcomes on a larger than usual scale for psychological intervention studies, evaluated and monitored treatment fidelity, and included follow-up, among other laudable features.

Key Considerations

In Chapter 6 I identified several characteristics that would be useful in a model of intervention delivery that could reach individuals in need of services and reduce the burdens of mental illness. Table 7.2 highlights the characteristics and lists models (covered in this chapter) in relation to those characteristics. For comparison purposes, the first row of the table includes the dominant model of administering psychotherapy. That model could be evaluated with other characteristics and "look" much stronger. Yet our goal here is to focus on models that can in fact have an impact on reducing the burdens of mental illness by reaching the large numbers of individuals in need who currently receive no treatment of any kind.

Task shifting in the second row of the table meets several characteristics that would foster widespread extension as a model of delivering treatment. Task shifting has several additional noteworthy features, including its applicability across countries (developed or developing) and across types of health care needs (e.g., prevention and treatment; physical and mental disorders). The approach emphasizes standardized treatments, a decentralized delivery model, and simplified treatment protocols. Standardized training is provided to lay counselors, and monitoring and evaluation are built into the system (e.g., to ensure integrity of treatment, to evaluate outcomes). As a model of delivery, task shifting is designed to provide interventions on a large scale and to reach individuals who otherwise would not receive services. These are key characteristics needed for mental health services in both developed and developing countries.

Task shifting is a multistage process that I have simplified to draw attention to the treatment delivery facet (see WHO, 2008a). The process begins with consultation of experts, stakeholders (e.g., patient population) in a given location (e.g., country), national endorsement by ruling government to permit the novel means of administering treatment and by whom, and attention to regulatory requirements on a temporary and more permanent basis that might preclude or limit delivery of treatment by lay individuals. In any given application, task shifting requires coordination among government agencies, nongovernment organizations, professional organizations, and local governments. This might make task shifting feasible and more easily implemented in developing countries where infrastructures (e.g., from local and national government, accrediting organizations) might be more amenable to change or at least rapid change. For example, in developed countries there are professional and legal restrictions (credentials, licensing, degrees, training) regarding who is allowed to provide treatment.

Table 7.2 Key Characteristics of the Models

Model	Scalability	Reach	Affordability	Expansion of Workforce	Expansion of Settings	Feasibility	Flexibility	Acceptability of the Model
Dominant model of psychotherapy	W	W	W	W	W-	W	W	?
Task shifting	?	S	S	S	?	S	S	—
Disruptive innovation	S	S	S	?	S	?	S	—
Unconventional settings	?	S	S	S	S	?	S	—

S = strong—the model could meet this criterion very well; *W* = weak—the model is not very good at doing this; ? = unclear—the model might meet the criterion but some qualification and not well tested in practice; — = the acceptability of a model is an empirical question and is unclear for the novel models.

Notes: All codes are estimates and can vary as versions within a model of delivery change (e.g., what type of disruptive innovation, such as apps versus urgent care centers). The initial model in the table is the dominant model of psychotherapy discussed in Chapter 6. That model included treatment that is delivered as in-person, one-to-one sessions with a mental health profession and in a special setting. The model is included in the first row merely as a point of departure for evaluating what other models add. The model is the only model listed with information about acceptability of the model. We know that many people find the delivery of psychotherapy acceptable among those who have received that; that is, they are very satisfied with the treatments delivered in this way (e.g., Consumers Union, 1995), but we also know from surveys that much of the general public does not think very much of psychotherapy, hence the "?".

Usually, lay individuals would not be able to routinely provide mental health care (e.g., in the United States), even though now the evidence is enormous that they can be just as effective as the highly trained mental health professional, as noted previously (see Chapter 5). Add to that the compelling evidence that by restricting treatment delivery to trained mental health professionals, the need for services cannot come close to being met.

In the United States, exceptions have been made to allow lay counselors to provide mental health support and services. For example, the US Veterans Administration has lay counselors (peer specialists) who are veterans and who themselves have and are recovering from a mental disorder (US Department of Veterans Affairs, 2015). They serve to provide support, intervention, and as-needed advocacy for other veterans in need of services. Before serving as a peer counselor, they receive brief didactic training that includes observing other counselors. After they are certified, they provide care for veterans in need of services in any of a variety of psychosocial intervention techniques (e.g., problem solving, symptom management, goal setting). As another example, peer-delivered services are in use to provide a variety of support services in relation to both physical and mental health (see Rogers & Swarbrick, 2016). Use of peers is not new from a historical standpoint and has a history of at least 40 years (Swarbrick et al., 2016). Yet the evidence at this point is relatively sparse, especially in relation to the administration of EBPIs for mental disorders. Even so, there is reason to expect from task shifting and other research on lay counselors that peers can effectively administered EBPIs.

Overall, task shifting has the demonstrated capability of the model to deliver physical and mental health services, to show positive outcomes on a large scale and in diverse circumstances, and to have an empirical base for guidelines about implementing the model. One does not usually speak of evidence-based models of delivery, but task shifting has been shown to meet that designation by having been implemented repeatedly (replicated) across many countries, settings, and types of dysfunction in relation to both physical and mental health. This one model might go far in making the leap from treating few to treating many in relation to mental illness. As with any model, tasking shifting will have its own set of limits. In the United States, for example, using lay counselors can conflict with state laws and professional organization positions regarding who can provide services. As I noted, the impact on reducing the burdens of mental illness is greater with multiple models given that any single model will have limits.

Task shifting emerged from concerns about administering physical health care services. Current efforts to extend this to mental health care are promising already, with emerging and consistent evidence for its impact on psychological disorders. I am suggesting much wider spread use of the model as one valuable way to extend the scalability and reach of services. The next model I discuss is much broader in its origins (not health care per se). Yet, as with task shifting, it has extended treatments to physical and mental health care.

DISRUPTIVE INNOVATIONS

Definition and Background

Disruptive innovation, or disruptive technology, emerged from business rather than from health care (Bower & Christensen, 1995; C. M. Christensen, 2003; C. M. Christensen et al., 2009). The concept pertains to a change in a product or service that is not a linear, evolutionary, or incremental step. Rather, the product or service often provides a disruptive, disjunctive, or qualitative leap and develops or extends a market that is not otherwise being served. The new product or service "disrupts" an existing market by changing who is served and how the service is provided. The disruption usually makes things simpler and more affordable.

The disruption does not refer to what happens to consumers (e.g., sacrifice in their lives, interruption of services), but rather refers to established companies or markets. For example, digital cameras and photography "disrupted" the market for and the business based on film (chemical) photography. Digital photography has not eliminated the use of film, which is not the issue in disrupting the market, but it has clearly led to a qualitative change in how most people take photos and the speed of access to the product (no need to develop film). Related, smartphones and tablets disrupted the business for personal point-and-shoot (rather than professional) cameras. Here, too, the purchase of cameras was not eliminated, and the technology of cameras evolved and continues to do so. Yet the availability and extremely widespread use of smartphones with high-resolution cameras, the ability to take videos, the ability to send files instantaneously through messaging and email, and other features changed photography in everyday life and the need for and utility of carrying a separate camera. If anything, the disruptive innovation of smartphones and tablets has "forced" camera companies to integrate the previously unique features of smartphones (instant sending of a photo over the Internet).

As my example conveys (as will others coming shortly), technology can play a major role in changes in products and how they are marketed or used. Understandably, *disruptive technology* was the initial term used, but it gave way to *disruptive innovation*. As illustrated with further examples, *innovation* better captures the breadth of products and services, some of which do not necessarily require a change in or even use of technology. In fact, it is important to consider the model of disruptive innovation more broadly. The model refers to the process by which products or services that are complicated, expensive, and less affordable move to novel delivery models and products that change these characteristics.

The concept of disruptive innovation may not be familiar, but the many innovative products and services that illustrate its application are part of our routine daily lives (C. M. Christensen et al., 2009). I have mentioned film and cameras and innovative products that altered taking photos and making videos. Other examples abound. For example, email, free video conferencing, text messaging, and various forms of social media are not mere extensions of earlier forms of communication (e.g., postal service, landline phones, chatting with others), but instead reflect leaps in new ways of staying in touch that are rapid, very accessible, less costly, and with novel advantages. As a related example, the development of cell phones made phone services available in many developing countries where service was lacking or quite restricted because of the limited infrastructure and resources to install and maintain landlines. Cell phone service "leapt over" the traditional barriers of providing phone services in novel ways. For example, a 2014 survey of several residents of seven African nations (Ghana, Kenya, Nigeria, Senegal, South Africa, Tanzania, and Uganda) revealed that almost no one had a landline (median of 2 percent), whereas 89 percent of adults had a cell phone or smartphone (Pew Research Center, 2015). Cell phone technology made unnecessary the need to develop the costly and long-term time frame of having land lines.

Disruptive innovations are evident in many domains, including manufacturing (e.g., interchangeable parts, assembly line in car production), business (e.g., smartphone, tablet), consumer purchasing (e.g., by credit cards, smartphones, and PayPal), social networking (e.g., Facebook, Twitter, LinkedIn, Instagram), and health care (e.g., home pregnancy tests, medical robotics) (see C. M. Christensen et al., 2009). These innovations often provide simpler, less expensive, or more convenient solutions to problems and often can be scaled to reach people who would not otherwise have access. Of course, simpler, less expensive, and more convenient in relation to health care services will address many of the characteristics (e.g., scalability, reach, affordability, feasibility) and surmount some of the barriers (e.g., cost, access to interventions) I noted if models of treatment delivery are to reach people in need.

Disruptive innovation in health care is not new. I mentioned telemedicine (see Chapter 5), which refers to the use of communication and information technology to extend the reach of medical practice. This is one example of a disruptive innovation that changed how and where some patients receive medical care (e.g., Roine et al., 2001). Early users of "technology" approximately 40 years ago when telemedicine emerged did not have access to the Internet and all the hardware and software platforms we take for granted today. Yet disruptive innovations go beyond the use of technology. For example, other disruptive innovations in health care have used nonmedical settings, such as drug stores and shopping malls, to provide a range of services to measure blood pressure or cholesterol, treat various illnesses (e.g., allergies, pinkeye, strep throat) and skin conditions (e.g., cold sores, minor burns, wart removal), and provide vaccines. Patient referrals can be can be made if the tests reveal the need for further diagnostic workup or intervention.

Direct preventive and treatment interventions can be provided to reach people more quickly than in traditional settings. Providing flu shots at drug stores and grocery stores and at schools (for children) is an illustration. An epidemic threat in 2009 (H1N1 virus, initially referred to as "swine flu" because of its resemblance to a virus contracted by pigs) led the US government to urge expansion of settings to include retailers where the flu shots could be administered

(Centers for Disease Control and Prevention, 2009). This was in recognition that the existing infrastructure and means of providing inoculations would not overcome the many barriers to reaching individuals in need and achieving the necessary level of community immunization (crowd or herd immunity) to protect public health.

Applications to Mental Health

Disruptive innovations could provide more accessible ways of delivering mental health interventions (see Rotheram-Borus et al., 2012). Many interventions have already extended to mental health care through the use of the Internet, smartphones, tablets, and video conferencing (e.g., Backhaus et al., 2012; Barak et al., 2008; Bennett-Levy et al., 2010). Delivery of treatment through the Internet or apps, as discussed in Chapter 5, falls under disruptive innovation; applications are disruptive in relation to the dominant model of administering psychotherapy. Self-help interventions through the Internet or phone apps may make the disruptive and qualitatively different features of treatment delivery and receipt especially obvious. Individuals have access to treatment 24/7 and may not require the use of a therapist at all (Bennett-Levy et al., 2010; Harwood & L'Abate, 2010). Already there are many apps that focus on mental health to help combat stress and anxiety, suicidal thoughts, getting to sleep, self-help and coaching in treatment techniques, and others (Kiume, 2013; Mohr, 2014).

Technology-based delivery of treatment is one type of disruptive innovation, and progress continues on those many fronts. The convergence of advances in hardware, software, and artificial intelligence already has us talking to and expecting answers from our equipment (smartphone, tablets). Advances related to treatment and assessment that can aid with treatment are dazzling but also changing quickly. Here are some samples yet to be routinely used in physical or mental health care but easy to envision in both contexts:

- The familiar wrist bands people use to monitor exercise, sleep, and the like are likely to advance remarkably in biological processes they can assess, and this will increase the options for evaluating psychological states with which these processes may be highly correlated (e.g., Cazalé et al., 2016);
- Smart clothes are available now to assess biological and emotional states, but these are relatively new and have not penetrated everyday life (at the time of this writing) (e.g., Chen et al., 2016);
- E-skin, a smart artificial skin, could be used to detect all sorts of health-related bodily functions and markers of biological and psychological states (e.g., Thakur, Dofe, & Jadhav, 2014);
- Touchscreen technology has advanced so that an epidermal touch panel can be placed on one's skin and used to play games, write, and control other devices (e.g., Kim et al., 2016);

- Exhaled molecules (one's breath) can be used to detect and distinguish among many different diseases (Nakhleh et al., 2016);
- Smart tattoos and digital tattoos are somewhat new and will be able to control other devices that may be integrated into treatment (e.g., Kao et al., 2016); and
- *Chatbots* and *messagingbots* refer to software that allows us to converse and text to manage many more aspects, activities, and tasks in our lives and to engage in more natural language exchanges resembling and mimicking social interaction, beyond what the various voice communication options (e.g., Siri, Cortana, Alexa) currently allow (e.g., Dale, 2016). These interactions might readily influence health (e.g., help provide support or manage stress).

As a further illustration of the fast tracking of many advances, consider wearable devices. Many are in development but still fairly far along, and some have been developed in the context of national defense (e.g., Hirshberg et al., 2014; Ranck, 2012). For example, a recently developed device is referred to as BACtrack Skyn (pronounced "back track," where "BAC" stands for blood alcohol content). The device is worn as a wrist band and detects ethanol molecules emitted by the skin; it provides continuous real-time monitoring of alcohol level that is sent and stored to another device, like a smartphone. This device is already commercially available in 20 countries and several thousand stores within the United States (Sachs, 2016). It is very likely that this will be a model for many devices to come in which array of biological and psychological states and conditions are evaluated based on molecules detected through sweat or breath. The technologies for many such conditions are available now, but are not implemented routinely at this moment and not scalable beyond demonstrations. Yet even scaling up may be on the near horizon. For example, one company plans to provide 50,000 employees with smartwatches to monitor indices related to their health and insurance benefits (Amini, 2016). This is a beginning for large-scale and personalized assessment of health conditions in real time.

For the disruptive innovations based on technology, certainly there is much more to come that will influence health care. For example, I mentioned smart tattoos in passing. It is easy to envision a smart tattoo that assesses critical bodily functions, that sends instructions to our smartphone or smartwatch to deliver some psychological intervention (coping skills, meditation or mindfulness instructions, emotion regulation strategies), and that sends an alert message, if needed, to our doctors by going directly into our encrypted medical records.[4] From that tattoo, it will be feasible just as we leave work to call ahead to our home and have our masseuse and spa ready, along with those iconic black round stones to place on our backs. Currently, the voice from our antiquated car GPS tells us, "You have arrived at your destination." It is a minor addition to include the phrase, "and your robe, slippers, three masseuses, and a glass of your favorite wine are waiting." (The three masseuses at my home said they would welcome an advance warning like this because warming those black stones needs some lead time.)

There are many other options that could be disruptive that are not necessarily based on technology. Some of these follow on the heels of success in physical health care. For example, increasingly, urgent care facilities are interspersed throughout a community and make walk-in access to immediate medical care readily available. These facilities can help patients receive the care they need, are more accessible than hospital emergency departments, and actually reduce health care costs—all characteristics we need in a model of delivery to address mental illness (e.g., Patwardhan et al., 2012; Weinick, Burns, & Mehrotra, 2010). Could we add to these facilities urgent mental health care? Integrated urgent care facilities would accommodate both mental and physical health care, in a preliminary way, with referrals to handle conditions in need of more intensive care. At such facilities, people could come in as needed or be brought to these facilities by relatives for immediate mental health intervention and planning (follow-up care if and as needed). Urgent care centers still require going someplace for treatment, but the "place" is much more convenient, user friendly, and accessible than a hospital or many private practice clinics. In fact, one of the obstacles to integrated health care services is that many of these facilities are in primary care centers (e.g., hospitals and clinics), and these locations still represent a barrier for many in getting to treatment, whether mental or physical services (Hefner et al., 2015). Integrated care in community settings could improve convenience and accessibility of services.

It seems like urgent care facilities for mental health problems would be feasible, whether integrated with physical health care or without the integration. Indeed, a large health care insurance company in the United States has added mental health care to its urgent care facilities (Kaiser Foundation; see http://khn.org/news/urgent-care-centers-opening-for-people-with-mental-lllness/). And separate (independent) urgent care facilities for mental health have emerged. For example, the Mental Health Urgent Care Center (Telecare Corporation, 2015) provides immediate relief for people in distress and helps them maintain stability in their lives and to avoid hospitalization, emergency department visits, and incarceration. Annually, more than 3,000 persons are served, who are 18 to 59 years of age and who suffer serious mental illness. Apart from providing access to psychosocial services and medication, referrals can be made as needed to other services.

Extension of mental health services for all or most urgent care centers or development of stand-alone centers would be a logical step for building on disruptive innovation and for extending treatment. Placement of such centers in areas of the city where many individuals are not otherwise well served might greatly extend the reach of mental health services. Many urgent care facilities are in a storefront-type setting and eschew all the medical, hospital, and psychological treatment accoutrements that might make them less attractive in relation to seeking mental health care. Thus a walk-in urgent care facility may mitigate at least some of the barriers of entering mental health treatment (e.g., scheduling and following through with a visit). Urgent care facilities, in conjunction with the use of lay counselors, mentioned previously in the context of task shifting, is an innovation that could change mental health services now and reach many more people in need.

A related development is the use of kiosks that are available to provide mental health assessment and screening (e.g., MindKare [Jacobs, 2016]; SimSensei Kiosk [DeVault et al., 2014]). For example, MindKare provides kiosks that can be placed in the community or workplace and allow individuals to self-assess anonymously to check on their mental health through a touchscreen interactive display. The screens are for anxiety, depression, posttraumatic stress disorder, bipolar disorder, eating disorders, and alcohol use disorders. After the questions are answered, the individual receives information about whether their results are consistent with a mental health disorder and information about local treatment resources. Screening for a variety of disorders is readily available on the Web, but with little quality control over the reliability and validity of the measure or over what information is provided and how. If these facets were addressed, the notion of a kiosk could make mental health information readily available, including information about access to treatment resources in the area. Presumably, there would be less stigma using a kiosk as an initial step, in comparison to seeking a diagnosis at a mental health facility. Also, kiosks could be such that physical and mental health and possibly other issues such as behavioral health (e.g., lifestyle behaviors) were included so that standing at a kiosk does not automatically signal that is one is trying to sort out for which of the hundreds of mental disorders one qualifies. As of this writing, MindKare kiosks have been set up in a few states and at least one college campus (Otto, 2015).[5]

As my examples convey, disruption is not a single model of delivery but a broad category of innovation with the characteristics in common being how they enter into the marketplace and exert influence. Disruptive innovations can leap over many of the usual barriers of receiving treatment and expand on the dominant model of in-person, individual psychotherapy at a clinic. Interestingly, when disruptive innovations first emerge (e.g., personal computer, cell phone), they usually do not compete head-to-head with the traditional product (e.g., mainframe computer, centralized computers in industry and on campuses; landline phones, pay phones). Over time the innovation may begin to compete and take over as the product develops and the use expands. Convenience, affordability, and novel features help the innovation begin to dominate or at least have major market share whether or not they replace other services or products. Perhaps innovative treatment delivery models that are disruptive will have that same course. Developing areas include computerized, online, and self-help therapies; extensions in the features of smartphones and smartwatches to assessing psychological states and conditions and then provide automated but individualized interventions; and new user-friendlier facilities (e.g., mental health urgent care centers or mental health services integrated with existing physical health centers).

Key Considerations

Table 7.2 summarizes key features of disruptive innovations as a broad model of delivery. There are many means of delivering treatment (e.g., technology, urgent care centers) within the overall model, but there are general characteristics worth noting. Typically, disruptive innovations make a product or service more affordable and accessible, and these are key reasons for presenting this as model of delivery of psychological services. When health care procedures (e.g., medical diagnostic evaluation and interventions) are first studied, they often require special skills. As the procedures develop and effects become reasonably predictable, their administration can be turned over to others (less expensive caregivers) and provided in settings (outside of hospitals and clinics) with equal or better quality than the higher cost counterparts (C. M. Christensen et al., 2009). An example from psychosocial interventions provides a relevant illustration. EBPIs for anxiety (e.g., systematic desensitization, graduated exposure, cognitive behavior therapy) initially relied on a small group of researchers and clinicians (with master's and doctoral degrees) who could implement the procedures. These are now well established and can be administered as self-help interventions or by lay counselors supervised by more trained individuals and with demonstrated effectiveness (e.g., Bennett-Levy et al., 2010; Dombeck & Wells-Moran, 2006). The larger literature on the use of lay counselors, such as highlighted previously in the discussion of task shifting, indicates that the quality of the interventions for many different disorders is not sacrificed when turned over to trained lay counselors. After quality is reliably established in a disruptive innovation, convenience is the next domain that is usually developed, which further increases accessibility (C. M. Christensen et al., 2009).

Disruptive interventions often (but not always) are brought to people where they are, and that certainly addresses convenience. In particular, technology and online services have allowed individuals to access services (e.g., assessment, intervention) in convenient, user-friendly, and immediate ways free from the usual barriers that can impede seeking or participating in treatment and are disruptive in that sense. The treatment outcome evidence for many technology and online services is improving, but it is still the case that many of the applications and convenient programs have no evidence in their behalf (e.g., Price et al., 2014). The pace of developing some innovations (e.g., apps) far outstrips the pace with which any small subset could be evaluated empirically in controlled studies. Technology can raise novel challenges for ensuring privacy. In short, innovations for treatment delivery are exciting and promising, but still require caution before considering them as evidence based, effective, and ready to deploy on a large scale.

INTERVENTIONS IN UNCONVENTIONAL (EVERYDAY) SETTINGS

A key impediment to reaching people in need of services is the feature of the dominant model that requires clients to come to special places (clinics, private practice offices, hospitals) to receive treatment. This requirement harbors several interrelated barriers, including physical restraints (clinics are often in urban areas but not in the inner cities), practical constraints of prospective clients (e.g., transportation, parking, finding babysitting, maybe squeezing in a session during a lunch hour for working parents), and attitudinal issues (e.g., stigma of going to a treatment facility where therapy or treatment of a "mental problem" is provided). Yet going to a special place is not an essential feature of receiving treatment for psychological problems.

Disruptive innovations already mentioned often are in settings (e.g., pharmacies, shopping malls), a person's home or at work in a private office (e.g., using the Internet), or in everyday life (e.g., smartphone apps). Yet a separate discussion of everyday settings as a model of delivery is warranted because interventions in such settings have emerged from different traditions (e.g., community psychology, community mental health settings, and even civil rights) and emphasis (i.e., setting) rather than the nature of change (i.e., disruptive) in the innovation itself. In addition, all disruptive (health care) innovations are not necessarily in natural everyday settings, and all interventions in everyday settings are not necessarily disruptive, as that term has been used previously.

Definition and Background

This model focuses on expanding delivery of care beyond traditional locales for services and into everyday settings where people regularly spend time. In this way, individuals who may need clinical services but are not receiving them through traditional venues can gain access to care. As a model of delivery, interventions in unconventional and everyday settings open multiple opportunities to reach people not otherwise served. The specific settings include schools, workplaces, homes, neighborhoods, prisons and juvenile retention facilities, churches, hair salons, barbershops, and gun shops, among others (e.g., Jürgens, Ball, & Verster, 2009; Linnan, D'Angelo, & Harrington, 2014; Luque, Ross, & Gwede, 2014; Vriniotis et al., 2015). This requires creative thinking to break down conceptual barriers about where treatment can and cannot be effectively presented, with assurances of privacy protections of both clients and anyone involved in administration of the intervention.

An example of a natural setting for physical health care is the beauty salon and to a slightly lesser extent the barbershop. As odd as it might seem at first, salons are an excellent setting for health education and interventions because of the large number of people who are regularly served there and because socialization and discussion of topics related to health and beauty occur regularly, including significant mental health problems (e.g., substance use and abuse) (Linnan & Ferguson, 2007; Sattler & Deane, 2016; Solomon et al., 2004). Moreover, many individuals see their stylists and cosmetologists as trusted and supportive, making them a potential source for important information (Cowen et al., 1979; Solomon et al., 2004). In the United States, several types of health programs (e.g., mammography for breast cancer screening, cardiovascular disease prevention, education for sexually transmitted diseases) have been based in salons and barbershops to promote critical health messages, specifically with ethnic minority groups (e.g., Lee,

Carvallo, & Lee, 2015; Linnan et al., 2014; Wilson et al., 2008).[6] Typically, salon employees (e.g., stylists, cosmetologists, beauticians) provide the intervention directly to clients after receiving focused training (e.g., Lewis et al., 2002; Sadler et al., 2000; Wilson et al., 2008).

As an illustration, a stroke education program for African American women was carried out through beauty salons in two urban areas. Beauticians attended a brief training (conducted at a one-time luncheon) and were provided with materials (e.g., pamphlets) to provide to their clients. They then educated their clients (during regular appointments) about stroke risks, warning signs, and appropriate responses to clinical scenarios. Women who received the intervention showed improved knowledge of the signs of stroke and appropriate responses (i.e., calling 911; Kleindorfer et al., 2008).

In a larger scale example, the Healthy Hair Starts With a Healthy Body Program included 700 stylists and more than 14,000 clients in eight communities (in the state of Michigan; Madigan, Smith-Wheelock, & Krein, 2007). Stylists attended two four-hour training programs about kidney disease, diabetes, and hypertension and were trained to conduct two "chats" with clients. Clients reported increased exercise, improved diet, and greater contact with medical professionals about related health issues. These and many other such demonstrations have shown an impact of laypersons in everyday settings administering health-related interventions. As in the example, the impact has been evaluated beyond improving knowledge of the clients and has led to pertinent behavior change, at least as self-reported.

Applications to Mental Health

Mental health care has been provided outside of traditional settings for many years, including correctional facilities, the workplace, and schools (e.g., Roman & Blum, 1996; Rones & Hoagwood, 2000; Smith, Sawyer, & Way, 2002). Indeed, school-based preventive and treatment interventions for children and adolescents are used routinely to provide services that focus on diverse clinical problems, including conduct problems, depression, stress, substance use, bullying, and suicidality. At this point, perhaps the use of schools is sufficiently common for preventive interventions to be considered a conventional rather than unconventional setting. Yet those foci usually are for school-aged children and adolescents; interventions for parents may also use schools because parents are familiar with the setting and usually these are conveniently located.

There may be multiple opportunities in less-well-used settings where underserved populations can be reached. As an example of a setting in use that might be expanded, emergency mental health services are provided through mobile crisis units often in conjunction with police (e.g., Lamanna, et al., 2015; Lancaster, 2016; Sentissi et al., 2014; Shannahan & Fields, 2016). As police respond to an immediate crisis, nonpolice mental health workers participate in the team, handle immediate mental health crises (e.g., trauma of a victim), and triage to other services if needed either at the time or later. Although controlled evidence is sparse, the impact has been more effective than standard care (e.g., hospital care) in reducing mental health symptoms and the family burden of mental health problems (Murphy et al., 2012).

Mobile crisis services focus on acute emergency episodes in the community. This form of care may be adapted to provide general, nonemergency care to individuals who can benefit from clinical interventions outside the context of a psychiatric emergency. For example, a family might call and schedule a visit with a mobile mental health unit because of concerns about behavioral problems at school; the unit could arrive at the family's home (or a different predetermined location) at a scheduled time for a consultation session to address these issues. Similarly, given the high sexual assault rates on college campuses, a woman (women are the vast majority of victims) might call a mobile unit to come to her immediately after the call. Immediate crisis management might be provided along with triage as needed for more intense care, support, and intervention.

Crisis units may be adapted to serve mental health needs during natural disasters, similar in form and function to how mobile medical care is provided to underserved populations during such emergencies (e.g., Krol et al., 2007). In this case, mobile units could provide trauma screening (and, subsequently, helpful resources and referrals) and general crisis management strategies to high-risk individuals. In either scenario, high-risk and underserved populations can be targeted, and mental health care can be brought directly to the individuals in their homes and neighborhoods. Mobile units can contribute greatly apart from a single event or crisis. For example, mobile units can bring hospital staff or lay people to remote settings and provide routine care and in the process reach people who would not otherwise be served (e.g., Cohen, 2015a).

The settings used in physical health care interventions discussed previously (i.e., beauty salons and barber shops) are good examples of some of the settings that the mental health field might use and where applications can be scaled up. Many of the characteristics that make such settings feasible for physical health prevention and intervention also make them suitable for mental health interventions. In fact, one program trained hair stylists to assess anxiety and depression symptoms and assisted the stylists in providing appropriate referral information to clients (Hanlon, 2011). Another such program trained stylists in domestic violence to help their clients receive the treatment they might need (Rousseau, 2017). This latter program has been enacted by state law (in Illinois) as an effort in domestic violence prevention. If programs like these were extended to the many beauty salons (approximately 86,000) and barbershops (approximately 4,000 in the United States) (Hair Care Services Industry Profile, 2016), the potential reach of treatment to people who do not seek or receive services would be a significant start.

One of the movements in mental health care is integrated care, in which mental health providers are integrated in physical health care settings such as hospitals and clinics. An even more promising addition would be to have integrated care in everyday settings or mobile units. Teams of mental and physical health professionals cannot be stationed in a beauty parlor, but they could be integrated with everyday settings by having them become part of the system to make referrals. A seamless or at least easy path from the beauty parlor, school, or shopping mall to a closely connected service nearby or available on call might facilitate delivery of services. In general, to reduce the burdens of mental illness, it would be beneficial to have more settings that are part of routine life (e.g., beauty salons, schools) and mobile units that bring interventions to people. More creative efforts to bring people to traditional settings (hospitals) are welcome but continue to represent a limitation of delivering care to those in the greatest need and suffering from the greatest neglect.

Key Considerations

There are many benefits of providing interventions in everyday settings, as summarized in Table 7.2. Perhaps most salient is their reach, that is, the possibility of reaching people who are unlikely to seek services through conventional resources and settings. With disruptive innovations, interventions often are brought to individuals rather than bringing individuals to the intervention (e.g., clinic, hospitals). Everyday settings might be conceived as a compromise of sorts—people still have to go places (beauty parlors, barbershops, nail salons, parks, playgrounds, restaurants, coffee shops, shopping malls, grocery stores, schools), but they go there anyway for other reasons. In some settings (e.g., shopping malls), attendance is declining for a variety of reasons, such the proliferation of online shopping. But online services do not replace everything (e.g., beauty salons, schools). Interventions and direct referrals to accessible care would be especially useful for those who are not seeking their primary care physicians for advice and, of course, for those who do not have primary care physicians. Everyday settings could be used to target special populations based on the settings that different groups are more apt to attend. Also, settings most people need to visit (e.g., grocery stores) tend already to exist in the diverse neighborhoods where mental health services tend to be sparse or nonexistent.

As a model of care, everyday settings offer several additional benefits. Among them is the use of lay providers (e.g., hair stylists, teachers) instead of mental health professionals. This reduces the costs associated with care and increases the ability to scale up a workforce to reach people in need, in keeping with the emphases of task shifting. It is possible that stigma would be reduced as well, in light of a departure of setting and of a person who provides the service, which would be different from the usual attendance at a clinic with a mental health professional.

There are challenges in moving interventions to everyday settings, related to the settings themselves (e.g., some settings are better suited to interventions than others) and to the interventions (e.g., some types of interventions may be more readily administered in natural settings). Promising intervention settings might include repeated contacts or visits (e.g., a location that people go to on a regular basis so that services and some follow-up can be included), reputable and reliable providers (e.g., individuals whom clients will trust and consider credible sources), and suitable duration and privacy of the interaction. Despite the challenges, this model has special opportunities to move interventions to people in novel ways and to target unserved populations based on the settings selected.

Two cautionary notes. First, natural settings might be well suited for providing information about mental illness and in that way help with barriers (e.g., mental health literacy, stigma). The information may be a useful point at which to start a process of obtaining an intervention, then to provide an easy transition to the next step (referral) for integrated care. However, knowledge, understanding, and consciousness raising are not very strong interventions on their own. Interventions in natural settings can and have done more, but the cautionary note is to underscore the emphasis. The goal is for novel models to help reduce the burdens of mental illness, and we look to a range of interventions and means of providing them that affect that in palpable ways. Knowledge and its friendly sisters (understanding and consciousness) are rarely sufficient to accomplish that. Second and related, the use of interventions in natural settings has undergone isolated studies in varied settings. Much more is needed in research and application to determine what settings, what interventions, and what mental health foci might be the most promising to reach people and produce important outcomes. All of that said, we have barely begun to exploit the potential of this model.

SUMMARY AND CONCLUSIONS

The models of delivery discussed in this chapter draw from many disciplines and influences. Task shifting and sharing, disruptive innovations, and treatment in everyday settings were grouped together because they serve as innovative ways of delivering interventions when the treatments are fairly traditional (i.e., EBPIs or variations), rather than delivering entirely new treatments.

Each model discussed in the chapter addresses limitations of the dominant model of delivering treatment (i.e., in-person, one-to-one sessions with a mental health profession and in a special setting). Related, each model includes one or more key characteristics outlined in Chapter 5 (e.g., scalability, reach) that are essential if we are to extend treatment to most or all of those in need and to reduce the burdens of mental illness. In proposing novel models, there is no suggestion that any one or two of these should replace the dominant model or that the dominant model should be eliminated. We are not looking for one other model that better addresses the challenge of reducing the burdens of mental illness. Rather we are looking for multiple models, each with slightly different emphases and benefits. If we are to scale treatment to help large numbers and to reach special populations in need, we will need multiple models. Thus the mindset of what we are trying to accomplish is to have multiple ways of providing effective treatments. This is quite different from contemporary intervention research, which has focused more on multiple treatments that can be used but cannot be delivered very well. In Chapter 8, we take up additional models of delivery, and these often involve changes to both the intervention and the model of delivery.

8

Novel Models of Delivery 2

Expanding Interventions and the Ways They Are Provided

The models in Chapter 7 draw primarily on new ways of delivering traditional psychosocial treatments, whether through using lay individuals (as in task shifting) or technology (e.g., Internet, apps) to deliver them or to move the interventions to everyday or more convenient settings (e.g., schools, beauty salons, urgent care centers). The novel models of delivery covered in this chapter tend to involve changes to the nature of the interventions from those in the prior models, and also are more population based. That is, the intervention not only provides evidence-based psychosocial interventions (EBPIs) in new and expanded ways but also changes what the intervention is and how many individuals are reached.

This chapter covers six models: best-buy interventions, lifestyle changes, use of social media, entertainment-education, socially assistive robotics, and social network interventions. Table 8.1 provides a summary of key characteristics for easy reference. As with the prior discussion, here I describe the models, provide examples, and explain how they complement and improve on the dominant model of psychotherapy as a way of reaching people in need of services.

BEST-BUY INTERVENTIONS

The first model begins with a focus on the problem—how to provide effective interventions to the most people in need. Cost and scalability are given special

Table 8.1 Novel Models of Delivering Treatment

Model	Key Characteristic	Examples	Sample References with Illustrations
Best-buy interventions	Interventions selected based on their cost-effectiveness, affordability, feasibility for the setting (e.g., rural, city), and other criteria Conceived as an economic tool to help countries select among evidence-based strategies to have impact, where impact is quantified (estimated) for different strategies	To reduce use of tobacco use, raising taxes, protecting people from cigarette smoke, warning about the dangers of smoking, and enforcing bans	Chisholm et al. (2007) WHO (2011a)
Fostering lifestyle changes	A range of behaviors individuals can engage in that are known to affect physical or mental health, including controlling diet, exercising, meditating, and interacting with nature	Exercise has a broad impact on health and physical health	Deslandes et al. (2009) Walsh (2011)
Social media	Use of widely available material that includes social networking (e.g., Facebook, Twitter, texting, YouTube, Skype) that bring people together in novel ways and to present information, to obtain assessment, and to provide feedback or delivery of interventions Use of interventions that can be brought to people wherever they are through these media connections	Writing regularly as part of blogging to draw on many evidence-based expressive writing interventions; meeting with a therapist or support group in a virtual social world	Baker & Moore (2008) Gorini et al. 2008)

Table 8.1 CONTINUED

Model	**Key Characteristic**	**Examples**	**Sample References with Illustrations**
Entertainment-education	Use of television or radio to deliver health-care messages and to model health-promoting behaviors. A culturally sensitive long-running series (e.g., TV series) in which different characters take on different roles, deal with the challenges related to the focus of the intervention, and model adaptive strategies.	An early application focused on reducing the birth rate and use of birth control in Mexico	Singhal & Rogers (1999) Singhal et al. (2004)
Socially assistive robots	Robots that interact with humans in some way Robots that can provide education and feedback, coach patients through activities and tasks, and provide companionship	Provide companionship to older adults to reduce loneliness, depression, social isolation, and cognitive impairment	Bemelmans et al. (2012) Rabbitt et al. (2015)
Social network interventions	Delineation of networks and using the networks to spread information or an intervention through individuals varying in degrees of separation from key individuals in that network	Use of peer groups to influence substance use and cigarette smoking	Christakis & Fowler (2009) Valente (2010)

priority in deciding what those interventions should be and how they are delivered. Right away with this overview, one can see the sharp contrast between this model and the dominant model of psychosocial treatment in which cost and scalability are huge limitations.

Definition and Background

Economics of health care (physical and mental health) have served as an impetus for the development of the best-buy model. As with other models I have mentioned, this one began with physical health care as the focus and moved into the overlapping area of mental health care. The economic impetus for this is underscored by concern with the broad impact of health care costs. This impetus was revealed in a survey of world business leaders by the World Economic Forum. The findings from the survey indicated that chronic disease (e.g., cardiovascular disease, cancer) was seen as a major threat to economic growth globally (Bloom et al., 2011; World Health Organization [WHO], 2011b). Disability and mortality exert a great economic impact not only on individuals, families, and households but also on industries and societies through consumption of health care services, loss of income, productivity, and capital expenditures that could otherwise support public and private investment. Best-buy interventions have emerged from this context to designate interventions for physical illnesses, particularly the control of chronic diseases and at a global scale (Institute of Medicine [IOM], 2010).

Best buy refers to an intervention for which "there is compelling evidence that is not only highly cost effective, but is also feasible, low-cost (affordable), and appropriate to implement within the constraints of a local health system" (WHO, 2011a, p. 2). The local health system is important because the focus is the opposite of "one size fits all." The orientation began with recognition that countries and areas within a country may well differ in ways that directly dictate what is a best buy. Consequently, the model includes features such as appropriateness for the setting (e.g., culture, resources), capacity of the health care system to deliver a given intervention to the targeted population, technical complexity of the intervention (e.g., level of training that might be required), and acceptability based on cultural, religious, and social norms. That is, given the features of this country or region, what would be the most cost-effective, affordable, feasible, but also acceptable way to reach people in need of services, that is, the best buy? In addition to best buys, "good buys" are occasionally distinguished and refer to interventions that do not meet all the criteria for feasibility of delivery and cost but still represent an expanded set of interventions that can be made available as resources allow.

Delineating evidence-based best buys was conceived as an economic tool to help countries assess how to achieve a given amount of change, given the number of eligible individuals in need of the intervention, the potential savings of that change, and the cost differences of alternative strategies, among other variables (e.g., Chisholm, Lund, & Saxena, 2007; Chisholm & Saxena, 2012; WHO, 2011a, 2011b). The best-buy interventions can vary for a given disorder and country because the cost of delivering a particular intervention in light of the health resources and infrastructure will vary. Even so, best-buy interventions have been delineated that are likely to have broad applicability across countries.

How to decide what interventions are likely to be a best buy is systematic and based on estimates of utilization and impact of a given intervention using mathematical models (e.g., Chisholm et al., 2007). Of course, math models make many assumptions, and these may or may not match the final application or effects of treatment delivery. Consequently, direct empirical tests follow to evaluate and ensure that well-intended, feasible, and scalable interventions yield the intended outcomes and in fact are best buys.

As an illustration, in one analysis four criteria (health impact, cost-effectiveness, cost of implementation, and feasibility of scaling up) were used to identify best-buy interventions that would have significant public health impact on noncommunicable diseases, including cardiovascular disease, cancers, diabetes, and chronic lung disease (WHO, 2011a). Best buys for cardiovascular disease and diabetes were counseling, multidrug therapy, and aspirin. These were selected in light of the reduction of disease burden (e.g., disability-adjusted life years [DALYs]) and very low cost.[1] A good-buy intervention was counseling for diabetes control for individuals older than 30 years whose risk for fatal events was especially high. The intervention would be quite cost-effective, but it has a higher cost (is less affordable) to deliver and is not feasible in many countries.

Applications to Mental Health

I mentioned previously the interconnections of mental and physical health. Several best-buy interventions for physical diseases often focus on domains of functioning that overlap with and are part of behavior, lifestyle, and mental health. Substance use and abuse are key mental health foci in intervention research and provide a good illustration.

Reducing tobacco and alcohol use and promoting healthy diets and physical activity are the foci of best-buy interventions for cardiovascular disease, cancer, diabetes, and chronic lung disease (WHO, 2011a). For tobacco use, raising taxes, protecting people from tobacco smoke (secondary smoke), warning about the dangers associated with tobacco, and enforcing smoking bans were estimated to save more than 5 million lives in 23 large low- and middle-income countries over a 10-year period (see WHO, 2003). Similarly, for alcohol use, best-buy interventions included enhanced taxation of alcoholic beverages and comprehensive bans on advertising and marketing, based on their favorable cost-effectiveness, affordability overall, and feasibility. Excessive alcohol use was identified as a critical focus for reducing the incidence of cardiovascular diseases and cancers, but in the process the benefits extend to other burdensome conditions (e.g., cirrhosis of the liver, depression, traffic injuries and deaths; WHO, 2011a). Clearly, the focus on substance use and abuse has direct implications and cost savings for physical health, while directly targeting problems (substance use and abuse) that are central to mental health.

Best buy has focused directly on interventions for select mental disorders. For example, for clinical depression, generically produced antidepressant medication, brief psychotherapy, and treating depression in primary care setting qualified as best buys (Chisholm et al., 2007). For psychoses, treating people with antipsychotic drugs and with psychosocial support was regarded as a best buy. Controlled trials of best buys demonstrating their utility, scalability, and impact relative to EBPIs or more standard treatments administered in the dominant model are not yet available from resources I could identify. Yet the usual reason for moving to best buys is that the costly versions of treatment delivery are not feasible. Direct head-to-head tests of treatments delivered by the dominant model versus the best-buy model may not be a high priority. The reason is that best buys are designed to reach many people, and treatments provided by the dominant model usually do not have that goal. From best buys, we need data to show that the interventions are having an impact.

Key Considerations

Several characteristics introduced earlier and applied to models discussed in Chapter 7 relate to the extent to which a given model is likely to reach people in need and have an impact on the burdens of mental illness. Table 8.2 highlights the characteristics of the best-buy model and for purposes of comparison lists all the models covered in this and in the Chapter 7. As the table makes evident, the best-buy model meets several characteristics that would foster widespread extension as a model of delivering treatment. Among the special strengths of the best-buy model are scalability, affordability, breadth of settings (e.g., blanketing an entire country, local conditions considered), and feasibility.

Clearly, economic considerations play a central role and constitute a special strength, given that these are major barriers in providing, reimbursing, and delivering mental (and physical) health care. For example, in an evaluation from the United Kingdom, an expenditure of 1 pound British sterling (£; approximately US$1.50) for intervention was estimated to save 5.0£ and 7.9£ (approximately US$7.50 and US$12.00) for early diagnosis and treatment of depression and conduct disorder, respectively (Knapp, McDaid, & Personage, 2011; costs not adjusted for current price inflation and exchange rates). Estimates such as these are based on long-range benefits and savings (i.e., over the life of the individual and for the period in which the intervention will be administered to the population). Scalability and feasibility also raise economic considerations. Can the intervention be delivered with available funding given the large swaths of people in need and to the local population and subgroups (e.g., rural areas, desert or mountain regions) where delivery is needed? Depending on the intervention, reaching many more people and in hard-to-reach locales could be expensive.

I mentioned that best-buy interventions rely on mathematical models followed by empirical tests to evaluate whether the intended outcomes were achieved and whether the interventions are best buys. As an example, best-buy interventions administered on a large scale have been used to improve health and educational performance in rural China (Rural Education Action Project, 2012). Rural youth have high rates of iron deficiency anemia, are nearsighted but do not have glasses, and are infected with worms—all of which have been associated with problems of concentration in class at school and lower cognitive functioning, which limit educational progress and contribute to the continued cycle of poverty. A best-buy

Table 8.2 Key Characteristics of the Models

Model	Scalability	Reach	Affordability	Expansion of Workforce	Expansion of Settings	Feasibility	Flexibility	Acceptability of the Model
Dominant model of psychotherapy	W	W	W	W	W-	W	W	?
Task shifting	?	S	S	S	?	S	S	—
Disruptive innovation	S	S	S	?	S	?	S	—
Unconventional settings	?	S	S	S	S	?	S	—
			*****************					
Best-buy interventions	S	S	S	NA	S	S	S	—
Fostering lifestyle change	S	S	S	NA	S	?	S	S
Social media	S	S	?	NA	S	?	S	S
Entertainment-education	S	S	?	NA	S	S	S	S
Socially assistive robots	?	?	?	S	S	?	?	?
Social network interventions	S	S	?	NA	NA	S	S	?

S = strong—the model could meet this criterion very well; *W* = weak—the model is not very good at doing this; *NA* = not applicable; ? = unclear or varied—model is dependent on specific variations and might meet the criterion, but some qualifications and not well tested in practice; — = the acceptability of a model is an empirical question and is unclear for the novel models.

NOTES: All codes are estimates and can vary as versions within a model of delivery change (e.g., type of robot for socially assistive robots). The models presented above the line of asterisks were covered in the Chapter 7. They are included here to provide a perspective on all models discussed in the book and to permit comparisons of the models. The initial model in the table is the dominant model of psychotherapy. That model included treatment that is delivered as in-person, one-to-one sessions with a mental health profession and in a special setting. The dominant model is included in the first row merely as a point of departure for evaluating what other models add.

intervention consisted of using lay individuals to counsel in nutrition practices. In addition, eyeglasses, multivitamins with iron, and deworming medication were provided. Randomized controlled trials (RCTs; with wait-list controls) revealed that the intended benefits were in fact achieved (e.g., Luo et al., 2011).

Best-buy interventions are large scale by design. In any intervention, even without the level of scaling to reach most of the population, sustaining the integrity of the intervention can be a challenge. Yet some best-buy interventions (e.g., selective taxes, bans on advertising to reduce substance use and abuse) differ from the usual psychosocial interventions and do not require compliance by clients or adherence to a specific treatment protocol by therapists. Of course, taxes and advertising have their own problems (e.g., black market sales that are not taxed, advertising that does not always reach the target population). However, the goal again is not to identify one model that has no obstacles or problems, but rather to have multiple models that together can reach people in need.

I have mentioned that acceptability is one characteristic to consider in devising a model. This is not a special problem of best-buy interventions. Yet best buys can include many different interventions. The use of taxes as one of these to control health-related behavior warrants comment. Again, taxes are not the mainstay or core intervention underlying best-buy interventions, but they have been used and have been implemented independently of adopting a best-buy model. Among the concerns is a conflict of individual rights and freedoms versus government control, as reflected in policy and law.

As an illustration, the WHO (2016) urged countries to impose a tax on sugary drinks as an effort to combat the global epidemic of obesity. The benefits would extend to other problem domains as well (e.g., diabetes, cancers, and heart disease). The case against sugary drinks is not new and also has been a source of controversy (see Brownell & Frieden, 2009). The WHO report makes the case strongly and elaborates the economic as well as health benefits internationally. Based on the WHO analysis one might readily regard such a tax as a "great buy" if the tax were imposed and showed likely benefits in obesity and the diseases I mentioned. The case is made that sugary drinks, like tobacco, are a public health issue, and the benefits achieved by taxing cigarettes (reduced consumption) ought to be applied to sugary drinks. In the United States, most states have adopted a policy on sugary drinks, but occasionally the tax has been enacted and later rescinded (Chaloupka & Davidson, 2010). Lobbyists from industries that sell the beverages have objected. Also, many citizens and other organizations object to government control of what one consumes. In the mix is the concern that the tax may be discriminatory because some groups as a function of socioeconomic standing, for example, are more likely to be taxed. I mention these points briefly, although they are part of a long-standing discussion to convey that we need multiple interventions and models. Any single intervention and model of delivery may have unique strengths but also unique obstacles. Acceptability of the model, as in the case of taxes, may limit application of a given intervention. The different profiles of strengths and limitations are precisely why we need multiple models of delivering interventions. No single model or small set of models is likely to reach the vast majority in need of services and be equally adept at addressing the characteristics noted in Table 8.2.

FOSTERING LIFESTYLE CHANGE

Our everyday habits in relation to eating, exercising, consuming substances (alcohol, cigarettes, "recreational" and illicit drugs), and socializing influence our health. This has been drilled into us by endless streams of information, recommendations, and public health messages. Yes, it is true that messages are inconsistent because new scientific findings often seem to contract old findings. Examples are numerous, and some of the familiar changing and conflicting messages include scientifically grounded advice that has recommended that we:

- Do not eat eggs because of the cholesterol; cancel that (for now)—eggs are fine, actually good for us;
- Stay away from chocolate; but wait, chocolate is very healthful, and even trumps many vegetables in the scope of nutrients;
- Stop using butter because of cholesterol and switch to margarine now! Wait, go back to butter because margarine has many problems (e.g., transfats). Wait again—dump both of them and try to use olive oil instead;
- Avoid avocados because of their fat; wait, eat avocados regularly as a way to protect one's heart;
- Drink a little bit of wine; but for maximum benefit with meals and be sure never to binge; and
- Follow the "food pyramid"; wait, forget the pyramid, follow the "food plate," and remember do not eat the plate itself, just the food groups that are represented (https://www.choosemyplate.gov/).

In fairness to science, finer-grained assessments and evaluation over time constantly expand and allow better understanding. That can readily lead to recent findings contradicting earlier findings. Also, many relations among variables (e.g., a particular food substance) are moderated (i.e., their effects are influenced by one or more other variables), so what was "good" or "bad" for our health with a clear message "depends." Even seemingly wonderfully healthful foods (e.g., grapefruit, some oranges) can be dietary no-nos and potentially dangerous to one's health, "depending" on whether someone is taking certain medications (e.g., Bailey, Dresser, & Arnold, 2013). In any case, new findings and views can be annoying or perplexing. (For example, are you old enough to remember when we learned that Pluto was a planet? Not anymore—scientists changed all of that!) Even so, several messages are clear (e.g., the Mediterranean diet is wise to follow; stress is wise to minimize or avoid). Lifestyle is known to influence health. It has not been harnessed as an intervention or model of delivery as part of a strategy to reduce the burdens of mental disorders in a systematic way and on a large national scale and involving multiple institutions (e.g., schools, workplace). Yet there is enormous untapped potential here.

Definition and Background

Lifestyle change or therapeutic lifestyle change refers to interventions that modify high-risk behaviors to reduce disease mortality and morbidity (American College of Lifestyle Medicine [ACLM], 2009; Egger, Binns, & Rossner, 2008; National Center for Chronic Disease Prevention and Health Promotion [NCCDPHP], 2011). The term *lifestyle change* is used broadly here to encompass a range of behaviors in which individuals can or do engage that positively affect health.

Lifestyle interventions have targeted behaviors such as diet, exercise, alcohol consumption, and cigarette smoking in light of their association with common chronic diseases and conditions, such as cardiovascular disease, diabetes, and obesity. Many physical ailments benefit from lifestyle change: cancer, chronic pain disorders, fibromyalgia, dyslipidemia, multiple sclerosis, osteoarthritis, osteoporosis, and rheumatoid arthritis (ACLM, 2009). For example, a review of several studies indicated that women who engage in exercise are much less likely to contract breast cancer (Wu, Zhang, & Kang, 2013). Often lifestyle changes are part of a larger treatment regimen (e.g., involving medication or surgery), or multiple lifestyle changes are included as a package (e.g., improved diet, exercise, and weight management) (NCCDPHP, 2011).

Lifestyle changes are a mainstay of medical practice as part of prevention of disease and secondary prevention, that is, reducing risk for further incidence after a problem has emerged. For example, individuals who have had a heart attack can reduce risk for a second attack and early death by engaging in lifestyle changes such as an exercise regimen (e.g., Piepoli et al., 2016); and men assigned to a lifestyle-change program (including diet, exercise, and stress management) are less likely to require conventional treatment for their prostate cancer than those receiving conventional care (Frattaroli et al., 2008). This a minute sample from a larger literature that makes the point that lifestyle change can play important and multiple roles in treatment and prevention.

Applications to Mental Health

Lifestyle changes have had a favorable impact on symptoms of many psychological disorders, including depression, anxiety, schizophrenia, eating disorders, body dysmorphic disorder, substance use disorders, and cognitive dysfunction in physical disorders (e.g., Alzheimer's disease), as attested to by multiple reviews (e.g., Jayakody, Gunadasa, & Hosker, 2013; Lopresti, Hood, & Drummond, 2013; Rosenbaum et al., 2014; Ströhle, 2009). The most frequently used lifestyle changes are exercise and nutrition as applied to physical health. Yet lifestyle has been extended to include a variety of other activities, such as spending time in nature, engaging in recreational activities, being involved in religious or spiritual activities, and volunteering and contributing to others, each with evidence on its behalf in relation to improving physical or mental health (e.g., Berman et al., 2012; Bratman et al., 2015; Countryside Recreation Network, 2006; R. Walsh, 2011).

Depression provides an example of how lifestyle changes can have a significant impact on clinical dysfunction. For many years, psychologists have incorporated some aspects of lifestyle change and various activities into treatment for depression (e.g., Dimidijian et al., 2006; Lewinsohn, 1975). The specific activities are individualized but usually focus on exercise, social engagement, and recreational activities (e.g., Leahy, Holland, & McGinn, 2012). Lifestyle changes alone or in combination with other interventions are effective for treating mild to moderate depression and are similar in their effects to those achieved by medication and psychotherapy (e.g., Rimer et al., 2012; Tkachuk & Martin, 1999). In fact, in one study, when compared with commonly used medications (selective serotonin reuptake inhibitors), aerobic exercise (40 minutes, three times a week) was associated with lower rates of relapse at 6-month follow-up (Babyak et al., 2000). Although much of this work has been conducted with adults, applications have extended to children, adolescents, postpartum adults, and older adults (e.g., Hamer & Chida, 2008; Larun et al., 2006; Sidhu, Vandana, & Balon, 2009). Each of these populations is among the group less likely to receive mental health services, so reach may be a special strength of the general model of fostering lifestyle changes.

Key Considerations

Table 8.2 conveys key characteristics of lifestyle changes. One of the most compelling advantages of lifestyle change is the broad impact that such change can have. For example, increased physical exercise can have multiple beneficial physical health outcomes (e.g., improved cardiovascular health, reduced risk for obesity, metabolic disorders, and cancer) and mental health outcomes (e.g., fewer symptoms of depression, reduced stress levels and anxiety, decreased substance use, improved neurocognitive functioning) (e.g., Bauer et al., 2016; Brown et al., 2010; Deslandes et al., 2009; Dunn et al., 2005; McMorris, Tomporowski, & Audiffren, 2009). The broad effects on general well-being and physical and mental health translate to reduced use of health services and are likely to make lifestyle changes a best-buy intervention.

Other noteworthy benefits of lifestyle changes are affordability (initial outlay of costs), cost-effectiveness (e.g., ratio of cost in relation to outcome relative to many other interventions), feasibility (no special equipment or professional service may be required), flexibility (e.g., lifestyle changes include multiple options that can be selected for convenience and personal preferences), and wide applicability (e.g., individuals with diagnosable or subclinical psychological problems can benefit; children, adolescents, and adults). Lifestyle changes may also remove barriers to treatment (e.g., stigma, lack of nearby services) for individuals seeking mental health services (Corrigan, 2004; Pescosolido et al., 2010).

Many distinct activities and practices are encompassed in the term *lifestyle change*; many psychological and physical health goals can be the targets of such changes; and individuals of different ages and stages (e.g., children, older adults) can benefit from them. That very diversity of activities and practices may make this especially important as a model of addressing mental health and reducing the burdens of mental illness. Also, lifestyle activities can be engaged in as part of one's daily routine (no special facilities required) or in facilities (e.g., gyms, parks, churches) that do not have the barriers (perceived and real) associated with seeking mental health treatment. Lifestyle interventions can be added to and offered in everyday settings (e.g., schools for children and adolescents, workplace for adults) and might be the first line of attack in providing large-scale interventions. Lifestyle changes, self-help interventions, and lay counselor–administered interventions are three viable intervention models that can be used before moving to specialized interventions that require costlier professional help and the dominant model.

Many of the challenges are familiar, such as getting individuals to adopt and adhere to lifestyle changes (e.g., exercising regularly). Perhaps the obstacles might be exacerbated by clinical dysfunction. For example, if an individual is experiencing a bout of depression or panic attack, is it feasible to think that person will run to some gym or jump on a home exercise machine? Perhaps not very likely given the base rate of individuals without depression engaging in exercise. Use of lifestyle changes like exercise might be well suited to control mild to moderate (subclinical) depression and in that way perhaps hold more severe depression at bay. Moreover, it might be easier to get individuals to engage in some lifestyle activity (e.g., with a partner or neighbor) than to go for psychological treatment or take medication for their depression.

There are novel aids (e.g., apps that facilitate monitoring activity in real time) that can assist in providing feedback, encouragement, and records of accomplishment for exercise. As an example, the National Institute of Aging provides multiple tools as part of a Web-based program (Go4Life) that provides sequences and types of exercises in which one can engage, interactive tools, and motivational features (e.g., goal setting, options for tracking), all aimed at helping individuals develop a personalized program of exercise and adhering to it (https://go4life.nia.nih.gov/4-types-exercise). Tools are readily available but not in very extensive use or even in the awareness of most individuals (e.g., in the United States). Indeed, some of the tools convey surprises. For example, exercise machines can conjure the video images of someone in a matching and fashionable exercise outfit walking, jogging, or sprinting with you through virtual representations of the famous cities and sites of the world. That exercise certainly "counts," but so do dancing and housecleaning (vacuuming, mopping, and dusting). (We have no excuses now—if you have no partner and your dancing is weak, grab the vacuum cleaner—and not the robotic one.)

Because lifestyle changes are not routinely seen as mental health treatment, basic questions of such treatments have few empirical answers (e.g., what lifestyle changes, for what problems, in what doses achieve clinically important changes?). Nevertheless, existing evidence conveys important mental health benefits, including alleviation of clinical dysfunction. The evidence has suggested moderate effects for the treatment of anxiety and depression, the clinical domains most well studied. Exercise is not invariably equal to those effects obtained with medication or psychosocial interventions (e.g., Cooney et al., 2013; Jayakody et al., 2013). Yet exercise is a viable option with demonstrated effects that could have an impact if it were scaled up systematically. Also, equal effectiveness is not necessarily the main issue in deciding what treatments to deploy. Reaching more people with a feasible intervention, as a first step in a set of interventions, would vastly improve on what we are doing now with the dominant model.

A cautionary note certainly is warranted. Not all lifestyle changes are equal, are equally effective, or have a strong evidence base that conveys their causal relation to outcome. For example, religiosity and spirituality are often associated with better physical and mental health and overall functioning (e.g., Jim et al., 2015; Rippentrop et al., 2005), but not invariably so (e.g., Cragun et al., 2016). Among the reasons no doubt are the many different populations studied and the obvious fact that definitions and types of religion and spirituality vary. But even more cogent is the type of research that is completed. One cannot easily do RCTs to evaluate religious beliefs and spirituality (randomly assign individuals to be religious) and see the effects on physical and mental health over time. With other lifestyle changes (e.g., diet and exercise), such work has readily been completed and also has drawn on nonhuman animal models to evaluate directly the biological and psychological benefits of exercise (e.g., Duman et al., 2008; Shirayama et al., 2002).

All that said, lifestyle changes represent a broad domain that could have a significant impact on mental and physical health. Also, it is likely that interventions within this domain (e.g., diet and exercise) would be among best buys or good buys, in part because they have low cost by not requiring trained health professionals and because their effects can be broad in terms of a range of positive physical and mental health outcomes. Lifestyle changes are easily considered as *transtreatments*, as discussed in Chapter 5, because they affect multiple disorders and outcomes. Getting people to engage in these is the challenge, but there is much more that can be done in that realm (e.g., Hansen, Skov, & Skov, 2016). We will return to the topic of implementation of models in Chapter 9. For now, it is important to add to our set of treatments and models of delivery those encompassed by lifestyle changes.

SOCIAL MEDIA

Technology has changed our everyday lives in so many ways and raises endless opportunities to improve physical and mental health. The different lines of work (e.g., smartphone apps, virtual reality, social robots) make grouping all uses of "technology" not very helpful. Consequently, I have singled out subareas to describe novel opportunities to deliver interventions. Social media represents a set of opportunities to provide treatment in new ways (models of delivery) as well as altering the interventions themselves. We know that our social relationships (quality and number) are associated with all sorts of benefits, including improved physical and mental health, better quality of life, greater longevity, less cognitive decline with age, an improved ability to ward off infectious diseases, and better prognoses when one experiences life-threatening illnesses (e.g., Cohen & Janicki-Deverts, 2009; Tay et al., 2013). The associations are not necessarily causal but certainly raise the prospect of considering improving social contacts as a critical facet of mental health. The value of social relations is well known and established, and certainly that basic finding is not new. What is relatively new is how people connect with each other through social media.

Definition and Background

Social media refers to content that is widely available to the public and includes, as primary examples, Web logs (blogs), social networking websites (e.g., Facebook), collaborative projects (e.g., Wikipedia), user-generated content communities (e.g., YouTube), virtual social worlds (e.g., Second Life), virtual games (Kaplan & Haenlein, 2010), and others (e.g., Grajales et al., 2014). These media vary in social dimensions (e.g., the amount of personal information that a user can disclose) and media richness (e.g., the type of media content allowed by the application). I have highlighted Internet-based applications to convey some of the possibilities from this large category in the discussion of current trends in intervention research and disruptive innovations. Social media have a broad range of options, and these options continue to proliferate. Among the endless ways to keep in touch are the various available (and growing) platforms (e.g., Twitter, Facebook, Instagram, LinkedIn, Tumbir, Flickr, Xing, Renren, Google+, Disqus; www.socialmediatoday.com/social-networks/2015-04-13/worlds-21-most-important-social-media-sites-and-apps-2015).

Advances in social and communication technology are increasingly part of daily life in light of an array of devices (e.g., smartphones, smartwatches, tablets), multiple options for communicating (e.g., texting, email, Facebook), and software of all kinds that bring immediate access to virtually every facet of human functioning (e.g., health care, religion, entertainment, work, news). These technological advances have fostered *cultural* changes in ways of communicating, socializing, obtaining information, and accessing resources (Campbell & Park, 2008; Ling, 2004). For example, social networking websites bring individuals into contact with one another in novel ways but also change the frequency and intimacy of those contacts. One can instantly share news, information, photos, and videos with large groups of people all across the world and quickly receive rich feedback on the shared materials. Meetings and connections are much more "person based" as individuals are accessed and engaged in interactions wherever they are (Campbell & Park, 2008). This is distinguished from "place based," such as meeting at one's home, at a social gathering, or coffee shop or restaurant. This is a useful feature to highlight here because bringing interventions to people rather than people to places is a valuable characteristic and was one of the strengths of disruptive innovations discussed in Chapter 7.

Social media clearly can enhance communication of health-related topics by making information more readily available, shared among individuals, and tailored to individual profiles on the Web (Moorehead et al., 2013). Increased accessibility to information and surveillance of requests for information may prove to be useful steps toward intervention. Yet, for present purposes, we would want to go beyond improved dissemination of information and social interaction surrounding that. We would want to look at more concrete outcomes that the social media produced, either directly (e.g., via social support) or indirectly, by prompting people to receive treatment and then to profit from that treatment.

Social media is frequently used to obtain information as the basis for intervening. For example, public health officials have used Twitter to track flu-like symptoms and predict patterns in influenza outbreaks, and have used that information to intervene to minimize danger and risk (Schmidt, 2012; Signorini, Segre, & Polgreen, 2011). In terms of direct patient care, social networking sites have been used to create thousands of different support groups for varied physical health problems (e.g., breast cancer, colorectal cancer, and diabetes) (Bender, Jimenez-Marroquin, & Jadad, 2011; De la Torre-Díez, Díaz-Pernas, & Antón-Rodríguez, 2012). Users can share messages with one another and increase awareness (e.g., prevention, early detection) of critical issues. The groups also provide access to support for individuals who might not otherwise have access to a support network or whose access might be limited by personal or geographical barriers.

Applications to Mental Health

Social media can provide interventions at the intersection of technology and social interaction. For example, blogging might be viewed as another medium for delivering one of the many evidence-based expressive writing interventions (e.g., for trauma; Frattaroli, 2006; Pennebaker, Mehl, & Niederhoffer, 2003).[2] Those who maintain blogs report having a large group of friends and high rates of perceived psychological support (Baker & Moore, 2008). Among adolescents with social difficulties (e.g., problems with peer relationships, inadequate support from friends), regularly blogging for 10 weeks (compared with a group keeping a non-blog computer journal or a no-treatment control group) improved self-esteem, reduced social-emotional distress, and increased engagement in social activities (Boniel-Nissam & Barak, 2013). Expressive writing is a well-studied intervention applied both to physical and mental health outcomes and now supplemented with blogging as a medium may have widespread applicability as part of social media interventions (e.g., Frisina, Borod, & Lepore, 2004; Krpan et al., 2013).

Twitter networks have emerged and provide enormous means and opportunities related to mental health care delivery and support (Cotton et al., 2014). Large networks have emerged and self-organized to include professional service providers as well as users. In time of need, one can find someone to help with concerns. For example, one site lists 40 Twitter accounts that encompass thousands of followers (Treat Depression, 2013). The sites encourage writing about mental health problems and offering advice and support. Another site lists 33 mental health experts and providers on Twitter who are also available for information and help (Medved, 2015). The scope of the use of Twitter is enormous. Based on 2016 estimates, an average of approximately 6,000 tweets are sent every single second, more than 350,000 per minute, and 500 million tweets per day) (www.dsayce.com/social-media/tweets-day/). Clearly just this one medium alone demonstrates the potential reach of a social-media based model of delivery.

The very nature of social networking websites (e.g., sharing thoughts, feelings, information with others) can make them an ideal forum for identifying high-risk individuals and those in need of mental health resources. For example, in Taiwan, a program used Facebook as a means of assessing suicidality risk among adolescents (Chiang et al., 2011). After authorizing the program to access some of their personal information (e.g., location, age, gender, email address), adolescents were prompted to complete a brief (five-item) questionnaire about suicidal feelings. This information was stored in a database, and adolescents who were deemed high risk were contacted by mental health professionals and were provided resources or ongoing services through the Internet. This use of social networking can facilitate case identification, screening mental health problems, and coordinating services for individuals who may not otherwise have access to care. This could be game-changing as a way of bringing people to treatment and bringing treatment to people.

A growing area of research focuses on the use of virtual social worlds (e.g., Second Life) as a "setting" for psychological intervention and support (e.g., Boulos, Hetherington, & Wheeler, 2007).[3] Some aspects of these treatment programs closely parallel in-person therapy. For example, a therapist and client can "meet" regularly for sessions in a virtual social world, with the client's avatar and a therapist's avatar interacting through such meetings (Gorini & Riva, 2008; Kim & Sundar, 2009; Pagliari, et al., 2012). This type of treatment offers some of the same benefits of other Internet-based treatments (e.g., increased accessibility to rural areas) as well as some unique benefits, such opportunities to easily create a community of supports in the virtual world. Outcome research, still relatively sparse, shows that effect sizes of virtual therapy are similar to those obtained in more well-studied person-based treatments (Yuen et al., 2013). Access to extensive support services (through the online community and not a mental health professional) is an important feature of some forms of virtual therapy. In fact, researchers are creating expanded support communities in virtual social worlds for patients with psychiatric diagnoses that have demonstrated significant benefits from support through a therapeutic community (Good et al., 2011).

Key Considerations

Social media has several characteristics that make it a valuable model of delivery (see Table 8.2). Among its unique characteristics is the opportunity for rapid connectivity. Blogs, social networking sites, and other uses of technology allow for information to travel quickly and be easily accessible to users. For example, when Facebook made it possible for users to easily see if other users were organ donors and, if interested, to sign up to be donors themselves, the number of organ donors increased substantially (by 700 percent in some states) within days (Goldman, 2012). One could envision how critical mental health information, such as depression screenings, might be made widely available through social networking sites. Furthermore, because of the opportunities for self-disclosure and general sharing of information and resources, several social media outlets provide opportunities to increase public awareness about mental health issues and may serve to destigmatize treatment seeking. There are few controlled studies that establish the impact of social media on health-related behaviors (Maher et al., 2014). The different media, the diverse health-related objectives, and the overall paucity of research make any recommendations premature.

The social component can positively influence behavior. Knowing that others can see and track one's activities (and seeking and tracking the activities of other people) can change attitudes, influence behavior, and foster seeking and obtaining support. For example, one Web-based health promotion program focused on helping people make small positive changes to improve their overall health (Poirier & Cobb, 2012). Users could make social connections (through the website) with other users. The individuals with more social ties were more engaged in the intervention based on self-reported behavior change and use of the website and its resources.

The pervasive use of social media and emerging technologies might make this model of intervention delivery rich in options going forward. Technological advances bring familiar and novel challenges. Among them are privacy protections, encryption of material, and use of information in ways not consented to or approved of by clients. These are significant challenges within but also outside the context of mental health and therapy, and these latter uses give new meaning to "identity theft." Technology will continue to advance in these areas. Social media as a model of delivery greatly expands the reach of psychological interventions, and expanding on both the intervention technique options within this model of delivery and the client protections is critical. Currently, the most critical information in relation to the present book is lacking. That is, we need information for utilizing social media strategically and specifically to alter mental disorders, and along with that, strong evidence that the interventions are effective. Data on scaling up are more readily available than evidence about treatment outcomes (Maher et al., 2014). Yet, for the present chapter, the goal is to identify models that could be used to deliver effective interventions. In all instances, we will need research to establish effectiveness.

OTHER MODELS BRIEFLY NOTED

Several other models are worth including here, in brief. Each has enormous potential to improve physical and mental health but is less well studied in those contexts than other models I have noted. Each is a mix of a novel intervention as well as a novel model of delivery.

Entertainment-Education

I have mentioned social media as a multifaceted opportunity to deliver interventions that could address mental health. It is worth distinguishing other media. Individuals often watch videos and programming from various video sources. The source of what we watch (e.g., traditional television, Internet, DVDs) and what we use to view the materials (e.g., smartphone, tablet, TV monitor) are not pertinent to the model I am highlighting.

The medium we use to view materials can be an effective way to implement widespread intervention with great capability to reach large segments of the population. *Entertainment-education* is a prominent example and refers to a model of delivery that provides an intervention through television (or radio if television is not available in the country or region of interest). The intervention is a television series with multiple episodes. Most readers can identify with that and may have current or past favorite TV series. The attraction of these series in everyday life is attested to by large audiences (tracked for marketing purchases), repeated "reruns" of old series on cable TV, and the sales of DVD collections of the "complete episodes" for a given series. Entertainment-education is a TV series but with a goal (of what to change) and a targeted population (e.g., a given culture or group within that).

The process of developing the series begins by studying individuals within a given culture (e.g., surveys, focus groups) and developing characters for an extended television drama that reflect local culture and people in their daily lives. Cultural relevance and features and lives of the target audience are taken into account from the outset. The characters take on different roles, deal with daily challenges of life within the culture, and model social change on the critical issues. The "issues" that are selected are based on the goals of the program. The intervention focus is integrated into realistic renditions of the lives of people in the relevant culture and how an issue emerges and is dealt with by the characters within the episodes of the series. The purpose is to develop an engaging series with multiple characters with whom the audience will identify and to integrate into the series dramatic events that will promote audience change.

The goal is to achieve concrete changes within individuals, communities, and societies. For example, one of the early applications in Mexico focused on family planning and efforts to reduce fertility rates (Singhal & Rogers, 1999). Family life, marital relations, and the daily drama and stressors were conveyed in detail as the televised series unfolded. The fictional family gained control over their lives and benefitted from family planning—all in realistic episodes that showed the struggles and decision making individuals and couples go through. In more psychological terms, the characters served as models and then as coping models that worked through the challenges related to the overall theme. Modeling is an effective method of learning; coping models also tend to lead to better change when compared with models that are masterful from the outset (without having to go through the coping with initial failure or obstacles). In any case, the episodes go well beyond providing information. The episodes make the decision making "up close and personal," realistic, and with characters (actors) the audience comes to know well over time. In terms of impact, in this initial program in Mexico, sales of contraceptives in the community rose dramatically, and there was a 34 percent drop in birth rates over a five-year period.

As another example, the model was used in an experiment designed to prevent the spread of HIV/AIDs in Tanzania (Vaughan et al., 2000). The entertainment-education program was delivered by a long-running radio soap opera. The impact of the program was reflected in a reduction of the number of sexual partners for both men and women and an increased use of condoms. More generally, the model has been used throughout the world on other social issues and has produced widely engaging shows (see Singhal et al., 2004). Ratings of shows are high, viewers or listeners become involved with the characters, and there is genuine change on the targeted social behavior, rather than just increased awareness.

The purpose here is not to review the evidence per se but to convey that the intervention can have a palpable real-life impact (e.g., behavioral measures) and goes beyond the usual appeals to increase awareness or knowledge of an issue. In addition to family planning and HIV/AIDS prevention, other behavior change target areas have included sexual abstinence for adolescents, parenting practices, and promoting a sustainable environment and mitigating climate change (Charles, 2009; Singhal et al., 2004; Singhal & Rogers, 1999). The model could be extended with a large-scale focus on mental health problems and handling stress, substance use, or depression. The model could be targeted to various groups and geographical regions and could have widespread reach, especially because this strategy has been successful on TV as well as radio. Specific domains of dysfunction could be targeted that are pervasive and have widespread consequences in both mental and physical health. Interventions directed at substance use and abuse (e.g., cigarette smoking) or depression meet those criteria. In addition, developing strategies that reduce mental and physical disorders through treatment and prevention (e.g., lifestyle changes) might be viable foci for the model.

I include the model here to suggest direct delivery of interventions to improve mental health and clinical dysfunction. The model may have several related uses that could indirectly affect delivery of mental health services. The term "education" in the name of the model immediately raises the prospect that the model could be used to communicate information related to mental health in novel ways. Merely providing information generally is not very potent as a way of changing behavior. Yet entertainment-education is rather novel, and its impact is as well.

For example, the model has been used to decrease barriers that keep individuals from seeking mental health treatment. A Spanish-language version of entertainment-education was designed to increase knowledge about depression and about seeking help and to decrease sigma (Hernandez & Organista, 2013). Reducing barriers could contribute enormously to getting people to mental health services provided by one of the other models I have discussed. However, in this particular demonstration and most others that focus on communication or reduction of barriers, the next step is not demonstrated, namely, whether reducing barriers in fact increases utilization of treatment and improved mental health outcomes (e.g., in DALYs) for those whose barriers were reduced. That step cannot be assumed. The examples I highlighted (in Mexico and Tanzania) had outcomes in direct impact on the behavior of individuals as well as the local society.

Table 8.2 conveys characteristics of entertainment-education in relation to key criteria that relate to reaching people in need of services. The model may be especially strong in scalability and reach. Television and radio, of course, can reach millions. Moreover, specific groups (e.g., within a population) can be targeted (e.g., by ethnicity, culture) to specifically reach individuals in need. It is not clear how affordable the intervention would be because of the outlay of producing an entire series (for TV and radio). This could be a major production. In terms of the cost-benefit impact in relation to the number of individuals reached per dollar spent and per dollar saved, the cost might be quite favorable, even if the initial outlay were expensive.

Perhaps one of the most compelling advantages of the model is the acceptability. Audiences very much enjoy the series and object when a series is terminated. That point is more than just about "high ratings" of some TV show. The context relates to points raised previously, namely, that mental health interventions (e.g., the value of psychological treatment) already are known to have fairly "low ratings" and that people often view "no treatment" as better than going to get treatment. Thus the acceptability of the entertainment-education model is enormously important. Within a given country and culture, the model might be used to change a domain that would be expected to have a broad impact. For example, increased physical exercise can have multiple beneficial physical health outcomes (e.g., improved cardiovascular health, reduced risk for obesity, metabolic disorders, and cancer) and mental health outcomes (e.g., fewer symptoms of depression, reduced stress levels and anxiety, decreased substance use, improved neurocognitive functioning). Entertainment-education with that focus would seem to be an excellent first line of attack to reduce the burdens of a variety of dysfunctions. When expended in this fashion beyond a single domain (e.g., mental health) or disorder (e.g., depression), the cost-benefit impact might make this a best-buy intervention.

Socially Assistive Robotics

Prior discussion of technology has drawn on computer and related apparatuses as ways of delivering treatment, using, for example, the Internet and apps. Entertainment-education utilizes television and radio, technology in some sense, but hardly what any one means anymore when the use of "current technology" is discussed. Technology is too broad of a category to be very meaningful given the many advances in areas that bear little resemblance to one another. An example with actual and even more potential for use in health care is robotics.

We are generally familiar with robots. Robots and automated devices increasingly are in the news and are becoming more and more integrated into our lives, as evident in robotic toy pets for children; robots that do chores in the home, such as robotic vacuum cleaners; highly specialized robotic surgical systems; drones that carry out surveillance and air strikes; drones that deliver online purchases; and robotic devices used in all types of manufacturing. Advances in artificial intelligence, as reflected in self-driving cars and unmanned (but robotic) space travel, constantly improve on the capacities and abilities of robots (e.g., in motor skills but also cognitive skills). The term *robots* and my examples belie the diversity of devices and applications in which robots play a role in our daily lives. The diversity is reflected in the many different types of robots and goals to which they are directed. Related, multiple disciplines are involved (e.g., robotics, artificial intelligence, engineering, medicine, communication, and psychology) in their development and application. The roles that robots play are enormous and continue to expand (e.g., guiding visitors through museums, checking in guests at hotels) and perhaps even surprise (e.g., robots as partners and friends, capable of intimacy, including sensing and responding to emotions, kissing with sensations [touch, smell] that can be transmitted digitally, and love and sex more broadly) (e.g., Cheok et al., 2017; Lazányi, 2016; Zhang & Cheok, 2016). Not all of these are ready to order online, but it is never too early to put them on one's online wish list.

In relation to the present discussion, the issue is whether or the extent to which robots could play a critical role and on a scale in the context of health care to provide services that would reduce the burdens of mental illness. Clinical applications in physical health care have been evident for some time as assisting in helping with physical exercise and activities for rehabilitation among stroke victims and with recovery for cardiac patients (e.g., Fasola & Matarić, 2010; Kang et al., 2005; Prange et al., 2006). Robotics is less familiar in the context of mental health.

Socially assistive robots (SARs) are those that interact with humans in some way and increasingly are used in health care (Broadbent, 2017; Feil-Seifer & Matarić, 2011; Rabbitt et al., 2015). The robots are able to provide education and feedback, coach patients through activities and tasks, assist with treatment compliance, monitor progress, and provide companionship. In fact, SARs have already been used in mental health care applications with some patient populations, primarily children with autism spectrum disorder and older adults with dementia (e.g., Moyle et al., 2013; Vanderborght et al., 2012).

One of the more commonly employed functions of SARs in mental health care has focused on robots in the role of a companion. In much of this work, SARs function in a way that is analogous to a trained therapy animal, such as the use of dogs in animal-assisted therapy (e.g., Fine, 2015). In animal-assisted therapy, of which there are scores of variations, the animal is brought into the treatment process and interacts with the client in ways that are considered to be therapeutic. Some practical as well as ethical (protective of animal and participant) concerns emerge with bringing live animals into clinical settings (e.g., therapy offices, hospitals, long-term care facilities), including issues related to animal welfare, patient allergies, and risk for illness or infection (e.g., Shibata, 2012). SARs are seen as a way of harnessing some of the clinical benefits associated with animal-assisted interventions while avoiding the challenges inherent in work involving live animals. A wide range of pet-like robots currently exist, although two have dominated: Paro, a robot designed to look like a baby harp seal; and Aibo, a small robotic dog (see Broadbent, 2017; Rabbitt et al., 2015).[4]

Paro has been used extensively in many countries, with a primary focus on the role of a companion and mostly with older adult residents and patients in nursing home or hospital facilities. Many of these individuals have been identified as having dementia-related cognitive impairment (e.g., Shibata & Wada, 2010) or are at high risk for depression (e.g., Banks, Willoughby, & Banks, 2008). Patients and residents report positive experiences and engage in interactions with the robots (e.g., Birks et al., 2016; Libin & Cohen-Mansfield, 2004; Marti et al., 2006). Several studies have noted improved mood and decreases in depression following the introduction of a SAR into a long-term care facility for older adults (see Bemelmans et al., 2012; Wada et al., 2005). In addition, patients spend increased time in public areas and around other patients and staff members after the robots are introduced (Wada & Shibata, 2006). Reductions in physiological stress levels (as measured by salivary and urinary hormones) follow interactions with a SAR (Kanamori et al., 2003; Wada & Shibata, 2007).

Controlled trials (RCTs) with older adults and with individuals experiencing dementia show reductions in loneliness, improved quality of life, and increased pleasure following interactions with Paro compared with control conditions (e.g., providing recreational activities, reading activities) (Moyle et al., 2013; Robinson et al., 2013). The benefits are not unique to Paro. For example, Aibo, the robotic dog, was tested in three long-term care facilities and compared with a trained live dog or no interaction with any dog (robotic or live). Aibo and the live dog led to greater reductions in loneliness than the control condition and were no different in the level of attachment they generated (Banks et al., 2008).

These examples do not convey the rich potential of social robots for mental health care. If their contribution were restricted to reducing loneliness, rather than a broad spectrum of psychiatric disorders, that alone would be huge. As I noted earlier, loneliness is associated with significant physical health and mental problems, changes in the immune system, and early death (see Cacioppo & Patrick, 2008). Of course, we do not know that experiences with social robots would change all of that. The reason to highlight social robots is their potential as companions and their use in health care. As a model of delivery, it is premature to place these next to something already in as widespread use as task shifting or best-buy interventions. Yet robots that could be companions and could interact with individuals could easily take on therapeutically relevant tasks, now used in apps and virtual reality, and much more.

Researchers studying robots are often quite careful to convey that the goal is not to replace humans. In the present context, in no way do I mean to suggest that robots could replace a professional mental health worker delivering therapy, although of course the benefits and differences among a live therapist, a virtual therapist, and a social robot represent an intriguing empirical issue. Yet the message of this book is to have a range of treatment options, and their head-to-head comparisons, for reasons I elaborate later, are not all that critical. Robots could be in places (the home, hospitals, schools, rural areas) and with individuals who are otherwise by themselves. Also, we have known for some time that social robots can recognize and respond to emotions of humans (e.g., through tone of voice; Breazeal, 2003) and that social robots can provide body language cues characteristic of human behavior (e.g., McColl & Nejat, 2014). I mention these examples to convey that the capacities of social robots are expanding, and social robots are likely to play an expanded role in mental and physical health care in the future. Of course, feasibility and acceptability of social robots and their roles in everyday life raise all sorts of issues that go beyond making further advances in hardware and software (e.g., Coeckelbergh et al., 2016). SARs can be expensive, and robots currently in use in research are usually too expensive to distribute on any scale or to hand out if a mental disorder is detected at some integrated care facility. But costs of technology for public use often fall drastically over time. Cost-effectiveness studies (e.g., cost of the SAR in light of how many patients can be treated and how many quality-adjusted life years [QALYs] are gained) would be needed. Yet, for present purposes, the goal is to provide means of reaching more people in need of services; social robots at an early stage are already doing that in the context of care for older adults.

Table 8.2 lists key characteristics of SARs and criteria that relate to reaching people in need of services and to other models we presented. As indicated in the table, the benefits and characteristics of SARs are not easily specified. Among the reasons is that the range of robots is large and breakthroughs in what given robots can do may well influence the applicability of any given criterion. At this point, one can say that therapeutic robots are not affordable or readily available to be dispensed widely for the treatment of mental disorders. Also, the criterion of whether SARs would be acceptable varies by type of robot and also by the type of activity in which the robot engages (see Rabbitt et al., 2015). As a model for delivering mental health services, this might be the least well developed and researched among the models I have covered. At the same time, SARs are used rather extensively with older adults and to help with loneliness and dementia. That is noteworthy because older adults represent one of the populations especially neglected in relation to mental health care and services. With the increased use of robots in everyday life, the fast-breaking advances in artificial intelligence, and the likely acceptability in light of further penetration into daily activities (e.g., drones, self-driving cars), I list SARs as a model to watch rather than as a feasible one that could be implemented now.

Social Network Interventions

In my discussion of social media I used the terms *networks* and *networking* in a generic sense and as used in daily life. I was referring to the practices of using various websites, applications, and means of communication to stay in touch, to connect with people, and to find others with similar interests. There is another use of the term *network* that is related but also more technical and readily distinguished. In this other sense, a network still refers to a set of social interactions and personal relationships that are connected. In addition, the more technical use invokes a set of concepts that elaborate specific features about how individuals are connected, the specific roles they might play in a larger group of individuals, the degree of separation (e.g., number of intermediaries between them) among individuals in that larger group, and how behaviors spread in a given network or cluster of individuals. The network can be represented mathematically and graphically to convey the connections and distance among various segments (clusters) of the network (Christakis & Fowler, 2009, 2013; Rogers, 2003).

Among the key features of this more technical use is the fact that influences among people can extend throughout a given network and beyond those we know and with whom we interact directly. In addition, there are formal properties, or rules that guide the structure and function of networks, and these can be represented computationally to understand the nature of the connections. In a broader contextual scheme, we are very familiar with various levels of analysis of factors that influence our lives. Biological (e.g., genome, brain development) and psychological (e.g., childrearing practices, personality) factors represent broad classes of influences on a variety of outcomes over the course of life. Social networks reflect another level of analysis and perhaps surprisingly are a critical source of influence. It is as if we are part of a "human superorganism" (Christakis & Fowler, 2009, p. ii), with information and influence freely being exchanged among the constituent parts, that is, throughout the network.

Social networks, how they can diffuse information, and their key features have scores of examples in business and industry where products or practice spread and circulate through the population (see Rogers, 2003). I mention those in passing because there is a broader literature and interest in how to have an innovative practice diffuse or spread through the population. This is obviously important in business and marketing, namely, how to maximize adoption of a product. The influence of social networks also has great relevance in relation to health and mental health—our emphasis here.

For example, a large-scale study focused on the spread of obesity (Christakis & Fowler, 2007). More than 12,000 adults were evaluated over a 32-year period and were assessed repeatedly during this interval. The goal was to assess whether weight gain (body mass index) in one person was associated with weight gain among his or her friends, siblings, spouse, and neighbors. Information was obtained about the connections (interpersonal and geographic) among individuals and evaluated over time. Several individuals who were obese were selected as a basis for examining connections and served as the target individuals. Contacts and connections of these individuals were measured in relation to all others from the network. Algorithms and computational models were used to evaluate data and identify and graph the connections and distance among individuals included in a network. The main finding was that obesity was related among individuals in a network, and this influence continued, but in reduced likelihood, as a function of degree of separation. Direct contact with the target individual (no separation) showed greater risk; this decreased with separation without direct contact, and so on. By the fourth degree of separation, there was no influence. Many hypotheses could be ruled out (e.g., just selecting friends who are also obese, influence of geographical proximity rather than network proximity, overall increases in weight in the entire sample). The net effect is that over time one's weight was influenced by others in the network and by proximity in the network (e.g., direct versus further removed from direct).

Social network research has addressed additional topics related to health and mental health. For example, the extent to which one becomes depressed is related to connections within the network (Rosenquist, Fowler, & Christakis, 2011). The connection extends up to three degrees of separation (i.e., one's friends, and one's friends' friends). Many other characteristics are influenced by one's network, including alcohol consumption, cigarette smoking, loneliness, divorce, happiness, and being a victim of gunshot violence, among others domains (see Christakis & Fowler, 2013; Green, Horel, & Papachristos, 2017). Also, the impact does not require direct person (in-person) contact. Using Facebook and other social networking services, for example, suicidal ideation, emotional states, and political action spread as a function of social networks (e.g., Bond et al., 2012; Coviello et al., 2014; Masuda, Kurahashi, & Onari, 2013).

The influence of social networks and how the influence operates are fascinating topics in their own right and have a long history. For present purposes in looking at novel models of intervening, the question is whether network influences can be harnessed toward therapeutic ends. Multiple steps have been identified that convey some of the complexities (Rogers, 2003; Valente, 2010, 2012). For example, Valente identified four key steps to guide network based interventions.[5] These include:

- Identifying a person or persons in the network who will be champions or opinion leaders and who will promote the change, or individuals who bridge different groups or parts of the network;
- Identifying subgroups of people who could change at the same time (e.g., based on their connections, or individuals with similar roles that might bring them together as a subgroup);
- Fostering peer-to-peer interaction to stimulate interpersonal communication (e.g., fostering word of mouth stimulation of adoption, helping the intervention to go "viral"); and

- Altering the network because networks are dynamic. Change may benefit by adding others to foster spread of the intervention, perhaps redundantly so that the paths to connect individuals are extended or linked in new ways.

These comments describe in general terms the approximate approach of identifying the network, selecting those likely to exert influence, and fostering communication or exchanges in the network. The process includes empirical evaluation of the network connections among individuals and use of multiple mathematical models to examine the optimal places to intervene (e.g., Carrington, Scott, & Wasserman, 2005).

My interest in mentioning social networks is in relation to models of delivering psychosocial interventions to reduce the burdens of mental illness. There have been intervention studies in relation to mental health, including interventions to reduce substance abuse and cigarette smoking among adolescents and physical activity among children (e.g., Valente et al., 2007; Zhang et al., 2015). Yet the projects at this point are more demonstrations of applications, even though often multiple individuals (e.g., hundreds) and settings (multiple) are involved. The intervention literature is not established or large in relation to altering psychological problems beyond a few studies.

The relevance and importance of networks in relation to mental disorders are not at all new (e.g., Mueller, 1980). Yet, at this point in time, three features converge to make it quite timely to use social networking as a model for large-scale change in mental health service delivery. First, the research on the importance of networks in developing and maintaining clinically relevant behaviors is now strong. Thus we know that networks are a critical influence for changing people in everyday life. Second, the ability to scale-up interventions by network analysis is already suggested by completed studies. For example, outside the context of mental health, a social networking intervention was used in an RCT involving 61 million people to mobilize political behavior (e.g., expression of views, seeking election information) (Bond et al., 2012). Third and most pertinent, the proliferation and use of social media in everyday life provide novel opportunities for connecting people. We know that networks do not depend on face-to-face or in-person interaction, so all the social media outlets that people use to connect with each other can serve as the basis for intervention. Thus, as a model of delivery, social networks have enormous and untapped potential and could spread interventions readily to promote mental health both for treatment and prevention.

MULTIPLE MODELS ARE NEEDED

The models highlighted in this and the previous chapter may seem like a very odd conglomeration with little overlap and connection. That is a fair characterization. Their connection does not come from their similarity in terms of delivering mental health interventions—the models are very different in how they work (interventions and delivery). Indeed, the goal is to bring them together precisely because they reflect diverse ways of addressing the challenges of reaching individuals in need and reducing the burdens of mental illness. This is a shift in orientation from the dominant model of therapy, with its emphasis of making therapy better (more effective), but with much less attention to reaching the scores of individuals for whom the very model is not helpful.

The diversity of the models is a key feature of what we are trying to accomplish. If we want to reach people in need, first and foremost, we need models that can be scaled up to connect with the enormous numbers who currently are unserved. Recall that in the United States alone approximately 50 percent of the population will experience at least one psychiatric disorder over their lifetime; that would translate to more than 160 million people. And we are developing interventions that can address the problem worldwide rather than just in a single country. Yet even if any particular model could be scaled up, its inherent features might well cause it to omit some segment of the population in need or to be deemed unacceptable to a population it could reach. That is why we want to emphasize having multiple models to deliver psychosocial interventions.

Optimizing Coverage

Figure 8.1 provides a pictorial illustration of what we are trying to accomplish and how multiple models play a critical role. Consider the top portion of the figure (A) to represent all individuals in need of mental health services. This would include individuals with clinical dysfunction, those with subclinical disorders, and others who are impaired in some way because of some aspect of their emotional, cognitive, behavioral, or social functioning (e.g., stress and distress, loneliness, suicidality) that somehow is not covered by the previous categories.

The middle portion of the figure (B) shows a small circle (a very small subgroup) covering up part of the larger circle. That circle represents the small portion of individuals who do receive treatment and receive that through the dominant model of individual therapy. An obvious feature of B is that the vast majority of individuals in need of treatment (A portion) still are not receiving interventions. As I have shown throughout the book, B is primarily where we are now. This book is about the bottom portion (C), where each circle represents a model of intervention delivery.

A few features of the C category are noteworthy. First, the various models of delivery (each model is a circle within the larger circle) overlap with one another, that is, occupy the same space in some places. This reflects the likelihood that individuals may be reached by more than one model. That is important because one model will have inherent limitations (e.g., vary in feasibility or acceptability to a given constituency). Also, we want multiple options to reach individuals, perhaps those who are especially neglected by current services.

Second, the dominant model of administering treatment (shaded circle from B and also now in C) is still present. There is nothing in this book that suggests eliminating that model. Lamentably, the dominant model by itself has very little

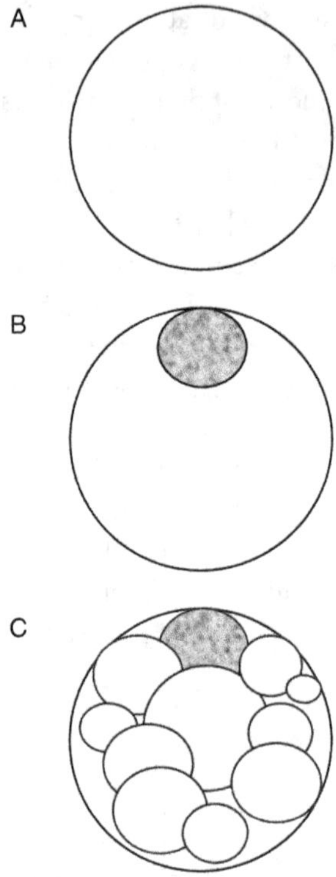

Figure 8.1 Representation of the role of multiple models for reaching individuals in need of services. The upper circle or pie (A) is intended to represent all those individuals in need of psychological services. The middle circle (B) consists of all persons in need of services, but with a small shaded portion (not intended to represent the scale) who receive the dominant model of psychotherapy. The lower circle (C) includes multiple models. Each model is represented by a circle and serves (provides intervention for) some segment of the population in need. The multiple circles obviously serve many more individuals in need of services. They also overlap (spill onto each other) a bit because for any single group that needs to be reached, more than one model is likely to be needed. Actually, C should have many overlapping models that would have even more overlap and more options. Finally, note there are still spaces in C not covered by one of the models. The reality may be that even with multiple models, some individuals in need of care will be missed. This means only that the goals to develop the models cannot be static and that new options will invariably be welcome and necessary. The models covered in this and the previous chapter (and listed in Table 8.1) are designed to reach a greater proportion of individuals in need. More models may well be developed beyond those I have highlighted.

impact on reducing the burdens of mental illness on any scale, but it may reduce the burden for a small portion (A in the figure) who need care.

Third, figure C conveys that even with multiple overlapping models, there are still "spaces" in the larger circle that are that are not covered. These spaces reflect people in need of treatment who will still receive none. Even with many models and overlap, we cannot be assured we will reach everyone in need. A realistic goal is to greatly reduce the burdens of mental illness rather than to eliminate them.

Consider what a remarkable accomplishment a simple "reversal" of this statistic would be. Currently, approximately 70 percent of individuals in the United States in need of mental health services receive nothing! What an accomplishment it would be to deploy multiple models of delivery so that 70 percent receive an EBPI! Of course, we would like the percentage to be much higher, but the bar is so low now that reaching most people in need and achieving 70 percent would be a virtual revolution in mental health services and in reducing the burdens of mental illness. The point is to recognize that we will be less than perfect in reaching everyone. But we could do vastly better as we approach the goal of reaching most, even almost all, individuals in need of services. Multiple models are available that make that feasible. Because most of the models I have discussed have yet to be implemented and evaluated in relation to mental illness, we could readily expect variations and creative offshoots of the models after implementation and evaluation began.

Clarification and Qualification

I have mentioned that these new models of delivery are separate from the interventions themselves. This is very clear when a given EBPI (e.g., cognitive behavior therapy) is administered by different models or means of delivery (in-person with a therapist, online self-help). In this chapter, many of the models include a change in both the intervention and model of delivery (e.g., entertainment-education).

Our goal should be to identify means of delivering interventions to reduce the burdens of mental illness. The interventions combined with the means ought to be evidence based. That is, the assumption is that we are seeking better ways to disseminate interventions that make a palpable difference in the lives of individuals. It is easy to see a danger emerging that could depart from this when the model is extended and becomes of great interest in its own right, but the evidence of the impact on delivery of treatment is not clear or not established.

To illustrate the point, consider Twitter. As I noted previously, Twitter communications have enormous reach and are used extensively in relation to mental health issues, for both delivery and receipt of information, support, and care (service). The vast majority of Twitter interventions for mental health (just as with the vast majority of therapy techniques administered with the dominant model) are not supported by evidence that they make any difference in the lives of people seeking help. That people like their Twitter experiences or believe they have helped is interesting and important, but liking an experience and believing that one is being helped are different from and not very related to actually being helped, something we have known for decades (Ankuta & Abeles, 1993; Lambert, Salzer, & Bickman, 1998; Pekarik & Wolff, 1996). My point is that we want the models to have reach and to be acceptable, and even liked, but we also must evaluate their impact to be sure the interventions they deliver actually help people in palpable ways.

I have singled out Twitter to make the point, but there is no reason to think Twitter is unique in this concern. Blogs and apps related to mental health care also have a paucity of studies in relation to the scores of options that are available.

There has been a similar problem of a longer duration in relation to self-help therapies. The problem is that there are at least a few thousand self-help interventions relying on written materials, apps, online programs, and many other media. In this haystack of interventions, there are only a small number of empirically based needles to be found, that is, self-help interventions with an evidence base. The difficulty with most social media–based interventions and self-help interventions is that there is no easy way for the public or indeed for the professional to readily discern which ones have empirical support. Another difficulty is that a model of delivery (self-help, Twitter, and social media more generally) becomes an end in itself, that is, a source of use and indeed pleasure perhaps, and the goal of providing effective interventions is somewhat lost. Here I am advocating EBPIs and models that can deliver them and intervention-model combinations that have an impact. As some models proliferate, the goals of having an evidence base and exerting a palpable impact on individual and social burdens of mental illness can easily become lost.

SUMMARY AND CONCLUSIONS

In this and the prior chapter, we have covered many different models of intervention delivery, which will allow overlapping ways of reaching people. The diversity of these models is of great importance because they provide many options on the delivery side (e.g., for society, for mental health services) and on the selection side (e.g., among prospective candidates for the intervention). Moreover, some of the models (e.g., best buy, Entertainment-education) do not require much effort in relation to what has to be done to "select" the intervention by individuals experiencing psychological problems. That feature is critically important because it is not very reasonable for many of those who experience various forms of psychiatric impairment to "shop" for treatments. Many of the models in varying degrees bring the intervention to people in need rather than requiring people to go to the treatment.

The multiple models also demonstrate that there are rich options available for presenting psychosocial interventions. Many of the models are not "just" promising or pregnant with undelivered potential; some already have been tried, evaluated empirically, and shown to have an impact. How to move forward to utilize the models and to have the needed impact? In the next chapter, several topics are presented that address this issue. We need more than models. How they are to be implemented and used? Different ways of thinking about mental health, as well as a variety of issues that place the model in a social context, all need to move forward. Stated more simply, having an array of novel models is a necessity, but is not sufficient to adequately affect and reduce the burden of mental illness.

PART IV

Extending Our Conceptual Views of Treatment, Research, and Interventions

9

Expanding Our Perspectives on Interventions, Models of Delivery, and Clinical Care

Chapters 7 and 8 discussed the availability of many models of delivering psychosocial interventions. The models vary in the extent to which they are ready to be implemented. Variations of some of the models, such as task shifting, disruptive innovations, and best buy, already have been used in some forms in the context of both physical and mental health and in both developing and developed countries. Moreover, these models already have evidence that they can affect health outcomes. Nevertheless, currently the models do not contribute appreciably to the proportion of mental health services in the United States and globally. Clearly, the availability of multiple models and evidence that some of them can be and have been applied effectively provides hope that evidence-based services might be used to reach the vast majority of individuals in need who receive no intervention at all.

Having viable models alone will not be enough to change mental health services. I have discussed barriers to intervention earlier in the book. Some of the models circumvent these (e.g., reduce or eliminate stigma by not being associated with going to treatment), but there are a variety of additional constraints in moving from models to implementation. The goals of this chapter are to address these constraints but in a constructive way. The chapter places models of delivery in broader contexts by expanding our thinking about mental health services and what is provided to whom, and ways of sequencing intervention and models of intervention delivery.

NOVEL FOCI FOR INTERVENTION DEVELOPMENT

The focus on novel models reflects a broader and overarching theme of expanding how we think about delivery of interventions for health care. From expanding interventions and models of delivery, the "expansion theme" continues in this chapter. However, this is at a higher level of abstraction and focuses on how we think about the means, goals, and foci of interventions and, by implication, changes in current priorities for research and practice. The overall goal has not changed, namely, reducing the burdens of mental illness. This can be enhanced by the way we think about how to achieve that overall goal and what we study to achieve that.

Weak and Strong Interventions

Obviously, we want interventions that have strong effects in the benefits they produce. "Strong" can be defined in many ways. Consider two ways to operationalize that as the amount of change that is produced on indices related to client functioning in everyday life and the proportion of individuals who receive the intervention and profit from the treatment or make those changes. In an idealized extreme to make the point, we would be elated if we had interventions that eliminated impairment among clients with a particular problem or set of problems (e.g., anxiety and depression) and if this intervention worked in this way for everyone or almost everyone. These would clearly be strong effects.[1]

When we obtain intervention effects, we want them to be strong. When they are not, we are likely to tinker in research by adding components to that intervention (e.g., homework assignments, booster [extra] sessions) or by adding an entirely different intervention (e.g., medication) to see if we can obtain even stronger effects. In addition, we may look at moderating variables (factors that influence outcome) to identify for whom effects are strong, weak, or nonexistent and see if we have leads there to improve the effects of intervention. Perhaps the effects of intervention *are* very strong, but the evidence of that is diluted because a special subgroup did not respond at all or became slightly worse. These approaches to surmounting weak interventions are standard in psychosocial intervention research more generally and are evident in the programs of research of individual investigators who are developing interventions over a period of time.

Needless to say, the search for strong interventions is important and obviously so; I am not challenging that. I am challenging the value of the dominance or almost exclusive focus on that search. In addition, perhaps we ought to consider and search for "weak" interventions—those that do not usually produce a large magnitude of change and do not affect very many people in ways that have a strong impact on their lives. Why search for weak interventions? We probably already have scores of them. Prominent examples might include public appeals from government agencies, educational efforts to "raise awareness," and advertisements to stop or start some behavior that will influence our health (e.g., engage in activities to reduce stress, exercise, have a better diet). We know from many different areas of research that rational appeals, providing information, and doling out advice are among the weakest ways of changing human behavior (e.g., Anderson, & Whiston, 2005; Maher et al., 2014; Snyder et al., 2004; Sweeney & Moyer, 2015). We know this well in health care more broadly, for example, by getting people to take their medication, to reduce sexual assault on college campuses, to use contraceptives for safer sex, to wear helmets (motorcycles, bicycles), to brush one's teeth and floss, to eat broccoli, so on. Of course, most educational and information appeals are never evaluated empirically and their impact is unknown, a topic to which we return later in the chapter.

Perhaps one of the more dramatic illustrations of efforts to raise awareness is reflected by the scores of days, weeks, and months devoted to individual causes (e.g., Suicide Awareness Month).[2] These efforts also might be some of the "weak" interventions we need, but we must have data to demonstrate that they have an impact in order to qualify for what I am suggesting. The goal is still to reduce the burdens of mental illness, and raising awareness or not in any given instance may or may not be effective. I am not asserting that the interventions are ineffective, but rather pleading for empirical demonstrations of their impact to evaluate and then develop them.

Given the disappointing results from weak interventions, by definition, why should we develop these further or establish their evidence base? I am so glad you asked. The reason is that it is often the case that weak interventions can be delivered inexpensively and reach large numbers, including those who otherwise might not receive treatment. Having some effect on clients with use of the media and Web-delivered messages, for example, would be great because not much in the way of effort is required. In other words, often weak interventions are or can be inversely related to cost and positively related to scalability. That is, the cost of some type of message usually is not very expensive, when contrasted with delivery of psychosocial interventions in some other way. And if the intervention is a message, there are vast options (e.g., Web, social media, smartphones and smartwatches) to reach many people in need of services and ways to ensure that the messages reach the intended people (e.g., via social networks). In addition, as individuals we may look up a particular psychological problem on the Web, perhaps because we have the proverbial "friend" who is concerned about it. After a few such searches or a profile of what we are seeking, those psychosocial health-related messages can be targeted to us in the way advertisements are individualized when we shop online.

The value of arguably weak interventions with a low cost can be seen in the context of what physicians say to their patients during routine office visits in an effort to reduce cigarette smoking. Physician visits are relatively brief (median of 13–16 minutes) in the United States (e.g., Peckham, 2016). During the visit, advice from the physician or nurse can have a small but reliable effect on cigarette smoking. The physician says something like the following, "I think it important for you to quit tobacco use now," or, "As your clinician, I want you to know that quitting tobacco is the most important thing you can do to protect your health." Perhaps we ought not to expect very much from passing comments that are not the reason for the visit. Yet this intervention leads to approximately a 2.5 percent incremental increase in smoking abstinence rates in comparison with no intervention, as supported from meta-analyses of multiple randomized controlled trials (e.g., Rice & Stead, 2008; Stead, Bergson, & Lancaster, 2008). A 2.5 percent improvement over intervention as usual (e.g., regular office visit without the physician or nurse comments) seems rather unexciting and weak! In a perfect world, we would want the special intervention to reach 100 percent abstinence and completely trump the control condition. Yet this is a low-cost intervention that can be used routinely by physicians and nurses during office visits of patients who smoke cigarettes. Indeed, internal medicine practice guidelines now recommend that physicians provide specific advice to stop smoking as part of standard care. Also, the 2.5 percent is deceptively simplistic and perhaps deceptively "weak." Cigarette smoking kills people and is associated with debilitating medical conditions (cancer, heart disease, chronic respiratory disease) along the way toward death, leaving secondary and tertiary consequences for others. The personal suffering of individuals and their families (e.g., disability-adjusted life years [DALYs], trauma of loved ones at the earlier than expected death of their relatives) and impact on society (e.g., cost for medical care and DALYs here, too) are greatly influenced by smoking cessation at virtually any level. In addition, that 2.5 percent may include a hundred thousand or a million patients, so the scale makes this weak intervention rather impressive. And more poignantly perhaps, if a life or a small handful of lives were saved, that might well be considered a huge (strong) effect.

The point of the example is to look for weak interventions that might be administered inexpensively and scaled to reach either many individuals or individuals who might not otherwise receive an intervention. Essential is the addition that the interventions have evidence attesting to their impact. It is quite easy to devise low-cost interventions that reach people and are well intended. That is not the goal. Rather, we want a new line of evidence-based psychosocial interventions (EBPIs).

Developing these interventions is *not* an alternative to seeking strong effects, but rather should augment our portfolio of ways of having an impact. And, of course, the point is not about cigarette smoking but rather to consider how we might have readily available interventions that could influence depression, anxiety, and self-injury on the clinical disorder side and that could influence lifestyle changes such as diet and exercise on the prevention side. But staying with the cigarette smoking example for a moment, one wonders whether the "genre" of that intervention might be expanded and with similar outcomes. For example, could targeted messages be provided during physician visits directed to patients (including children and adolescents) with other conditions that would affect physical and mental health? For example, one would hardly expect physician comments to adolescents about a risky behavior or two (e.g., driving while intoxicated or in a car where the driver has been drinking) to have much of an impact. But if it could have an impact and be made (constructed, designed, and tested) to have that impact, that would be an enormous contribution.

At visits to our doctors and dentists, we often complete some measure that is a medical history of various conditions and an update on any new symptoms. Perhaps that measure or a slightly expanded measure could be administered that provided a brief screen for stress, anxiety, and depression, just to identify possible domains. If "just" depression were the focus, that would be extremely important given the enormous prevalence of that disorder worldwide. Based on this expanded assessment, we might have physicians or nurses immediately alerted to give us a targeted statement analogous to the one related to cigarette smoking. This alert is especially easy to do with the increased use of electronic records and our physician's glance at a computer screen right after the initial greeting as our appointment starts. The message might alert the doctor or nurse to say, "The best thing you can do for your health now is to [begin to exercise three days a week, go for walks in nature, take up yoga, meditation, or tai chi]." As with the cigarette smoking example, we want evidence that such statements make a difference, but the point here is about the genre of interventions, all designed to have some effect even if not huge and all relatively simple to deliver.

I hasten to add that providing messages to change behavior, whether in written or oral form, rarely draws on what we know from research on how messages should be presented. By "should" I am not drawing on any moral imperative, but rather on the evidence on how to increase the likelihood that the message will have an impact. For example, *message framing* consists of the way in which something is presented (Rothman & Salovey, 1997). The same message might be given in many different ways. Two of the more common ways are presenting the outcome as positive (what one will gain by engaging in the behavior) or negative (what one will lose by not engaging in the behavior). Message frame is well known and utilized in the context of advertising, but not clearly as prevalent in relation to health messages designed to change mental and physical health-related behavior on a large scale. Nevertheless, in health contexts, we have learned from research that message framing has an impact on individuals' attitudes and actions (e.g., Gallagher & Updegraff, 2012). And in research, message framing has been used in many different contexts (e.g., fostering vaccinations, dental care, better driving behaviors, use of environmentally friendly products).

Social norm messages also can greatly influence behavior and can be more frequently used to promote health. *Social norms* rely on the fact that we are greatly influenced by what our peers and others are doing in relation to a particular behavior (Schultz et al., 2007). Messages that convey that most people engage in this or that behavior can be mobilized to change what people actually do. This approach already has been used for a variety of health-related behaviors (e.g., cigarette smoking, alcohol consumption, HIV/AIDS, bullying) (e.g., Rivard & Butler, 2017). There is more here than my passing comments, but the overall point remains. Certainly, empirical findings about how to maximize the impact of messages could be better incorporated into in-person as well as media-delivered messages to have an impact on health and specifically mental health.

There may be many other interventions that are "weak" and highly scalable. "Nudging" people by influencing choice is something already well practiced in marketing and somewhat in health care (Hansen et al., 2016; Thaler & Sunstein, 2008). This refers to "choice architecture" and how possible actions are presented to individuals and in ways that greatly influence decisions. That is based on what we know from cognitive psychology; people can be nudged into decisions that can improve their health. The primary context to convey nudging work is in the context of choice.

Choice is always presented in some way that is not truly neutral (e.g., always within a context in which it is presented and whether a default option refers to one way of acting versus another). For example, when people are asked whether they wish to enroll in a company retirement plan, often the default position (not enrolling) means that most do not enroll. Enrollment, even despite the added incentive of receiving matching (free) money from an employer, is infrequent, even though, when explicitly asked, people say they want a plan. There is a strong tendency to opt for the status quo or default position, which is captured nicely by the statement that one should never underestimate "the power of inertia" (Thaler & Sunstein, 2008, p. 8). If the default position is reversed, that is, if doing nothing leads to enrollment or if one has to choose explicitly (and there is no default position), then enrollment is much higher.

Among the advantages is that nudging is an alternative to regulations (e.g., taxes, laws) that take away choice. Essentially, what nudging does is make the healthier choice easy or easier than the alternative (Hansen et al., 2016). In relation to the present discussion, nudging can be (and has been) used in ways that might promote exercise and activities (like bike riding, walking, eating small food portions), discourage deleterious health-related habits (cigarette smoking, overuse of alcohol), and participating in programs (such as prevention checks for physical and mental health) (e.g., Hansen et al., 2016; Marteau, Hollands, & Kelly, 2015). Currently, evidence is limited in terms of impact and large-scale extensions in relation to mental health and substance use, but applications continue to draw on the underlying concepts.

Nudging has its own challenges, including worries about abuse by policy makers and the ethical issues of exerting control over people in this way (see Hansen et al., 2016). Yet in relation to the present discussion, nudging ought to be on the table in presenting information and choices that relate to health. This may or may not be a strong intervention, but it raises the question of what can be done to make engaging in behaviors that promote mental and physical health easier and on a large scale.

There are many other interventions that could promote behaviors related to physical and mental health. Apps and wearable devices might send not only messages but also animated figures or even games that promote mental health–related behaviors and indeed even encouragement to seek intervention. We might not expect any of them to have a dramatic effect on reducing the burdens of mental illness. Yet weak interventions that can be delivered widely could be a valuable addition to our armamentarium of interventions that reach people. There are not too many programs of research in clinical psychology and psychiatry establishing the evidence base of weak interventions.

Weak interventions are not part of our conceptualization of how to develop strategies that make a difference, but could make a very constructive contribution. Perhaps a question to guide us would be: What are low-cost, relatively easily implemented interventions that are scalable and that would be expected to have some effect on reducing the burdens of mental illness and related woes? Such interventions should at least be on the table in light of whom we wish to reach. Later in this chapter I discuss stepped care, in which more intensive, effortful, and costly interventions are implemented only after less costly efforts have been exhausted. In that context, weak and low-cost interventions could play a critical role as a first line of intervention attack.

Special Attention to the Few

In clinical practice, the clients are individuals in need of treatment or who perceive themselves as likely to profit from treatment for some help with their lives. Typically, they self-select, that is, go to the trouble of initiating treatment for themselves or loved ones. Of course, I have no objection to any of that. Yet there are additional ways of deciding to whom treatment is applied that are likely to help in reducing the burdens of mental illness.

The 80/20 Rule

Consider for a moment that all individuals with mental illness are occupying a pie chart or circle. Everyone with mental illness is in the circle. Among all individuals with mental illness, it is very likely that not all individuals contribute to and experience the burdens of mental illness equally. It is more likely that a small proportion, or small slice of that pie, accounts for a high portion of the burden of mental illness. That burden could be defined in different ways (e.g., suffering, cost, DALYs, years of life lost [YLL], and so on). Perhaps we could give much more attention to that small proportion in our research and practice.

Let us take a very brief excursion as background by moving to Pareto's principle, more commonly known as the *80/20 rule*. The rule is named after Vilfredo Pareto (1848–1923), who was an engineer, economist, sociologist, political scientist, and philosopher. Pareto made the observation that in Italy, where he worked, approximately 80 percent of the land was owned by approximately 20 percent of the population. This proportion of input or cause (20 percent) to output or effect (80 percent) has been examined and applied well beyond the original context.

The primary applications have been in business and economics (e.g., marketing, sales, procurement, stocking of goods, distribution of wealth) but has been extended to sports, science, safety, health, and other areas (Evans, 2014; Koch, 2011).[3] Consider three quite different facets of human activities to sample application of the principle. First, global income (wealth) follows the rule. Globally, approximately 83 percent of income goes to approximately 20 percent of the people (United Nations Development Program, 1992). Second, utilization of health care does as well. For example, in the United States, approximately 20 percent of patients use 80 percent of health care resources (Weinberg, 2009). Third, use of library books follows the rule. In libraries, approximately 80 percent of books that circulate (are checked out) involve only 20 percent of holdings (Buckland, 1975). In the many other contexts in which the rule has been applied, the goal is to understand utilization of resources (i.e., the 80 percent) and where the focus might be to have maximum impact (i.e., the 20 percent). One wants to identify the 20 percent as the recipient of effort, money, or personnel to reach the larger majority, or the 80 percent. That does not mean neglecting those who are not in the 80 percent, but it does mean focusing effort where the effect is likely to be the greatest in terms of reach or impact.

For present purposes, the general principle is a useful guide in relation to the focus of intervention research. As I mentioned before the brief excursion, it is likely that a small proportion (whether 20 percent or not) utilize a large proportion (whether 80 percent or not) of resources that reflect the burdens of mental illness. Another way to frame this is not to mention "use" as if it were a complaint, but rather to say that a small proportion need, draw on, and utilize a variety of services, which places a heavy burden on resources. A key area that is neglected in the context of the psychosocial intervention research is this group or rather, perhaps, this small set of groups. The guiding unknowns are whether we can identify which individuals are suffering and experience the greatest burdens of mental illness, and then whether we can use that information to develop effective interventions for them. From a health care perspective, we know well how to identify the many groups who receive the least attention in relation to services and whose costs are likely to be the greatest. Consequently, providing resources to those groups would be possible; it is just that much of the psychosocial intervention research has neglected a focus on those groups.

Proportionate Universalism

Providing attention to special groups would not be at the expense of drawing (depleting) resources from others. The task is to raise the level of care for all citizens. Services are paltry for most people in the United States and worldwide, and there is no implied endorsement here to draw from those who receive care (already a tiny group) to those who need it even more.

A policy in health care to address inequities in service delivery and to provide a way of allocating resources is referred to as *proportionate universalism* (see Benach et al., 2013; Macdonald, Beeston, & McCullough, 2014). This consists of providing improved services to all, but allocating the proportion of resources and services in relation to the level of disadvantage, burden, or need. That is, services are universally available but at a scale and intensity proportionate to the degree of need. Explicit policies would be adopted to ensure that allocation of resources would be provided to the subpopulation with poorest rates of health (mental or physical) and experiencing the poorest outcomes.

As an illustration, a recent study identified 14 differentially disadvantaged neighborhoods and evaluated different levels of investment they were receiving (Egan et al., 2016). The goal was to evaluate whether greater investment in the neighborhoods made a difference in mental and physical health outcomes over a five-year period. In fact, higher investment in disadvantaged neighborhoods, compared with lower investment, was reflected in better mental and physical health outcomes. Perhaps what makes this especially interesting is that the allocation of investment was not directed at health care services. Rather, the investment was allocated in terms of improved housing (such as heating improvements, kitchen improvements, reroofings, and dwelling protectors [overclad]). Greater allocation of resources for housing in neighborhoods with greater need indeed was associated with improved outcomes. Nonmental (or physical) health interventions can indeed have broad impact.

Proportionate universalism focuses on where need (burdens, poorest outcomes) is the greatest. That need can be determined empirically and may expand on the groups we might expect to be identified. For example, clearly in relation to health care in the United States, ethnic and cultural minorities are at a disadvantage, with enormous disparities that remain to be rectified. Interestingly, the total burden of poor health (in the United States) often is greater among nonminority individuals of low socioeconomic status because there are more people within that demographic (absolute numbers). The policy focuses on where need is and no doubt in that process would address ethnic and cultural disparities as well as address other groups as empirically determined.

The point of proportionate universalism is not only to provide services and resources on the basis of need but also to lift the overall level of care for all. In relation to my focus here, that is a valuable guiding principle to address the "reach" criterion of models of delivering treatment. That is, we want to be sure not just to scale up treatments (universalism) but also to ensure we reach people in special need (proportionate). The concepts of universal and targeted interventions are often used in discussion of prevention. In that context, too, the focus is on providing interventions for all and special interventions to individuals at high risk. Proportionate universalism is more focused on allocation of resources and services but has aspects of both the universal and targeted.

General Comments

The idea of providing more intense concentration and use of resources where they are needed most is not new and may not seem very inspired as a result. But what is new, and what has made the model more feasible and focused, is better assessment and use of data to identify where services are needed. For example, police usually know where crimes are likely to be committed—that part is not new. However, predictive policing is used to integrate collection of extensive data (big data), use of mathematical models (some of which, interestingly, draw on models derived from the study of earthquakes), draw information from social networks of people to identify likely perpetrators and victims, and in general focus on "hot spots" where crime is likely (Hvistendahl, 2016). This information is fed to laptops in real time with predictive maps to police patrolling in their cars. The large-scale impact of the model is not yet well studied. Yet the model illustrates the larger move toward harnessing data in ways not heretofore available to focus resources where needed.

In the context of providing mental health services, the models I have highlighted come with both caveats and nuances. First and foremost, there is no single measure of burden that reflects all types of burden. There is individual suffering defined subjectively and through other measures such as DALYs; YLLs would identify different people. Second, burden varies as a function of particular time frame (e.g., in one's most productive years as an adult or lifelong). Third, burdens and need can vary by disorder or domain of dysfunction. Substance abuse and depression or adult- versus child-onset disorders conceivably could identify different groups that are poorly served rather than just one group (e.g., individuals of lower socioeconomic status). Yet this need not be a constraint—there are clearly groups whose health care disparities are obvious and whose burdens and suffering are the least well served. This means that we do not just provide vacuous claims that more services and money as needed to address health care disparities. Rather, there is a genuine allocation of services and resources to those whose burdens are especially great.

In terms of research on treatment, the vast psychological literature on EBPIs is not addressing the topic of interventions for individuals who suffer the greatest burdens. In general, research on psychosocial treatments has pretty much neglected the matter of the burdens of mental illness, its many measures, and where an impact might be needed and achieved. And in terms of clinical services, when budget cuts are made there is usually the equivalent of what might be called disproportionate discrimination; that is, those in greatest need are most likely to see funding cuts to services.

Attending More to the Physical and Mental Disorder Connections

The distinction between physical and mental disorders is clear among professionals and lay people alike, and at the margins classifying a source of disability as either a physical or mental disorder would have enormous reliability. So, in the brand-new Kazdin Disorder Classification System (invented just a few seconds ago), most people would classify strep throat (from streptococcus bacteria), athlete's foot, broken leg, and HIV as physical disorders or physical health problems, and depression, fear of spiders, being sexually attracted to socially inappropriate objects, and hearing voices that compel one to hurt other people as mental disorders or mental health problems. Even at the margins and with seemingly clear conditions, my system breaks down. Many of the mental disorders and characteristics I casually listed have underlying physical links and bases. When we look at the full range of physical and mental disorders, the classification system unravels, and physical and mental health problems are not so clearly separate. There are quite strong connections between mental and physical disorders, and given many of these connections, it is unclear if the distinction is valuable or eventually (with more research findings) will even be defensible.

There is a long history of challenging the distinction between so-called diseases of the body versus those of the mind (see Kendell, 2001). Past and current examples convey how the distinction seemed sound but became blurred or just vanished. Perhaps the most well-known example goes back to the 18th and 19th centuries. During that time, a condition known as *general paresis* was considered to be a mental disorder in light of a variety of psychological symptoms (including depression, delusions, mania, apathy, and impairment in memory, judgment, and concentration). This was not a minor disorder and indeed constituted up to 10 to 25 percent of patients in public mental asylums (e.g., Davis, 2012; Hum, 1998). Eventually, general paresis shifted from being considered a mental disorder to the other column, that is, a physical disorder. Laboratory studies identified the bacteria involved, and applied studies demonstrated that the disease could be treated—that is, it became clear that the mental disorder really was a physical disorder.[4] The psychological or mental symptoms were the result of late-stage syphilis and essentially a brain disease resulting from it. By the early 1900s, the illness became treatable (with penicillin) and not regarded as a mental disorder.

In more current research, there has been increased recognition that several mental disorders are fundamentally physical disorders with genetic and other contributors that ultimately affect brain functioning. For example, schizophrenia has been considered a brain disease for some time (e.g., Chua & McKenna, 1995; Henn & Nasrallah, 1982). What is new are the enormous advances in evaluation of genetic and brain structure and functioning, at fine-grained levels (brain circuits, neurons, molecular and cellular structures) and over the course of development antedating and through onset (including studies of the placenta, neonates, infants through teens), and how these underlie core psychological processes (cognition and affect; learning, memory, perception) and symptoms (e.g., Cannon, 2015; Fornito & Bullmore, 2015; Klauser et al., 2017). Similarly, chronic fatigue syndrome, once viewed as psychosomatic (biological problems resulting from something psychological), now looks much more like a physical disease (perhaps an autoimmune disorder) (Wadman, 2016). Now many disorders have been added to the list of mental disorders that are conceived as physical disorders (genetic, brain disorders), including bipolar disorder, major depressive disorder, and autism spectrum disorder (e.g., Johnston-Wilson et al., 2000; Marshall et al., 2008). Other disorders are fundamentally biological, but their symptoms include psychiatric disorder symptoms. For example, a rare tumor among children masquerades as attention-deficit disorder (Batsis et al., 2016). Many children who have the tumor meet criteria for and previously received a diagnosis of attention-deficit disorder, well beyond the expected base rate. In preliminary work (with a small sample size), after the tumor was removed the symptoms remitted—intriguing at this point and clearly revealing the connection of physical and mental disorders, with the latter possibly coalescing into the former.

It is well recognized that many disorders (such as anxiety and eating disorders, substance abuse disorders) have both biological (e.g., genetic) and environmental factors that confer risk. Consequently, calling a disorder a genetic or brain disorder does not eliminate the role of other factors (e.g., social and physical environmental factors) or indicate that an intervention has to focus on one domain (biological or psychosocial) rather than another. It is important to keep in mind that many physical disorders have biological and environmental factors (e.g., air and water pollutants, insecticides, overexposure to the sun, poor diet) that confer risk as well (e.g., cancer, cardiovascular disease, Alzheimer's disease). These initial comments merely are designed to show one way in which physical and mental disorders belong in the same discussion; that is, they overlap, and what is classified as mental may well be a physical disease in which the emphasis has been given to symptoms in psychological domains (e.g., cognitive processes, socialization, perception, memory).

Other connections between mental and physical disease are readily apparent and have implications for intervention. Three in particular should be noted: (1) instances in which a physical disorder increases the risk for the onset of a mental disorder, (2) vice versa, and (3) when a physical and mental disorder tend to be comorbid (having one currently increases the likelihood of having the other currently). The poster child and well-studied example is the relation of heart disease and depression. As I mentioned in Chapter 2, individuals who are depressed are much more likely to have a heart attack than are those who are not depressed (Lichtman et al., 2014; Nemeroff & Goldschmidt-Clermont, 2012). And among individuals who have a heart attack, those who are also depressed are approximately three times more likely to die from a future heart attack than those who have had the attack but are not depressed (Bush et al., 2005). Similarly, individuals who have a stroke are much more likely to become clinically depressed than if they had not had a stroke (Jørgensen et al., 2016). Finally, women who are depressed early in their pregnancy are twice as likely to develop diabetes, and women who have diabetes during gestation are more likely to report postpartum depression within 6 weeks after giving birth (Hinkle et al., 2016). With just these examples, the connections and bidirectional influences of physical and mental disorders are striking and intriguing.

Perhaps the most dramatic and lamentable finding in relation to the connection of mental and physical illness is that serious mental illness is related to contracting a variety of physical disorders and an earlier than expected death. As mentioned earlier, those with mental illness die earlier than expected, with reviews showing an average of 15 to 30 years earlier (e.g., Hert et al., 2011; Nordentoft et al., 2013; Thornicroft, 2011). Some of the connections between mental disorder and early death might be obvious. For example, we know that some disorders such as substance use and abuse have all sorts of mortality-breeding risks (e.g., overdose, exchanging infected needles, higher rates of suicide, and weakened immune system also associated with mental disorders). And individuals with mental disorders have higher rates of cigarette smoking, which on its own predicts early death (e.g., Smith, Mazure, & McKee, 2014). Moreover, individuals with mental disorder are less likely to follow intervention regimens for their physical health problems. For example, depression among individuals with HIV/AIDS predicts not adhering to medication, and this could also lead to early death (e.g., Kalichman, Ramachandran, & Catz, 1999; Magidson et al., 2015). There are other influences that explain the connection (e.g., poverty is related to both mental and physical disability). The reasons and influences are important to understand because having that information better guides our interventions.

I wish to make a point that relates to the goal of extending intervention in ways that might reduce the burdens of mental illness. Given the strong connection between physical and mental illness, are there ways to consider novel foci of interventions? Instead of fostering the intervention by disorder type and by the professional disciplines that provide them, can we reach out with approaches that select broader targets (physical and mental health disorder combinations) or health more generally? Some leads for how to proceed are in the next sections.

Targeting Transmechanisms

In an earlier chapter, I introduced the terms *transdiagnosis* and *transtreatment*. Transdiagnosis refers to findings that showed commonalities (e.g., biological and environmental risk factors) that span multiple psychiatric disorders. Research with a focus on transdiagnoses usually begins with recruiting and identifying samples with different disorders and then showing common features and characteristics or dimensions that might group disorders into to broad categories that combine what heretofore have been conceived as mostly separate specific disorders (e.g., depression, anxiety) (e.g., Cross-Disorder Group of the Psychiatric Genomics Consortium, 2013; Kendler et al., 2003). Many disorders have been known to go together for some time (e.g., depression and anxiety; bulimia and anorexia), and looking for commonalities (and often finding them) makes great sense conceptually. And now, many empirical investigations have supported the value of a transdiagnostic approach. By showing commonalities among etiologies and risk profiles, better methods of diagnosis and intervention may emerge.

Transtreatments were identified as those interventions designed to apply broadly to many different disorders. Indeed, if many different disorders share several features, can they be treated with variations of a single intervention? Transtreatments have been developed, and as I discussed, these are mostly variations of cognitive behavioral treatments and exposure-based treatments, and are applied primarily to various forms of depression and anxiety. The transtreatments I highlighted were based on a conceptual view about how to change affect, cognition, and behavior (e.g., via altering cognitions) as well as research on how to eliminate anxiety (e.g., via extinction-based procedures such as exposure therapy). What has been missing in much of the psychosocial treatment literature in general, not just transtreatments, EBPIs, or the interventions as usual, is a deeper understanding of how disorders come about and the precise mechanisms of action through which interventions affect those core processes and lead to change (Kazdin, 2014). We might consider, as we move forward in intervention research, expanding our focus in another but related way that looks at processes leading to disorders rather than (or in addition to) taking effective treatments and determining the scope of dysfunctions to which they can be applied.

I introduce a term here to clarify that expanded focus, namely, *transmechanism*. We know that a mechanism usually refers to the underlying process that explains how a particular effect occurs and the steps leading from those processes to the outcome. I refer here to transmechanism as an underlying process that may be at the core of many different disorders. In our thinking about interventions, I suggest that we move to this broader or higher level of abstraction and focus on common initial pathways or common pathways of origin.[5] Transdiagnostic work does focus on common elements (e.g., gene characteristics), and these will be elaborated no doubt to explain how they unfold through additional processes (e.g., brain circuitry) that influence those characteristics we call mental disorders. The focus here is similar, looking for common features, but different enough to make a distinction.

As a point of departure, we begin with the question: Are there processes we know that serve as a common precursor or early pathway leading to mental and physical disorders? I am calling those transmechanisms and suggest that we target them. Of course, in the abstract the idea may seem reasonable, but are there any clues as to what these foci might be? I highlight some examples just to illustrate the category I have in mind when referring to transmechanism, and to foster thinking about intervention targets in a way that departs from our current emphasis with transtreatments.

The immune system, especially a weak and compromised system, appears to be strongly implicated in the onset and course of physical and mental illness.[6] Among the many functions of the immune system are to ward off and respond to infections, toxins, and foreign agents in the body. As part of our reaction to infection, there is temporary inflammation as cells migrate to areas, and several changes in the surrounding area occur, all where the immune reaction is needed. The inflammation is short lived as the infection is addressed and the cells return to their normal state. Yet inflammation can be triggered by one's own cells (autoimmune diseases) and also may not return to a normal state. Inflammation that does abate can lead to a series of biological processes that influence mental health outcomes, including depression (unipolar and bipolar), autism spectrum disorder, schizophrenia, and chronic fatigue syndrome (e.g., Berk et al., 2013; Danese & Baldwin, 2017; Goldstein et al., 2009; Morris et al., 2016). We know that immune responses have genetic components but also can be influenced by environmental events (e.g., early exposure to violence, loneliness, stress, pollutants in the air and water). We also know that a compromised or challenged immune system occurs before the disorder, so we know the timeline. For example, maternal exposure to viral or bacterial infections during pregnancy increases the likelihood of mental illness in the offspring (e.g., Estes & McAllister, 2016). Multiple mechanisms are proposed as influencing development, including immune responses and their impact on the fetal brain (e.g., Ratnayake et al., 2013).

Research on the immune system and psychiatric disorders has gone well beyond showing that there are correlations or predictive relations. For example, the research on depression has shown that induction of mood dysfunction (in healthy individuals) and responsiveness or failure to respond to intervention (e.g., via antidepressant medication) are related to challenges to and normalization of immune responses. Also, depression is associated with various autoimmune physical disorders such as diabetes (types 1 and 2), inflammatory bowel disease, psoriasis, rheumatoid arthritis, atherosclerosis, lupus, and multiple sclerosis (Maes et al., 2011), which are connected through immune and autoimmune system dysfunction.

It is one thing to identify possible mechanisms or early pathways leading to many disorders, but are there viable and feasible options for intervening at that stage or any evidence that disrupting the pathways reduces the onset (incidence) of some untoward physical or mental health outcome? Research on the immune systems and immunotherapy (e.g., in relation to physical disease) has proliferated enormously and has elaborated several other systems (e.g., microbiota in the gut, neurohumors) that are intricately intertwined. While we know of interventions that can decrease inflammation (e.g., anti-inflammatories such as aspirin!), this is not likely to be specific enough to disrupt pathways leading to mental disorders. On the other hand, aspirin actually has been proposed as a viable avenue of research, with evidence suggesting that it might well have direct impact on the underpinnings of various psychiatric disorders (Berk et al., 2013). I am not arguing for a particular intervention but rather for the broader effort of identifying mechanisms and processes that have multiple deleterious physical or mental health outcomes.

The pathways underlying psychiatric disorders are likely to be elaborated increasingly at the molecular and cellular levels to provide targets that are better known to lead to critical outcomes. Nonhuman animal models will continue to be needed to elaborate the steps from molecules to symptoms and then feasible targets to interrupt or controvert those steps (e.g., Tung et al., 2012). In such models, interventions could be shown to interrupt processes leading to a compromised immune system and inflammatory response. We are certainly not there yet, but we do know that social influences can materially harm or help the immune system. On the harm side, loneliness, ostracism, stress, and prolonged exposure to violence or abuse can compromise the immune system (e.g., Segerstrom & Miller, 2004). On the help side, social support and strong social networks can mitigate the effects of a compromised immune system (e.g., Eisenberger & Cole, 2012; Uchino, 2006). Here, too, we are hardly close to having recommendable interventions with an evidence base, yet my purpose is to promote further thinking about our intervention targets.

Current research in psychosocial interventions tends to focus on symptoms, key constructs that the conceptual approach dictates (e.g., self-defeating cognitions), some of which are known to correlate with dysfunction. We know so little about the mechanisms that explain precisely how interventions lead to change. Thus we are at a bit of a loss as to what elements of treatment can be optimized in what ways to promote therapeutic change. My aim is to redirect our focus from the mechanisms of treatment to mechanisms that predict multiple clinical dysfunctions, that is, transmechanisms. Inflammation and a compromised immune system certainly qualify as promising foci, given their relation to a variety of mental and physical health outcomes. Other broad targets of intervention might serve as well. For example, chronic stress has been known for some time to be linked to physical and mental disorders and substance abuse disorders (e.g., Brady & Sinha, 2005; Danese & Baldwin, 2017; Staufenbiel et al., 2013). Similarly, sleep and dysfunctional sleep play a perhaps surprisingly major role in the onset of multiple physical and mental disorders (e.g., Koffel et al., 2016; Ray & Travis, 2016). Here, too, I wish merely to raise the issue of targets that might precede the onset of multiple deleterious outcomes.

It is premature to suggest that we immediately turn to interventions targeting common origins of many different disorders. We do not have the evidence that making changes in the processes I have highlighted (e.g., immune system, stress, sleep) can be feasible or scalable, or will have a palpable impact. Also, the complexities of the immune and stress reactions and changes in sleep patterns and their interactions with other systems are now being elaborated in ways made possible by novel technologies. As advances are made, more research might give attention to broad antecedents to physical and mental disorders.

When "early intervention" is discussed, it usually refers to intervening in childhood or even before to prevent or minimize later clinical dysfunction. Typically, prevention efforts have targeted multiple risk factors for identifying children at risk for particular untoward outcomes and then trying to alter those risk factors that are malleable (e.g., exposure to abuse or neglect, cognitive stimulation and development, school, exposure to TV and video violence). Intervening on risk factors may be prudent, but risk factors are not necessarily involved in the causal sequence (Kraemer et al., 1997). I am arguing for early intervention in a related but slightly different way, namely, on common origins for which we are further along in our knowledge that they play a causal role in the unfolding of multiple dysfunctions later in life. We are looking for not only common risk factors but also one or more mechanisms by which the later dysfunction may emerge. Some of that information is likely to come from nonhuman animal studies, in which processes can be looked at carefully (e.g., gene knockout studies, tracking and interrupting brain circuitry). Common initial origins could have a broad impact on the burdens of both mental and physical health. I am arguing for targeting processes we know a bit about that have untoward physical and mental health outcomes. This is a step further than and provides a complement to focus on risk factors. This is also a step often neglected among researchers developing and testing psychosocial interventions.

Improving the Background or Base Level of Health

The immediate prior discussion focuses on potential pathways leading to broad and multiple outcomes of mental and physical disorders. This discussion is related but is broader in scope; it is about efforts to improve the general health of a nation. This is not separate from the search for transmechanisms and processes that we can target. Rather, this point focuses on the fact that we have sufficient information in some areas to make a difference in improving mental and physical health. Here, the target is not disorders per se but rather the overall level of health of a population or subpopulations. The rationale is obvious. If we can improve health, ideally there will be less need to contend with disorders and illnesses and less disability. This is a win-win situation because improved health would benefit individuals and also society at large (fewer DALYs, more reduced cost of acute and chronic care). Proverbs about prevention and its importance apply here, as reflected in the 1735 quote by the Benjamin Franklin (1706–1790), "An ounce [or 28.35 grams] of prevention is worth a pound [or 453.59 grams] of cure" (see Keil, 2011). The underlying rationale has served as the basis for services and funding for physical and mental health care and education that continue more than 280 years later. The value and logic of the approach are not at all new (e.g., Hatch, 1982) and continue to be promoted (e.g., Howell et al., 2016).

Three points deserve special emphasis in relation to the goals of this book. The first is whether there are interventions that could improve the overall health of a nation. Of course, there are several, and the most frequently discussed in the media but also in government resources (e.g., Centers for Disease Control and Prevention, WebMD) relate to diet, exercise, substance use and abuse, and meditation-mindfulness activities (e.g., yoga, tai chi, qigong). In terms of this first point, do we have options? Yes, the benefits of each of these has been demonstrated, at least in small-scale clinical trials.

The second point to emphasize is that we need know whether implementation of one or more general population health interventions is feasible. Feasibility might include whether special requirements (e.g., skilled instructor or trainer, special equipment, access to facilities that people must attend) are needed to deliver the intervention to individuals in everyday life. Each intervention I have mentioned varies in the extent to which someone else (e.g., special trainer) is needed both to motivate the participant and provide the needed expertise, but that maybe surmountable (by delivery using apps or DVD, which is the case, for example, with both diet and exercise). That "someone else" could be a virtual therapist who lives in "the cloud."

The third point is that we need to know whether we can make the interventions effective and feasible on the desired scale. This part is less clear and most relevant to the goals of this book. Many lifestyle interventions that could change the overall health of the nation are not promoted in a way that makes them optimally effective or scalable. Low-cost appeals and information are provided (e.g., bulletins from various government agencies, claiming a national day to stop or start some unconstructive or constructive habit). These are weak as interventions go. And for reasons discussed earlier in the chapter, we want weak interventions that are low cost, scalable, and have an impact (empirical evidence that they make a difference). Yet, in this context, we would want the intervention or one of a few interventions to diffuse throughout the population to actually reach large numbers and then to show some effect. "Diffuse throughout the population" suggests that social networking interventions would be especially useful in this regard (Rogers, 2003).

Exercise has some very valuable characteristics that may give this special status as an intervention to foster and promote health on a large scale. Among its characteristics are that:

- Benefits come from relatively small amounts of exercise;
- Many different activities qualify (e.g., from chores around the house to sports);
- Exercise can be used throughout the life span (at least childhood through old age);
- Individuals can choose and vary over time (e.g., within a week, over decades) what form the exercise will take; and
- Exercise can be done by oneself, in pairs, or in a group context, and any mix and match combination is fine.

I mentioned previously that in the United States, regular exercise is routinely omitted from daily activities in schools. Could we do more to make engaging in exercise easier (such as incentives, reduction in health care costs, reductions or elimination for copayment for medications, tax rebates, free memberships in health clubs that are conveniently located, food stamps redeemable for fresh produce, more "nudging," as that concept was discussed previously)?

Large-scale implementation can draw on policy, law, and legislation. Yet there can be a backlash if the intervention is perceived as too controlling and an infringement of individual rights. For example, taxing unhealthful foods and subsidizing healthful ones so that the latter are more affordable has been evaluated as a viable means of improving diet and decreasing obesity (with likely impacts on diabetes, cancer, and heart disease). The practice in various forms has been effective (e.g., Powell et al., 2013; Thow, Downs, & Jan, 2014). In some cases, special sales taxes have been widely adopted. For example, in the United States, 34 states and the District of Columbia (Washington DC) levy taxes on sugar-sweetened soda sold through food stores, and in 39 states stores levy taxes on the soda sold from vending machines (most recent available data as of January 2014). Many other countries have instituted such taxes as well (e.g., France, Hungary, Mexico, Norway, South Africa, United Kingdom; WHO, 2016).

The policy of taxing foods is controversial to say the least. The weight of the evidence supports the finding that consumption decreases with the taxes (WHO, 2016). Yet the primary public concerns are not about the data but reflect how the policy interferes with individual freedom, choice, and autonomy (Kuchler, Tegene, & Harris, 2005; Pratt, 2012). Feasibility depends on acceptability of the intervention, actual adoption, and implementation. How the intervention is couched, presented, and rolled out, as well as the intervention itself, might influence whether we can expect adoption and therefore benefits from any large-scale intervention designed to help.

Many political and public considerations are involved in large-scale efforts to improve the health of a nation. A success story might be taken from cigarette smoking in the United States, in which taxes and prices of cigarettes have had an impact on overall rates of cigarette smoking. This might be a partial model for how such change comes about, although the campaign to decrease smoking involved many factors (e.g., litigation against cigarette producers for allegedly hiding information and for making cigarettes more addictive). Also, there was much in this particular story that was inherently adversarial. Perhaps most general health-improving interventions would not be able to draw on that model (e.g., whom does one sue for not making broccoli or Brussels sprouts widely available?). And when that model might be relevant (e.g., promotion of fast foods to children), industry can mount formidable resources to thwart departures from current practices. Indeed, the tax on soda with sugar led to predictable industry campaigns to fight the tax or reduce its scope.

The broad question is: What are the many everyday practices and lifestyles that might be fostered to improve both mental and physical health? All sorts of potential interventions are on the table: prenatal diet and health care, child care, wellness care, increasing breastfeeding, making some things much easier over the course of life (e.g., exercise opportunities, healthier eating), and more. These examples emphasize those interventions that might be provided in early child development. Of course, we would want viable alternatives that could reach diverse people at any and all points in their lives, including general health practices and options for one of the fastest growing subpopulations, older adults. But for any point in life, we want to identify interventions that can be scaled and reach people usually not served.

Practices in everyday life that might be mobilized to improve health are an insufficient criterion for guiding policy and indeed could present enormous problems. For example, engaging in sex and eating chocolate are two separate practices (i.e., not necessarily simultaneously, a study yet to be done) that have enormous health benefits. No doubt efforts to foster and increase these on a large scale might well be popular but slam into many other obstacles and problems. Obviously, I am not suggesting or implying all practices that might enhance health should be advocated, promoted, or used in the service of the goal of reducing the burdens of illness, both mental and physical. We would need guiding principles about what is a legitimate focus, what is acceptable within the values of a culture, as reflected in beliefs, policy, and law, and what ancillary consequences might influence the wisdom of their adoption. In addition, we would probably want to draw on two of the many steps that have guided the selection of best-buy interventions. Those steps include math modeling to estimate benefit to the target population, cost, affordability, and feasibility and then empirical evaluation to check if the model was a good approximation and whether in fact benefits accrued. By using a best-buy approach, we are selecting not merely seemingly good ideas but also evidence for their impact and evidence that they are feasible and can be scaled. A variety of reasonable ideas might not meet these criteria (e.g., broccoli for everyone, Mediterranean diet lunch packs for all schoolchildren, treadmills at all bus stops so people can exercise while they are waiting, under-the-desk elliptical trainers in the front of seats on busses, metros, trains, and airplanes).

General Comments

In summary, in an effort to reduce the burdens of mental illness, it is likely we would profit greatly from:

- Systematically developing weak, low-cost, evidence-based interventions that could be scaled;
- Considering physical and mental health together in developing and selecting interventions;
- Studying potential interventions that target common initial paths that lead or are linked to mental and physical disorders; and
- Improving the base level of health on a large social scale for drawing on a variety of interventions we know already to have great benefits (e.g., diet and exercise).

Broadly, we must expand our thinking in terms of available means to reduce the burdens of mental illness. For this latter purpose, the previous specific points are only samples to illustrate sweeping domains of what to consider. In fact, many of the specific points (improve diet and exercise, maternal nutrition of a nation) are not new at all. However, they are not integrated in an overall plan to prioritize those likely to have the most impact, to use interventions that are likely to maximize outcome, and to place them in an evaluative context (e.g., best-buy). There are new options to pursue, but the first line of attack is applying much more systematically and effectively those interventions for which we already have some evidence.

In passing I also wish to mention other avenues to improve the base level of health of a nation. There are within health care several influences that direct attention to positive and adaptive functioning rather than just the absence of physical or mental health problems. Concepts such as well-being and happiness are two examples of such foci. Both well-being and happiness are associated with health and longevity and adaptive functioning in everyday life (e.g., in social relations, employment, improved physical health care, social support) (e.g., Diener & Chan, 2011; Howell et al., 2016). A similar concept, referred to as *recovery,* connects directly in recommendations for evaluating treatments for physical and mental disorders (Leamy et al., 2011; SAMHSA, 2012). We want not only reduction or elimination of symptoms of disorders but also improved functioning, as reflected in having a purpose in one's life, being involved in meaningful relationships, and having optimism about the future. Indeed, these criteria may even be more relevant than symptom reduction in cases of chronic or debilitating conditions for which there can be little or no relief, in light of current knowledge about interventions.

I mention well-being and happiness here because they are relevant and would be a suitable focus for improving the base level of functioning in the global population. Yet the emphasis of this book is on reducing the burdens of mental disorders, and as part of that, my focus is on interventions with more direct application to those conditions and ways to actually deliver the interventions to reach people. This does not at all gainsay the significance of promoting well-being, but such stark untreated conditions (e.g., depression, substance abuse, suicide) demand that I give their care greater attention.

STEPPED CARE: HOW TO DEPLOY INTERVENTIONS AND MODELS OF DELIVERY

Stepped care is a term frequently used in the context of interventions and in both physical and mental health care. Stepped care is the notion that less intensive, less costly, and more readily applicable interventions are the place to begin, and one moves to more aggressive, costly, and specialized intervention only when needed. The concept of stepped care has been around for some time and continues to be advocated as a model for providing psychological interventions (e.g., Clark, 2011; Draper & O'Donohue, 2011; Haaga, 2000; Newman & Howard, 1986). In this section, I discuss stepped care in the familiar context of interventions but extend this more broadly to models of delivery.

Interventions and Their Sequencing

In many intervention studies, stepped care is used. Previously I mentioned an example of stepped care for the treatment of depression (Patel et al., 2010, 2011). The interventions and sequence included:

1. Psychoeducation;
2. Antidepressant medication or interpersonal psychotherapy for those who did not respond;
3. Both interventions if individuals do not respond to just one of those; and
4. Continuation of both interventions and referral to a specialist as needed.

From this and many applications, we know the model of stepped care can be used effectively as a way of sequencing different interventions. Yet routine care in the context of mental health services does not systematically include stepped care beyond gross and accidental exceptions. By gross and accidental, I mean they are blunt and not programmed or used systematically. Here is one variation on the steps. A person may begin by speaking to a friend about a psychological problem (anxiety, sadness), then perhaps to one's general practitioner for support or medication, and then to a mental health professional, most likely in the context of the dominant model of therapy. This is extremely haphazard and depends on the initiative, resolve, and persistence of the person with the problem or his or her close relatives. Yet one can see the approximate "steps" to more intensive, effortful, and likely costly care.

An informal and haphazard stepped care can also be seen in relation to the use of inpatient hospitalization for someone with a mental disorder. Here is a variation of that. First we try to treat a given individual with a mental disorder (when intervention is applied at all) in an outpatient setting in individual or perhaps group sessions and with medication. If that fails, then the intervention is augmented with (or completely switches to) placement of the individual in a community living setting where he or she can be monitored and receive a variety of services and continued medication. The community settings are less expensive to run than are hospitals and are staffed with individuals who are not as costly as medical doctors in fully staffed hospitals. Medical and mental health professionals oversee the facilities but are usually not on the premises full time. If that intervention fails because the patient needs more intensive services, then hospital care might be added (day treatment in a psychiatric hospital, but return at night to the community setting). In the day treatment setting, many more intensive interventions can be provided (multiple medications, psychological services, activities intended to be therapeutic). Finally, if that still is not sufficient, the patient may be hospitalized as a full-time resident. In principle, the sequence I have noted is roughly accurate, but there is rarely any systematic progression or oversight of that progression. Also, the sequence entails more costly and restrictive interventions but lacks evidence that an intervention later in the sequence is any more effective. Indeed, it is likely that the sequence will stop completely because a step (service) is not available or is too costly.

The progression from one mental health intervention to another also is interrupted and ended by the patient's entry into other systems. For example, it is possible that an individual will be pulled out by the criminal justice system in light of some crime and be placed in jail or prison or be out on the street as a homeless person, coming under occasional social service care or just neglect. In short, there is stepped care in mental health at some broad conceptual and obvious level, where in principle one can obtain less intense before more intense services, but there is no formal systematic execution that is in place routinely. And, of course, the whole notion of care begins with the problem of there being no first step for most people, that is, the vast majority of individuals in need of care receive absolutely nothing for their mental health problems.

Among the problems for implementing stepped care is that mental health services in the United States are analogous to zone defense in basketball or football rather than "man-to-man" (person-to-person) defense. In zone defense, one is responsible for anyone (e.g., the patient) that enters one's zone (e.g., comes to one's clinic or hospital), but after they are out of one's zone, they are in someone else's (zone) and become their responsibility. And when treatment stops in my zone, that other zone (e.g., no care at all, homelessness, prison) I am not even likely to know. Zones can work great in athletics. They do not serve patients very well. In contrast to zones, person-to-person care would be following patients wherever they went and then helping them be placed in the next intervention as part of stepped care. Someone (e.g., a case worker) should oversee the patients to make sure they are placed where needed and placed into another care service if one service is not working. There might be zones (e.g., if a patient leaves the state or province and there is not continuity of services or organizations in the new setting). Here, we would be concerned about passing the baton, a separate matter.

Integrated care, discussed in Chapter 5, would enable focus on the person and avoid the problems with a zone defense approach. Integrated care is still not the rule, and all integrated care services do not serve all needs. Even so, integrated care, if the rule rather than the exception, would be a suitable place to begin stepped care for the group that attends such a setting.

Let us return to psychotherapy and the dominant model of its delivery and how stepped care fits there. Currently, for individuals seeking treatment for depression, cognitive therapy and interpersonal psychotherapy are two EBPIs. Typically, these are individually administered by a professional in a clinic setting (dominant model). The dominant model reaches so few people, and delivery of these interventions at a clinic is hugely expensive. So we asked a stepped-care question: "Are there opportunities to intervene to reduce and treat depression effectively without moving to these individually based therapies, at least as an initial point (step) of departure?" Stepped-care would consider a range of interventions that could be applied as needed if a less costly intervention did not achieve change.

Where can we begin with low-cost interventions that might reach large swaths of individuals and be effective? Two come to mind merely to make the point and again in the context of treating depression. In addition, we can draw on concepts from prior discussions, such as one about weak interventions. Perhaps in a stepped-care model, a psychoeducational intervention might be systematically tried as the initial point of departure. This would consist of telling people about depression and what they can do about it on their own, including activities in which they engage; it would be easy to add an app to provide information, assessment, or even more. We know already that information and education in relation to the intervention of disorders (or as behavior-changing techniques more generally) typically are weak in the magnitude of change and number of individuals affected, as interventions go. Yet in a stepped-care model that is not necessarily problematic at all, it is likely that some number of individuals in need of intervention would be helped sufficiently with systematic efforts to provide psychoeducation. Psychoeducation can be delivered widely through many media (e.g., smartphone, TV, brochures, the Web) that capitalize on social networks, provided where people are in everyday life (e.g., grocery stores, shopping malls, doctors' offices), adapted culturally (e.g., language, customs, models of person pictured on the medium), made available 24/7, and if needed disseminated by lay individuals rather than professionals. These methods of delivery are not merely ways to provide psychoeducation but can also draw on behavior-changing tools such as individualized feedback (on smartphone), a personalized avatar, praise, feedback, and small talk from voiced programmed to help, and so on. In short, psychoeducation can be provided and bolstered by technology and make this more than just dolling out information. If that is not sufficient, an easy and logical next step would be to move to Web-based intervention exercises, perhaps with a little help from a lay counselor or completely by self-help.

As another possibility, physical exercise might be promoted as a first or early line of attack to intervene for depression (but other domains of mental disability as well). There is already some evidence about its effectiveness clinically in humans, as well as basic nonhuman animal research to suggest some of the mechanisms through which exercise operates in depression (e.g., Deslandes et al., 2009; Duman et al., 2008; Wolff et al., 2011). Also, as mentioned earlier, exercise can take many different forms to suit individual tastes and preferences and can vary across the developmental spectrum (e.g., children through older adults). Again, we would not expect exercise to eliminate clinical depression for all or even most individuals, but it may have a place in a stepped-care model. With accumulated data on responsiveness, individuals for whom this step might be especially effective (or not) could be identified and predicted. I have discussed stepped care as if one began with a single intervention (e.g., psychoeducational communication or exercise), but there might well be a package (combination) of a couple of low-cost interventions that are combined for that initial step and ideally the opportunity for people to choose their own first step.

Stepped care develops a sequence of interventions that vary in effort and cost. Other considerations need to be taken into account in how they are sequenced and implemented. The nature of the clinical problem as one consideration is critical. A given client might not necessarily go through the sequence in order, or through the steps from a low-cost "lite" intervention to one that is costlier, effortful, and intensive. For example, we do not take a depressed suicidal adolescent or adult and say, "Let us see what a couple of brochures about depression and suicide could do for you first—read these and then we will talk to see if you need more." Criteria would be needed to place individuals at a given point on the continuum of the interventions included in the steps for a clinical problem or to meet criteria to be out of the continuum altogether. Moderator research might well be helpful in deciding where in a stepped-care sequence of intervention is an optimal place to begin a client given the larger profile of the client's full set of clinical problems, impairment, and resources (e.g., family, friends). These are all important clinical research topics. What is missing now is stepped-care thinking in routinely providing clinical services and programs of research designed to establish the steps themselves, their effectiveness, and under what conditions to jump from one step to another. Again, psychosocial intervention research, working in the dominant model, has neglected the focus on a sequence of interventions that could be applied.

In one sense, it might seem true that most people currently receive the least costly intervention to administer, that is, nothing.[7] On those rare occasions in which one does receive formal psychological treatment, the path is a leap (rather than stepped) from no intervention to the dominant model of care, which is way too expensive and unavailable to have much effect on very many people. Much could be done to treat and reduce the burden of mental illness by moving to expanded, more disseminable, and stepped-care interventions.

Models of Delivery and Their Sequencing

Stepped care involves dual considerations of not only the intervention technique but also the model of delivery. That is, models of delivering a given intervention may vary considerably in effort and cost. For example, we can consider an intervention (e.g., cognitive behavior therapy) and, holding that "constant" for a moment, consider the different ways that might be provided. The different ways, or models of delivery, can be conceived in a stepped-care fashion and be deployed as such. Thus the intervention might be provided by self-help (e.g., online, DVDs, an app), partial help with a lay counselor (e.g., on line, in person), and then at the extreme if and as needed with a professional mental health worker. I kept the intervention constant for this example, just to isolate the model and to help conceptualize stepped care beyond using different interventions.

Novel models I mentioned often include novel interventions, so the distinction is not always clear, and it need not be. For example, we might consider models I covered (e.g., best buy, task shifting, entertainment-education) as varying in cost or effort. In terms of making policy or reimbursement decisions, stepped care might favor beginning where feasible with models that are less costly and effortful (e.g., in terms of professional time) and more scalable. There are multiple dimensions in characterizing the cost and effort of a model, and lining them up for a clear sequence of what model to use before another is not at all straightforward. Yet the thinking of stepped care in developing models is a useful way to expand our thinking about exerting impact.

For example, developing interventions that can be provided by visual media (movies, DVDs) would initially be costly but would be applicable to millions as a model of delivery. Entertainment-education discussed previously was one model that was adaptable to different problems (e.g., in relation to health) and cultures. As a model, entertainment would be costly to produce but low cost when averaged over time and across people exposed to the intervention after the materials were prepared. That might vary on the problem focus (e.g., depression or physical and mental health at once in some way). Web-based self-help models of delivery might be lower in cost to produce and, like entertainment-education, could be quite scalable. Finally, changes in social policy, law, advertising, and taxes have characterized some of the best-buy interventions. These are institutional interventions put into place and by their nature are quite scalable. Changes in social policy and law have costs and effort that can vary greatly because they may involve delivery, enforcement, and mechanisms of implementation.

In short, models of delivery also should be considered from the perspective of cost, effort, and scalability. A given intervention might be provided in different ways, and ways that they are selected might be sequenced. Considering options among the interventions and among the models of delivery and adapting these to local conditions mean that adopting stepped care is not straightforward. Yet efforts to implement stepped care themselves could be sequenced in a stepped fashion. A given model could be trialed on a relatively small scale (e.g., a state or province) or in some unit controlled by local, state, or federal governments and then revised and extended more broadly with initial data about the cost, feasibility, and impact.

SUMMARY AND CONCLUSIONS

The use of novel models of providing clinical services that actually reach people in need is one way to expand our perspectives on reducing the burdens of mental illness. There are other ways to expand our thinking, perspectives, and research on interventions toward the same end, including developing weak treatments that are low cost and scalable, giving special attention to individuals who contribute to the greatest burdens of mental illness, implementing interventions that are likely to have an impact on both physical and mental health, identifying and focusing on transmechanisms that underscore many different outcomes, and improving the base level of health in society. Stepped care was introduced as a way of proceeding not only in the usual way this is discussed (stepped-care interventions) but also in how these interventions are delivered (stepped-care models of delivery). Considering stepped care more routinely in the provision of mental health services was part of the rationale for advocating more attention to weaker but scalable interventions. Stepped care requires much more research to identify at least a few steps, showing that a later (costlier, intensive) step is needed and makes a difference, as well as how to sequence the steps based on the disorder and other characteristics the clients present. Although stepped care is not a new idea, it has yet to be well studied in research or systematically implemented in clinical practice, beyond the blunt and haphazard ways I have mentioned (e.g., outpatient treatment before hospitalization; medication for depression before electroconvulsive shock therapy). We would profit from programs of intervention research that were designed to identify evidence-based interventions along a stepped-care continuum.

In this chapter, very concrete ways of expanding our perspectives were provided on the investigation and implementation of interventions. The next chapter looks at the overall goal of reducing the burdens of mental illness more broadly. The challenge is conceptualized in ways that reveal its complexities and relation to other social ills, but also in ways that will help to suggest possible remedies.

10

Conceptualizing the Challenge and Moving to Solutions

Novel models of delivering treatment and novel foci of intervention development and implementation could have a great impact on scaling up interventions and reaching people in need of services. These subjects of the previous chapters call for a move away from the dominant means of delivering treatment but also the dominant way of investigating treatment (e.g., more research on weak treatments and on sequences of treatments to develop stepped care). Yet more is needed to reduce the burdens of mental illness.

In the present chapter, the challenge is addressed at different levels, beginning with broad conceptualizations of the challenge of reducing the burdens of mental illness. The conceptualizations alert us to context, complexities, and characteristics that influence how to proceed to solutions. From these conceptualizations, the chapter moves to more concrete actions to reduce the burdens of mental illness, including some initiatives in place and already underway. Additional ways are suggested, with the goal of moving to palpable solutions that can have an enduring impact.

CONCEPTUALIZING THE CHALLENGE

Reducing the burdens of mental illness can be conceptualized in multiple ways that place the goal in broader contexts and also help frame how we might proceed toward solutions. The two perspectives presented here are referred to as "wicked problems" and "grand challenges." They provide context, sensitize us to many issues beyond the context of mental illness and its challenges, and also reveal steps that may have impact.

Wicked Problems

The challenge of reducing the burdens of mental illness is broad, global, and multifaceted and requires more than merely extending some new models of treatment. Our understanding of the challenge can be further informed by introducing the notion of *wicked problems* (Horn & Weber, 2007; Rittel & Webber, 1973). The term is used in policymaking, social planning, and business and captures the novel features of many challenges. Wicked problems are likely to have several of the characteristics highlighted in Box 10.1. What we gain by referring to a challenge as a wicked problem is clarity about the fact that it requires novel ways of thinking in relation to problem formulation, evaluation, and intervention strategies.

One characteristic of a wicked problem is that it is likely to be related to other challenges that themselves may also be wicked problems. Table 10.1 samples some familiar challenges in society that are wicked problems and related to reducing the burdens of mental illness. Challenges listed in the table (again, only a sample of those that might have been listed) have diverse and dynamic interrelations with mental illness and its care. Thus some are associated (correlated) with mental illness; others exert a causal role in or are consequence of mental illness. And still others may show bidirectional effects and multiple relations because they include multiple components.

For example, consider victimization by violence as a challenge (in Table 10.1). Actually, victimization takes many different forms (e.g., domestic violence by an intimate partner, child physical and sexual abuse, bullying), each of which might well be distinguished here as it is in research as its own challenge (or as its own wicked problem). However, various forms of interpersonal violence are quite interrelated. For example, a person who is a victim of one type of violence or abuse is at much greater risk for being a victim of another type of abuse. And a perpetrator of one type of violence or abuse is at greater risk for being a perpetrator of another type of abuse. For present purposes and to make the point about one challenge being related to the burden of mental illness, consider the broader class without the many sources of victimization from violence.

Victimization in its many forms is associated with all sorts of later mental health problems, including increased risk for depression, posttraumatic stress disorder and other forms of anxiety, substance abuse disorders, psychoses, eating disorders, criminal behavior, and suicidal ideation, attempt, and completion (e.g., Coker et al., 2002; Holt, Buckley, & Whelan, 2008; Jonas et al., 2014; Lindert et al., 2014). In addition, children exposed to one or more forms of violence in the home (e.g., witnessing domestic violence, being physically or sexually abused) have a greatly elevated risk for psychiatric disorder later in life (e.g., Franzese

Box 10.1

Salient Characteristics of Wicked Problems

- There is no single, definitive, or simple formulation of the problem;
- The problem is not likely to be the result of an event (e.g., tsunami, hurricane), but rather a set of intersecting trends that co-occur and coinfluence each other;
- The problem has embedded in it other problems—including other wicked problems;
- There is no one solution—no single, one-shot effort that will eliminate the problem;
- The problem is never likely to be solved;
- Multiple stakeholders are likely to be involved, and this fact leads to multiple formulations of what "really" is the problem and therefore what are legitimate or appropriate solutions;
- Values, culture, politics, and economics are likely to be involved in the problem and in possible strategies to address the problem;
- Information as a basis for action will be incomplete because of the uniqueness of the problem and the complexities of its interrelations with other problems; and
- The problem is likely to be unique and therefore does not easily lend itself to previously tried strategies.

Note: These and other characteristics emerged in the context of urban planning (see Rittel & Webber, 1973) but have been extended to business, social, and public policy and to many familiar social problems, such as poverty, delivery of health care, crime, the HIV/AIDS epidemic, and terrorism. The list draws from multiple sources (Conklin, 2006; Horn & Weber, 2007; www.strategykinetics.com).

et al., 2014; Geffner, Igelman, & Zellner, 2014). This is barely the tip of the iceberg of the impact of violence on psychiatric disorders and complexity of the relations and spread of effects (e.g., victimization and violence are passed on intergenerationally, victimization greatly increases risk for physical disorders and early death later in life, and individuals with mental disorders are at greater risk for being victimized). Yet this demonstrates my point about the interrelation of broad challenges. We can look at reducing the burden of mental illness on its own merit, but we can see even with these brief comments that the challenge is connected to another challenge.

Violence exposure leading to or associated with mental health problems may be intuitive in part because they are stereotypically connected in the minds of many people (i.e., the myth that all or most mentally ill individuals are more violent than non–mentally ill individuals). Consider another challenge that at first blush might seem to be more of a stretch: climate change, which has strong and multiple connections to mental illness (Clayton et al., 2017). Climate change encompasses

Table 10.1 REDUCING THE BURDEN OF MENTAL ILLNESS AS A WICKED PROBLEM RELATES TO MANY OTHER CHALLENGES AS SAMPLED HERE

Challenge or Other Wicked Problem	Brief Sample Connecting This to Mental Illness	Sample References of Support
Poverty	See text for a description	See text
War	Increased posttraumatic stress disorder (PTSD), depression, and suicidality among soldiers who participate in war Increase of these mental disorders among civilians who are victims in war-torn areas, including rape of women, displacement from one's home (e.g., loss of home, migration), loss of loved ones, and physical disability from being a casualty	Berntsen et al. (2012) Loncar et al. (2014) Pompili et al. (2013)
Climate change	See text for a description	See text
Overpopulation	Associated with climate change, poverty, crime, and victimization (other challenges) and their consequences and including less adequate living conditions, increased poverty, food insecurity, victimization, more neighborhood crime, and poor access to physical health care, all of which increase the rates of mental disorders, including trauma, depression, and others	El-Sayed & Galea (2015) McMichael & Butler (2011)
Pollution (both air and water)	Increase in a range of psychiatric disorders, including autism, as a function of air pollutant concentration Low lead levels (water, air) are associated with attention-deficit disorder and intellectual disability	Grandjean & Landrigan (2014) Oudin et al. (2016) Shiue (2015)
Terrorism	Trauma to civilians from illness, injury, and death Being displaced from one's home, witnessing and experiencing violence (e.g., killing of one's relatives, rape), exposure to torture, loss of basic living resources such as food, water, and health services Increased risk for PTSD, depression, and acute stress disorder	Bleich et al. (2003) Canetti et al. (2014) Steel et al. (2009)

(*continued*)

Table 10.1 CONTINUED

Challenge or Other Wicked Problem	Brief Sample Connecting This to Mental Illness	Sample References of Support
Displacement and refugee status of children	Trauma, stress, associated disruption in all living circumstances, low resources for health, unsanitary conditions, victimization, and lack of protection all increase risk for mental and physical disorders later, especially PTSD and depression	Fazel et al. (2005, 2012) Taylor et al. (2014)
Crime	Crime and mental disorders overlap in many risk factors and correlates, including low socioeconomic status, homelessness, lack of jobs, substance abuse, and victimization Victims of crimes experience trauma, acute stress, and disability	Kilpatrick & Acierno (2003) Lorenk et al. (2012)
Victimization from violence (e.g., domestic violence, bullying of children exposure to violence, abuse, and neglect)	See text for a description	See text
Single-parenting and birth of child to a solo parent	Often associated with other challenges in this table, such as poverty Increased risk for physical and mental disorders, substance abuse, and suicide of the child; fewer resources, more stress, and more poverty among single parents	McMunn et al. (2001) Weitoft et al. (2003)

NOTES: This table abbreviated in many ways to make the point about the interrelations of multiple challenges. More challenges could readily be added; also the associations with mental illness (center column) would be expanded as well with more disorders and different disorders over the lifespan. Each challenge is a major area of research and many connections and types of studies have elaborated multiple facets beyond the scope and goals of the table.

many stressors, including increases in ambient temperature (warming), more extremes of weather (e.g., severity and number of hurricanes, flooding, and draughts), food shortages and hunger related to weather extremes, and rising sea levels (leading to forced migrations, loss of homes and income). The food shortages and forced migrations alone are expected to increase violent conflict, a connection well described elsewhere (Brinkman & Hendrix, 2011). Violent conflicts are associated with displacement from one's home, but other consequences of climate change also have that effect (e.g., from rising sea levels, increased weather catastrophes). These consequences "cascade" or spill over to other challenges (e.g., see poverty, war, displacement in Table 10.1) and greatly reduce mental and physical health care services for those who are displaced (e.g., Barnett & Adger, 2007). Climate changes are already known to be associated with a range of mental disorders, including posttraumatic stress disorder, depression, psychoses, suicidality, and others (e.g., Bourque & Willox, 2014; Chand & Murthy, 2008; Doherty & Clayton, 2011; Padhy et al., 2015). Many of the facets of climate change (e.g., draughts, hunger, hurricanes) were studied in relation to mental health problems long before climate change became a public concern. For example, climate change is strongly associated with increases in air pollution, which is already known to influence brain development, increases in physical and mental disorders, and early death (e.g., Calderón-Garcidueñas et al., 2015; D'Amato et al., 2014; Ramanathan & Feng, 2009). Perhaps the impact of climate change on physical health would be intuitive, but the impact is even broader than we might expect, leading to increases in mental disorders and decreases (from displacement) in needed services.

As a final illustration of related challenges, poverty is among the more well-studied challenges because of its very broad impact on physical and mental health, educational attainment, employment, adaptive functioning, and earlier than expected death. *Poverty* is a huge umbrella term for a variety of conditions: malnutrition, food insecurity, lack of access to clean water, living in polluted environments, inadequate housing, stress associated with lack of finances, frequent accidents, and other risk factors associated with poor physical health or safety protections—each of these is consistently associated with mental disorders (Lund et al., 2011; McMillan et al., 2010; Patel & Kleinman, 2003). The full range of disorders is evident, including depression, anxiety, schizophrenia, substance abuse disorders, suicidal ideation and attempt, and more. These relations have been demonstrated across diverse ethnic groups within the United States and among people from many different countries. (e.g., Gavin et al., 2010; McMillan et al., 2010). The multifaceted disadvantages of poverty in relation to child physical and mental health and psychological development more broadly (brain, cognitive processes) have been studied extensively and well known for some time (e.g., Bradley & Corwyn, 2002; Korenman, Miller, & Sjaastad, 1995).

Each challenge (in Table 10.1) is a multifaceted topic studied by many experts from multiple disciplines, and each has scores of distinguishable subchallenges. For the purposes of my argument here, the idea is that the challenge of reducing the burdens of mental illness often is connected to many other challenges and social ills. I have simplified the nuances of the challenges here. For example, I did not discuss the fact that each of the challenges listed in Table 10.1 has a huge physical health impact in addition to its impact on mental health.

That reducing the burden of mental illness, a huge challenge in its own right, is intertwined with other challenges could be a cause for dismay and hopelessness, so how can we proceed in ways that will have an impact? After all, with this book I have focused on one fairly daunting challenge, only now to make explicit that this one challenge is intertwined with other challenges that arguably are as or indeed much more daunting. (Perhaps with this book we should include a coupon for antidepressants.) I could have downplayed the connections by mentioning multiple challenges and saying that many challenges overlap like multiple Venn diagrams, avoided further comment. Yet naming the reduction of the burdens of mental illness as a wicked problem provides helpful insights into how to proceed and what to expect along the way. It is not the case that to have an impact on the burdens of mental illness we need to address all the other challenges. Yet knowing that multiple challenges are interconnected has value as we proceed.

Here are some of the features of a wicked problem that may be useful as a point of departure. First, the nature of wicked problems, as I noted, is that there will be no single solution. I have conveyed the importance of using multiple models of delivering interventions that can reach people in need of mental health services. Multiple models are in keeping with the nature of wicked problems, that is, drawing on multiple solutions rather than expecting one to have a sufficient impact. The thinking from a wicked problem is even more expansive in keeping open the search for multiple solutions and strategies to intervene (avert, prevent, treat) mental health problems. One caution the wicked problem conceptualization raises is that we ought to be wary about arguing about the "best way" to proceed, if that will delay actually proceeding. The best way to proceed is not to look for the one best way; we need multiple solutions, none of which will be up to the challenge on its own.

Second, with a wicked problem, whatever solutions we implement are likely to be tried under conditions in which our data are not sufficient (see Horn & Weber, 2007). This point is critical, too, because we want the best data and the most pertinent data to guide us, but it will always be possible to ask: "Do we really know enough to act in ways that will have an impact on the problem?" In everyday life, we are familiar with this frustrating state of affairs—a treatment for a serious disease often involves so many unknowns, including the basic question of whether the treatment is really effective. Usually, we do not forgo treatment for ourselves or our relatives because of incomplete data, especially when the options can come down to proceeding on incomplete, poor, or no data or dying relatively soon.

Decision making is more complex and diffuse for wicked problems than for individual life decisions, so many more parties might be involved with different perspectives, agenda, and expectations for success. Moreover, the dire consequences that may result from not acting are not as clear or agreed on as someone dying, as noted in the everyday example I used previously. Thus wicked problems usually lack a sense of urgency or agreed-on urgency for those not directly experiencing consequences on a day-to-day basis. And policymakers who might be making the decisions can be extremely far removed from the day-to-day unless they have a personal stake in the matter. In any case, addressing the wicked problem of reducing the burdens of mental illness invariably will have the same incomplete data problem; we will not have the luxury of complete data, nor the understanding we would like as the basis of making critical decisions. We must move forward with what we have because not acting has its own deleterious consequences. This is the challenge of setting social policy and law, but that has strong other interests (e.g., lobbyists, industry) that can exert huge influence.

We must proceed knowing that by the nature of the problem and its scope, we will not seek the level of certainty of the data we would like. We proceed because of the significance of moving to action and the philosophy that it is better to light one candle than to curse the darkness. With wicked problems, we know at the outset that multiple candles need to be lighted if we are to expect an impact. But we can also anticipate multiple perspectives, disagreement, and competing views about how to move forward. That means that what some see as lighting one candle others may see as starting an uncontrollable fire with dire consequences. Wicked problems alert us to expect quite competing views on how to proceed, and perhaps to the fact that having the information we want is a luxury that should not serve as a basis for delaying. While those competing views are aired and discussed, with government officials often calling for a task force report of some kind, action is delayed, and often the apparent urgency that may have been felt is delayed and diluted by time. In general, the notion of a wicked problem helps us to see that reducing the burdens of mental illness is enmeshed with many other significant social problems, and to watch for potential mine fields in proceeding and enacting conclusions. We cannot expect to resolve the natural tensions and competing views before proceeding. Indeed, a broader social issue might be to develop guidelines further in terms of when and how to proceed (guiding principles) that weigh the uncertainty of the evidence, the likely impact of delaying action, and the benefits of specific strategies that could be tried now.

Grand Challenges

Another way to conceptualize the goal of reducing the burdens of mental illness is the concept of *grand challenges*. There is no single definition, but there are key characteristics, summarized in Box 10.2. Delineating a problem or focus as a grand challenge has several implications, including focusing attention on a major problem, setting that problem as a priority among many questions and challenges, identifying the specific barriers or the components that need to be addressed to meet or mitigate the challenge, identifying the needed resources (e.g., in personpower, agencies, funding), and helping to build collaborations among those who could help make an impact (e.g., business, political leaders, scientists, the public, the media). In addition, these features imply that progress can be made and that an impact is achievable after some critical barriers are resolved. In short, delineating a grand challenge makes clear the commitment needed to address a problem, to mobilize collective action, and to foster innovation.

Historically, the notion of a grand challenge is attributed to the mathematician David Hilbert (1862–1943), who listed a number of unsolved problems in mathematics (the number varied on his reflections and reconsideration but was 23 or 24) (Gray, 2000). Many of those mathematical problems have since been

Box 10.2

Key Characteristics of a Grand Challenge

- Selecting a well-defined problem often global in scope;
- Identifying breakthroughs, barriers, and obstacles needed to solve or overcome a significant problem;
- Focusing attention and mobilizing resources directed toward that problem (e.g., resources from many organizations, input from scientists and business leaders, involvement of multiple countries);
- Specifying the components that may be needed (subchallenges) to make progress on the larger problem;
- When possible, providing resources (funding, prizes) to incentivize further the focus on aspects of the challenge;
- No single, definitive, or simple formulation of the problem; and
- A problem that is not likely to be the result of an event (e.g., tsunami, hurricane), but rather a set of intersecting events.

For additional information, other sources are available (Grand Challenges, Canada, 2011; Varmus et al., 2003).

solved, but what is instructive for present purposes is the notion of delineating these problems as challenges. That delineation focused considerable effort among mathematicians and set the critical challenges as a priority.

The notion of grand challenges has been picked up extensively by international, national, and more local governing bodies and organizations, as well as by many disciplines and fields of study. Arguably one of the most, if not the most, prominent of these was initiated by the Bill & Melinda Gates Foundation, beginning in 2003, which was developed in collaboration with the National Institutes of Health. The Grand Challenges in Global Health initiative began with a process of selecting scientists and public health experts from multiple countries and soliciting broad input. More than 1,000 submissions from 75 different countries were obtained to identify the key questions. Through an extensive process of deliberation, further input, and more, the massive number was whittled down to a small list of 14 grand challenges, mostly focusing on infectious diseases. Box 10.3 lists these challenges to provide a view of their generality and specificity (see Varmus et al., 2003). Of course, identifying the challenges is an initial step. Moving toward their solution requires multiple collaborations and mechanisms for applying and receiving funds to address the challenges and then moving toward solutions. In the case of the Bill & Melinda Gates Foundation, a mechanism is well in place to fund promising work and to move to larger scale applications for the work that looks promising. The Foundation notes that Grand Challenges is a family of initiatives fostering innovation to solve key global health and development problems (http://gcgh.grandchallenges.org/).

Box 10.3

Grand Challenges in Global Health

To improve childhood vaccines:

1. Create effective single-dose vaccines that can be used soon after birth;
2. Prepare vaccines that do not require refrigeration; and
3. Develop needle-free delivery systems for vaccines.

To create new vaccines:

4. Devise reliable tests in model systems to evaluate live attenuated vaccines;
5. Solve how to design antigens for effective, protective immunity; and
6. Learn which immunological responses provide protective immunity.

To control insects that transmit agents of disease:

7. Develop a genetic strategy to deplete or incapacitate a disease-transmitting insect population; and
8. Develop a chemical strategy to deplete or incapacitate a disease-transmitting insect population.

To improve nutrition to promote health:

9. Create a full range of optimal bioavailable nutrients in a single staple plant species.

To improve drug treatment of infectious diseases:

10. Discover drugs and delivery systems that minimize the likelihood of drug-resistant microorganisms.

To cure latent and chronic infections:

11. Create therapies that can cure latent infections; and
12. Create immunological methods that can cure chronic infections.

To measure disease and health status accurately and economically in poor countries:

13. Develop technologies that permit quantitative assessment of population health status; and
14. Develop technologies that allow assessment of individuals for multiple conditions or pathogens at point-of-care.

See Varmus et al. (2003) for a discussion of these and the processes involved in their selection.

Often a grand challenge includes many components or subchallenges. For example, a consortium of organizations from multiple countries has taking on global mental health as a grand challenge (e.g., National Institute of Mental Health [NIMH], Global Alliance for Chronic Disease, Wellcome Trust, and other partners). This is referred to as the Global Mental Health Challenge and includes many subchallenges that form the overall goal. Various possible challenges submitted by individuals from many countries were rated by panels using an extensive process of input and repeated surveys. Morethan 40 challenges were identified as top priorities to improve global mental health (e.g., develop interventions than can be used by non–mental health specialists, strengthen the mental health expertise of all health care personnel) (see www.nimh.nih.gov/about/organization/gmh/grandchallenges/index.shtml). Box 10.4 presents a sample many of these to convey the types of challenges selected; many relate to issues we have discussed in the context of delivering treatments in novel ways (e.g., use of lay counselors for treatment, providing interventions in everyday settings).

Box 10.4

A Sample From the List of 40 Grand Challenges in Global Mental Health

1. Integrate core packages of mental health services into routine primary health care;
2. Reduce the cost and improve the supply of effective psychotropic drugs for mental, neurological, and substance use disorders;
3. Train health professionals in low- and middle-income countries to provide evidence-based care for children with mental, neurologic, and substance use disorders;
4. Provide adequate community-based care and rehabilitation for people with chronic mental illness;
5. Develop treatments for mental disorders for use by nonspecialist health workers with minimal training;
6. Develop school-based mental health promotion programs for children and adolescents;
7. Develop sustainable models to train and increase the number of culturally and ethnically diverse lay and specialist providers to deliver evidence-based services for mental, neurological and substance use disorders;
8. Improve access to evidence-based interventions (i.e., screening and treatment) for mental, neurological, and substance use disorders in populations affected by conflict and displacement;
9. Develop an evidence-based set of primary prevention interventions for a wide range of mental, neurological, and substance use disorders;
10. Integrate mental, neurological, and substance use disorders into the chronic disease agenda at all levels of government;

11. Reduce the duration of untreated illness by developing culturally sensitive early interventions for mental, neurological, and substance use disorders across settings;
12. Conduct screening for mental, neurological, and substance use disorders during routine primary health care visits;
13. Develop locally appropriate strategies to eliminate childhood abuse and enhance child protection;
14. Increase capacity in low- and middle-income countries by creating regional centers for mental health research, education, training, and practice that incorporate the views and needs of local people;
15. Develop mobile and IT technologies (e.g., telemedicine) to increase access to evidence-based care for mental, neurological, and substance use disorders;
16. Establish and implement minimum health care standards for mental, neurological, and substance use disorders around the world;
17. Develop national child and adolescent mental health policies;
18. Redesign health systems to integrate mental, neurological, and substance use disorders with other chronic diseases;
19. Develop methods to improve parenting skills and promote secure attachment with caregivers in infancy and childhood; and
20. Develop interventions to reduce the long-term negative impact of low childhood socioeconomic status on cognitive ability and mental health.

Note: This list is only a sample of the 40 challenges. Perhaps noteworthy is how many of the challenges relate to other significant social (wicked) problems, including violence against children (#13) and poverty (#20). (For the full list of the 40 challenges, please see www.nimh.nih.gov/about/organization/gmh/grandchallenges/index.shtml.)

I mention the Global Mental Health Challenge, but of course there are many challenges facing societies around the world. These are frequently delineated specifically as grand challenges and placed on the agenda of worldwide organizations (e.g., World Health Organization, United Nations), government agencies (e.g., within the United States, the Centers for Disease Control and Prevention [CDC], US Aid From the Americas), and many nongovernment foundations and institutes (e.g., Bill & Melinda Gates Foundation, Kavli Neuroscience Discovery Institute). Examples of the foci of grand challenges include global climate change, crime, sex and drug trafficking, cancer, overpopulation, premature births, teaching all children to read, and eliminating the HIV/AIDS epidemic. Many disciplines and fields of study (e.g., engineering, robotics, ecosystems and the environment, agriculture and farming, preservation of wildlife, economics and social sciences, and many other areas) also identify grand challenges as a way to set priorities for the next several years among the many areas studied within that discipline. I draw attention to the notion of a grand challenge because global mental health is already part of international priorities. As important, I mention the concept because of what it is designed to accomplish, namely, mobilizing effort, expertise, and resources toward a goal or set of goals. That is certainly important in the goal set for this book of reducing the burdens of mental illness.

MOVING FORWARD TOWARD CONCRETE SOLUTIONS

The notion of wicked problems hovers at a high level of abstraction and alerts us to the interrelations among various challenges, multiple perspectives in framing the challenges and therefore the solutions, the incompleteness of data, and other features that are useful as we move forward to solutions. The notion of grand challenges is much more focused and in ways that convey precisely what is needed to have an impact on a specific target. As evident in this discussion, both perspectives provide useful information.

Illustrations of Models and Progress

Among the benefits of the grand challenge approach is that scores of subchallenges are often identified. These become more specific subgoals and questions that narrow the focus and goals. There now have been efforts to take up many more health challenges, with a primary emphasis on physical health. I provide three examples that move from circumscribed, to broader, to very broad efforts to address health burdens.

ZERO SUICIDE

The first illustration and most circumscribed of my examples addresses suicide. Suicide is the 10th leading cause of death for all Americans (CDC, 2015), and our overall rate of suicide is increasing (Curtin, Warner, & Hedegaard, 2016). Apart from the direct tragic loss that suicide reflects, family members of individuals who commit suicide are at much greater risk for serious mental and physical disorders and earlier than expected death, including suicide, following a relative's suicide (Erlangsen et al., 2017; Mueller et al., 2015; Pitman et al., 2014).

Zero Suicide is a collaborative program (the US Surgeon General and the National Action Alliance for Suicide Prevention, Suicide Prevention Resource Center with support from the Substance Abuse and Mental Health Services Administration [SAMHSA]) to make reduction of suicide a national priority (SAMHSA, 2016). Box 10.5 summarizes the goals and priorities of the program. The table shows that a specific target goal has been selected. The Zero Suicide program begins with the view that suicide deaths for individuals under care within health and behavioral health systems are preventable (http://zerosuicide.sprc.org/about). In addition, to have impact a system-wide approach is needed that goes well beyond that context.

The program includes several essential elements (see Box 10.5). Several sources of support to help implement these elements are provided and include providing a toolkit, which consists of a collection of information, tools, resources, and

Box 10.5

The Mission of the National Action Alliance for Suicide Prevention

Vision: The National Action Alliance for Suicide Prevention envisions a nation free from the tragic experience of suicide.

Mission: To advance the *National Strategy for Suicide Prevention* (NSSP; Office of the Surgeon General, 2012) by:

- Championing suicide prevention as a national priority;
- Catalyzing efforts to implement high-priority objectives of the NSSP; and
- Cultivating the resources needed to sustain progress.

Goal: To save 20,000 lives in five years.

Essential Elements of Suicide Care
Seven essential elements were selected:

1. Lead—Create a leadership-driven, safety-oriented culture committed to dramatically reducing suicide among people under care. Include survivors of suicide attempts and suicide loss in leadership and planning roles;
2. Train—Develop a competent, confident, and caring workforce;
3. Identify—Systematically identify and assess suicide risk among people receiving care;
4. Engage—Ensure every individual has a pathway to care that is both timely and adequate to meet his or her needs. Include collaborative safety planning and restriction of lethal means;
5. Treat—Use effective, evidence-based treatments that directly target suicidal thoughts and behaviors;
6. Transition—Provide continuous contact and support, especially after acute care; and
7. Improve—Apply a data-driven quality improvement approach to inform system changes that will lead to improved patient outcomes and better care for those at risk.

Source: http://actionallianceforsuicideprevention.org/about-us.

activities for health care leaders to assist them in implementing the seven elements of Zero Suicide (http://zerosuicide.sprc.org/about). An annual meeting is held to provide training in the seven elements and to support organizations that might adopt and adapt the tools and resources. Technical consultation is readily available to help programs get started or move forward with the tools. Special workshops are available to support work on specific facets of the problem. For example, an online course is available for health care professionals working in emergency departments. The course teaches workers how to conduct screening, assessment, and brief interventions, such as safety planning and lethal means counseling. Thus setting priorities and goals is followed by extensive practical guidelines and hands-on assistance.

The scope of the effort and involvement of many resources are impressive. A sample includes separate efforts to provide materials and interventions to reach high-risk groups (e.g., veterans, Native American and Alaskan Native youth), to implement programs in settings in daily life (e.g., the workplace), and to involve several segments of society that could have an impact (e.g., faith leaders and the clergy) (SAMHSA, 2016). There are also extensive grant programs to fund efforts to reduce suicide and attempts in youth, including 50 states and 47 Native American tribes. NIMH also has a grant program (referred to as Zero Suicide) to support large-scale projects, cost-benefit analyses of various interventions, and evaluation of stepped care—all aimed at reducing risk.

Among the advantages of delineating a priority at a national level is to mobilize multiple agencies and resources. Also, materials and interventions are available that can be deployed as suited to the various conditions evident in individual states and their services. The range of services and interventions is extensive. For example, SAMSHA has a 24-hour confidential hotline (National Suicide Prevention Lifeline) that has helped more than 6 million people; individuals can text or chat live with a crisis counselor. Also, SAMSHA has provided a free app (Suicide Safe; http://store.samhsa.gov/apps/suicidesafe/) to help clinicians address suicide risk. I cannot elaborate the full range of materials available, but my comments convey an extensive effort to scale the interventions (e.g., all states, territories) and to reach high-risk and neglected groups and people in everyday settings, as well as those who are seen in health care facilities. An independent evaluation of facets of the program (counties conducting legal service trainings) showed reductions in suicides among youth compared with matched comparison counties (SAMSHA, 2016).

Winnable Battles

An excellent example of an effort to reduce burdens of many problems emanates from the CDC and is referred to as *Winnable Battles* (www.cdc.gov/winnable-battles/). This initiative "focused on several high-burden areas with known, effective, evidence-based strategies where progress could be made in a relatively short timeframe" (CDC, 2016b, p. 4). The foci included

- tobacco use;
- nutrition, physical activity, and obesity (increase breastfeeding, reduce childhood obesity);
- food safety (reduce foodborne illness);
- motor vehicle injuries;
- teen pregnancy;
- HIV in the United States; and
- health-care associated infections (e.g., contracting infections while in a hospital).

Criteria for selection included a health problem that caused a significant burden, affected many people, and incurred costs, for which there existed effective strategies that could help, and which had the prospect of achieving an impact within a relatively brief time frame (e.g., within one to four years). This was a program conducted in conjunction with all 50 states, Washington DC, and the US territories.

For example, tobacco use was selected because it is the leading cause of preventable death in the United States. Currently, approximately 40 million people in the United States smoke cigarettes; approximately 480,000 deaths per year result, with approximately 41,000 of these resulting from exposure to secondary smoke. The CDC worked with states in multiple ways to help with existing programs involving public awareness using a Tips From Former Smokers (TIPS) campaign that fostered use of quitlines, working with states to enforce bans on tobacco advertising, promotion, sponsorships, and raising tobacco taxes. Comprehensive programs were viewed as a "best buy" and focused on diverse facets of the problem (e.g., promoting cessation of smoking, preventing initiation of smoking, eliminating exposure to smoke). Essentially, public education bolstered by policies and laws as part of a large package of interventions was conducted state by state. Targets were set in relation to reductions in smoking but also in promotion of policies that would encompass more of the states and territories. Over the course of the program, cigarette smoking among adults fell from approximately 21 percent (in 2008) to 15 percent (in 2015). Even greater decreases were achieved for smoking among adolescents (from 20 percent to 11 percent). Also, when the program began, 37 percent of the US population were covered by (subject to) smoke-free laws; this increased to 59 percent by the end of the program.

A few points are especially noteworthy. First and importantly, the CDC was responsible for the program, which means that remarkable expertise, financial and administrative resources, and a long history of evaluation and intervention were available to influence public health. The Winnable Battles program was a special effort within that agency to identify specific challenges, mobilize assessment and intervention resources, and work with the states, all of which had been in place in various ways. Also, efforts were made to work with individual states, their unique policies and laws, and what could be implemented as best buys. Worth underscoring is the availability of extensive assessments to permit monitoring of individual states, providing feedback to the states and Winnable Battles program. Second, many states (32) that adopted the Winnable Battles plans mobilized resources to operate independently of the centralized CDC structure that began the program. This is an excellent outcome because the Winnable Battles program of CDC was a time-limited effort and a model. Third, although the program is not permanently in place, in a brief period it demonstrated a clear impact on critical health problems. To have this as a more enduring solution to challenges such as reducing the burdens of mental illness, the infrastructure for implementation, intervention, and data collection need to be built in and sustained. Finally, the program was not intended to be a research project or demonstration. This is not a criticism. The important tasks were to implement multifaceted and feasible interventions and track changes over time. The process does not preclude research, but this was not a public health or clinical trial. Extensive databases from the Winnable Battles program are made available (CDC, 2016b), and research can readily be done.

Overall, the Winnable Battles program provides a model of what can be accomplished. The scale of intervention and its adoption and assessment are precisely what is needed. All the "battles" that were selected were not equally successful, and all the goals were not met. On the other hand, palpable progress was made on certain measures (e.g., number of cigarette smokers, number of health care [in hospital]-associated infections, teen pregnancy rates). These measures are obviously critical in their own right, but they also have implications for the consequences that follow from them (e.g., death from smoking, child disadvantage in development from conditions into which children are born with teen mothers). The Winnable Battles program was already conducted on scale. The next step would be to continue the foci and develop the infrastructure and support that would keep the program or the next iteration in place.

Healthy People 2020

The prior illustrations move from one to a few foci (Zero Suicide, Winnable Battles, respectively). A broader and enduring initiative is referred to as Healthy People (www.healthypeople.gov/). The program is overseen by the Office of Disease Prevention and Health Promotion (ODPHP), which was created by the US Congress in 1976 to lead disease prevention and health promotion efforts.[1] Healthy People is a program within that and identifies goals for improving health of all people in the United States. The effort is comprehensive in scope by selecting a wide range of health goals for the nation, identifying baseline data related to the goals, selecting 10-year targets, monitoring the outcomes with objective data, and evaluating improvements (Koh et al., 2011).

The program began in 1990 with release of the 10-year forward-looking program (Healthy People 2000). For each decade since then, the program has set objectives and evaluated progress made. The emphases have been on diseases and other conditions of health. These continue to be included in the current version, but the focus expanded to encompass social determinants that include social, economic, and environmental sources of disadvantage because these underlie health and well-being and also contribute to disparities in health care. (In the terminology of this chapter, the inclusion of social determinants is recognition that health and disease as a wicked problem are related to several other problems [e.g., poverty, homelessness, crime].)

The goals of the program are selected by a complex process involving advice from multiple disciplines including business, social policy, public health, health economics, health communication, and many others and that drew from public, private, and community organizations. In the end, four broad goals were selected (Koh et al., 2011, p. 554):

1. Attain high-quality, longer lives free of preventable disease, disability, injury, and premature death;
2. Achieve health equity, eliminate disparities, and improve the health of all groups;

3. Create social and physical environments that promote good health for all; and
4. Promote quality of life, healthy development, and healthy behaviors across all life stages.

These overarching goals led to a focus on 12 high-priority health issues that represent a major threat to public health and with that 26 *Leading Health Indicators* organized under the topic areas to assess the health of the nation and to motivate action at national, state, and community levels. Leading Health Indicators at once convey the objectives and the indices or measures that will be used to evaluate the goals. Table 10.2 conveys the topics (goals) and the Leading Health Indicators used to evaluate them.

Healthy People 2020 is a resource for federal, state, and local governments and organizations. The resources provide information as well as a model for proceeding to make an impact. The model begins with an overall four-step framework to help communities move forward on the goals. These steps are to

- Mobilize partners;
- Assess the needs of the community;
- Create and implement a plan to reach objectives; and
- Track the community's progress.

Each of these is made more concrete with toolkits, lessons, webinars, and step-by-step guides on how to move forward. Each state and territory in the United States has a Healthy People Coordinator who serves as a liaison to ensure that the plan of the state or territory is in line with Healthy People goals and objectives.

Critical to the program is providing science-based (objective) measures to evaluate progress, and these were noted in Table 10.2 as Leading Health Indicators for each goal. The National Center for Health Statistics (NCHS) serves as the Healthy People data support team and provides funding for the major national data sources used to track the measures. As for the interventions, more than 500 reviews of evidence-based interventions (treatment and prevention) are provided for physical disorders (the main emphasis), mental disorders, substance use and abuse, and a range of lifestyle and health-related issues (e.g., activity, exercise) for diverse age groups and populations (e.g., adolescents; lesbian, gay, bisexual, and transsexual individuals; older adults). The reviews also provide an evaluation of the weight or strength of the evidence. In addition, examples of interventions and progress are provided online to showcase what communities have done and are doing to achieve changes. In general, Healthy People 2020 provides the infrastructure for assessment, training, and resources for selecting among interventions. Needless to say, not all states and territories select all objectives. And one can track progress within a given locale as well as see what they are doing or have done to effect change. Progress is tracked over time in relation to the overall goal and specific targets for improvements (e.g., www.healthypeople.gov/2020/data-search/Search-the-Data#statemap=1).

Table 10.2 Topic Areas and Corresponding Measures (Leading Health Indicators) to Evaluate Progress for Healthy People 2020

12 Topic Areas	**26 Leading Health Indicators**
Access to health services	Persons with medical insurance
	Persons with a usual primary care provider
Clinical preventive services	Adults who receive a colorectal cancer screening based on the most recent guidelines
	Adults with hypertension whose blood pressure is under control
	Adult diabetic population with an A1c value greater than 9 percent
	Children aged 19 to 35 months who receive the recommended doses of diphtheria, tetanus, and pertussis (DTaP); polio; measles, mumps, and rubella (MMR); *Haemophilus influenzae* type b (Hib); hepatitis B; varicella; and pneumococcal conjugate (PCV) vaccines
Environmental quality	Air quality index (AQI) exceeding 100
	Children aged 3 to 11 years exposed to secondhand smoke
Injury and violence	Fatal injuries
	Homicides
Maternal, infant, and child health	Infant deaths
	Preterm births
Mental health	Suicides
	Adolescents who experience major depressive episodes (MDEs)
Nutrition, physical activity, and obesity	Adults who meet current federal physical activity guidelines for aerobic physical activity and muscle-strengthening activity
	Adults who are obese
	Children and adolescents who are considered obese
	Total vegetable intake for persons aged 2 years and older
Oral health	Persons 2 years and older who used the oral health care system in the past 12 months
Reproductive and sexual health	Sexually active females aged 15–44 years who received reproductive health services in the past 12 months
	Persons living with HIV who know their serostatus
Social determinants	Students who graduate with a regular diploma four years after starting ninth grade
Substance abuse	Adolescents using alcohol or any illicit drugs during the past 30 days
	Adults engaging in binge drinking during the past 30 days
Tobacco	Adults who are current cigarette smokers
	Adolescents who smoked cigarettes in the past 30 days

SOURCE: Office of Disease Prevention and Health Promotion Publication No. B0132. November 2010; www.healthypeople.gov.

Healthy People represents a comprehensive health program for the United States. An especially interesting facet of Healthy People 2020 is attention to social determinants. The overall theme is that the health of individuals is related to the health of the larger community and that the communities influence the health of individuals (US Department of Health and Human Services [USDHHS], 2000). This is an especially interesting addition to the conceptualization of how to have an impact. I noted earlier the often-cited claim that there is no health without mental health. The Healthy People 2020 initiative extends this further by noting that there is no health without community health. This focus conveys the importance of addressing social woes (e.g., poverty, crime—other wicked problems) to have an optimal impact on health as well as ensuring that health benefits reach all Americans, including those who have suffered the greatest disparities.

General Comments

These three initiatives share many characteristics, including a strong infrastructure to implement interventions in many ways (e.g., in response to local conditions), involving both centralized (e.g., government, national organizations) and localized control over implementation. Also, each includes multiple interventions and multiple ways of delivering them. A critical feature I have glossed over, but will return to later, is assessment and tracking. Well-funded, well-intentioned, and multifaceted programs for a significant health problem are not enough—we are doing all of this to have an impact, so an evaluative component is essential.

Other examples are available in which a major national effort is made to make one or a few domains related to health change a top priority. Prominent among these is a recent report emanating from the US Surgeon General on alcohol, drugs, and health (Vivek & Murthy, 2016; https://addiction.surgeongeneral.gov/). The Office of the Surgeon general provides reports on the nation's health, and these receive major (though regrettably temporary) attention in the news, but are more enduring in setting priorities for action. One report, *Facing Addiction in America: Surgeon General's Report on Alcohol, Drugs, and Health,* was the first on the topic on alcohol and drugs (Office of the Surgeon General, 2016). The report evaluates the scope of the problem, what is known (e.g., prevalence and consequences), and what can be done (e.g., policy, evidence-based treatment). A general vision for what is needed is stated: "embedding prevention, treatment, and recovery services into the larger health care system will increase access to care, improve quality of services, and produce improved outcomes for countless Americans" (https://addiction.surgeongeneral.gov/vision-future). Yet the strength of the report comes from many specific suggestions delineated by key stakeholders, including individuals and families, educators and academic institutions, health care professionals and professional associations, health care systems, communities, industry and commerce, and federal, state, local, and tribal governments. For example, recommendations for individuals and families include that they should reach out if they think they have a problem, be supportive (not judgmental) if a loved one has a problem, show support toward people in recovery, advocate for the changes needed in their community, and talk to their children about alcohol and drugs. The guidelines suggested that researchers should conduct research that focuses on implementable, sustainable solutions to address high-priority substance use issues; consider how scientific research can inform public policy; and promote rigorous evaluation of programs and policies. For these recommendations and those to other stakeholders, more specific detail is provided as to what should be done. They draw on evidence-based practices where available. I mentioned recommendations to convey that a report is more than just a statement of the problem but also provides action plans for many constituencies who could make a difference. This initiative will no doubt have an impact on mobilizing resources given the heft of the government support. Yet specific funding, sets of government and private organizations, and formal monitoring will be needed to evaluate the impact of any initiatives. One has to move from an excellent report with recommendations to an infrastructure like that illustrated by the Winnable Battles and Zero Suicide programs.

EXPANDED FOCI TO HAVE AN IMPACT ON THE BURDENS OF MENTAL ILLNESS

Each example I highlighted and others like them reflect remarkable efforts with palpable gains on many key health issues. The examples include foci on domains of mental illness, including substance use, eating disorders, and suicide, in keeping with the goals of this book. There are priorities I would like to underscore here to give special attention to issues and foci we have discussed to reduce the burdens of mental illness.

First, more concentrated attention is needed that focuses on depression and anxiety. Although one might select any number of disorders, they are highly prevalent conditions, exert enormous cost, affect people in childhood through older age, have evidence-based interventions, and directly affect morbidity and mortality. For example, careful analyses across 36 countries noted that untreated depression and anxiety cost approximately $1 trillion (US) per year (Chisolm et al., 2016). Moreover, the return on investment (benefits of treating the disorders in relation to costs) is enormous; that is, it pays to treat rather than to neglect. Depression and anxiety deserve to be placed high on the list of national priorities—indeed, international priorities. Apart from the availability of evidence-based psychosocial interventions (EBPIs), there are already many models of delivery (online, self-help, Web-based) that could be centralized and mobilized systematically to be scaled up. The benefits of scaling up for "just" these two disorders are likely to be reflected in accumulated years of life (millions of years!) and huge financial savings (Chisolm et al., 2016). There is attention to depression in the examples I have provided. Healthy People 2020 uses two Leading Health Indicators (suicide and adolescents with a major depressive episode within the past year) to reflect goals and measures of progress. Extensions to depression and anxiety in the population nationally would be a high priority.

Second, more attention is needed to ensure that services are reaching those who are the least likely to receive them. It is obviously important to chart progress on targets (e.g., number of individuals who abuse substances), but we want to be clear about whether services are being delivered where need and neglect are greatest. It is important that there be equal access to care in principle but also in practice. In the Zero Suicide program, for example, several facets of the initiative focused on high-risk groups for suicide, including youth, Native American, and Alaskan Native samples. At the outset of any initiative identifying both high-risk groups and groups whose disparities in receiving care are great should be a priority. As part of the effort to reach those in need, it is important to track not only progress in the outcome (e.g., reductions in prevalence and incidence) but also who is and is not being served.

Third, more attention may be accorded to improving healthy lifestyles among citizens that would be expected to have broad payoffs. For example, a national initiative on exercise could be extremely valuable. We would want to increase exercise on scale, have targets, monitor the effects of what we do on rates of exercising, and ensure that cultural and ethnic adaptations were addressed. Here, the monitoring procedures would include data both on the adoption of exercise and on key indicators of the many outcomes that might be affected. For example, prevalence of exercise and the various outcomes (e.g., disability-adjusted life years [DALYS], quality-adjusted life years [QALYs], or particular disorder and disease entities) would be important. In short, some of the priorities selected for intervention should be actions of the public that would be expected to have a broad impact on multiple health outcomes.

Exercise is one example that, if improved on a large scale, would be likely to have sweeping benefits to both physical and mental health. Similarly, eating a nutritional diet appears to be related to mental and physical health as well, and perhaps that is another place to intervene as a means to achieving multiple outcomes (e.g., McMartin, Jacka, & Colman, 2013; O'Neil et al., 2014).[2] There are many other lifestyle changes (e.g., walks in nature, meditation) with broad effects (e.g., Walsh, 2011). Overall, the guiding question is whether there are some strategies or interventions (means) that can be expected to have benefits on multiple challenges or problem domains. This suggestion here includes three components: (1) Add more "means" as part of the many challenges and foci (e.g., Winnable Battles, Leading Health Indicators); (2) select these based on their likely breadth of impact across multiple challenges, and (3) monitor adoption of the means (e.g., prevalence of activity) as well as multiple outcomes for which an impact would be expected. Selection of which means and for what outcomes are not mere guesses; they can be modeled and then evaluated empirically, similar to the way in which best-buy interventions have been selected and evaluated.

There are many excellent initiatives to address physical health challenges and, to a lesser extent, mental health challenges, a few of which I have mentioned as illustrations. Goals are set, objective measures are used, and progress can be seen (e.g.,

Healthy People 2020; Winnable Battles). New challenges are constantly emerging, not so much because a prior challenge has been resolved, but rather because new priorities come to light and occasionally the opportunity looks promising that something might be accomplished by shifting a focus a bit (e.g., as adding the focus on social determinants in Healthy People 2020). The scope of the challenges itself raises critical issues and is a challenge of its own.

To begin, resources to address and enact strategies to combat various challenges are limited. Obviously, not all health and social challenges can be addressed, and for any given challenge, not all promising solutions are feasible to implement. This raises questions about how to set priorities and to make decisions. Healthy People 2020, for example, conveys the challenge. To improve the health of the nation, more than 42 topic areas of health were selected, with nearly 600 objectives and 1,200 measures to evaluate progress. In the end, this list was reduced (see Table 10.2). Deciding top priorities means ignoring or delaying many others. Obviously, there is much to do, and priorities need to be set because of all sorts of constraints (e.g., funding, as well as feasibility of having an impact but not diluting efforts too much).

Because of the number of challenges and their likely interrelations, I suggest according more attention to challenges that are means (activities of everyday life, exercise) that would be expected to affect a number of challenges and outcomes. I do not suggest this as a way to replace selection of important problem domains but instead as a way of seeking greater efficiencies. Some foci might spill over and affect multiple problem areas. More attention to those would be an excellent addition.

ASSESSMENT AND MONITORING OF PROGRESS

Assessment as Central to Intervention

When one considers efforts to remedy any challenge, attention usually is drawn to the interventions or what will be done to achieve change. What will be the interventions: EBPIs, changes in policy and law, models of delivering services, and so on? Much less attention, at least in the eye of many stakeholders and the public, is drawn to measurement and the quality of the information that will be used to evaluate progress. The examples I have provided (e.g., Zero Suicide, Winnable Battles, Healthy People 2020) have very strong assessments in place, including scores of measures to evaluate impact. By selecting programs with broad governmental and nongovernmental agency support, I may have unwittingly implied that assessment is routine in program evaluation.

Assessment is an essential ingredient underlying intervention but is often omitted from efforts to effect change when large-scale central oversight with a broad funding base or access to other agencies to collect the data is not available. We need sound data and indices of the problem to evaluate progress and to track changes, leaving aside for the moment whether or not these can be attributed to our interventions. Occasionally, the importance of measurement is recognized formally on par with other challenges. For example, I mentioned the Grand Challenges in Global Health (see Box 10.3). The final two grand challenges focused on *assessment* and included the goals to develop technologies that permit quantitative assessment of population health status and to develop technologies that allow assessment of individuals for multiple conditions or pathogens at point-of-care. And in Healthy People 2020, the measures to reflect change (Leading Health Indicators) are absolutely central to the entire program from the very outset and conceptualization. These examples underscore the fundamental importance of evaluation.

The critical role of assessment and monitoring progress is obvious but often is viewed as a low priority or even not a good use of funds in relation to many programs that are not at the level or scale of those in my illustrations. In our society, there is an endless array of programs to prevent or change a problem. These programs include interventions to address virtually every facet of life, such as developing skills in preschoolers, preventing substance use and abuse among teens, encouraging safer driving among all of us, improving safety in business and industry, decreasing errors in hospitals that lead to death, treating trauma in veterans, increasing exercise in older adults, decreasing bullying, preventing suicide, and so on. For example, virtually every school at every grade level has a set of programs with some goal in mind. Perhaps in our positive evaluation of constructive efforts to help—often with a focus on genuinely important problems, we extend this positive gloss to the assumed likely outcome that these efforts will generate. Yet we know all too well that when evaluations are included, programs and well-intended interventions do not always work.

For simplicity's sake, consider three outcomes that are possible with any intervention, implemented on a small or large scale:

1. The intervention may make a difference and help some or many people exposed to it;
2. The intervention may make no difference and not be any better than doing what was done before or not intervening at all; or
3. The intervention may make people worse and despite the good intentions cause some harm compared with what was done before or with no intervention.

I state these "for simplicity's sake" because all three outcomes can occur within a given program. And the value of a program may be determined in part by the proportion of each of the three outcomes among all those who received the intervention and the consequences of the worst outcomes. We know from instances in which evaluations are done that all three options I have outlined can and do occur. One might consider that only the third option is a genuine problem—people became worse. Yet the second option is a genuine problem as well because of the cost in funds to deliver that intervention and in lost time among persons who might have been treated effectively with another intervention. That is not academic or merely an intellectual point. If a person received an ineffective treatment (outcome #2) for posttraumatic stress disorder or depression, or for pancreatic cancer or HIV, the person was not just sitting idly by hoping for improvement—these problems are life-and-death matters. The loss of time in receiving an effective intervention could be disastrous (e.g., suicide, death through the course of the disease, spreading HIV to others).

While we as citizens love programs and efforts to help, assessment and evaluation of the impact of any of these programs do not engender the same positive views. The very thought of evaluation raises doubt—after all, evaluation might show that the program is not working very well, or not at all. In addition, if evaluation did not show the positive effects that were expected, this might well have negative consequences in terms of lost funding, jobs, and programs. Understandably, evaluation is left out of most programs that are implemented to effect change. Some of the reasons may be the added expense, the need to have expertise to conduct the evaluation, and the delays that planning an evaluation can introduce into any program. Yet we proceed blindly and only in the short term when we do not include an evaluation.

As an example, in an adjacent city to where I am living and writing at this moment, three new programs are being implemented to reduce adolescent substance abuse in public schools. Interventions with an evidence base, although available, were not selected. But maybe the programs will be effective anyway and even better than other options. If so, maybe we will have new programs with an evidence base. The problem is that the great enthusiasm (and financial support) for implementing the programs has no evaluation built in to determine whether there is any impact at all. It is not likely that suggestions for a rigorous evaluation (for the sake of the children) would be welcome or, if welcome, would be funded. Yet implementation of three new programs that might have no impact or make people worse would be a strong argument for evaluating their impact. Evaluation is not a luxury, and it is also not "just" a research issue; it is critical precisely because individuals are so important and we need to know whether they are helped or harmed.

Three Critical Assessment Domains

Reducing the burdens of mental illness requires assessment in at least three domains. First, assessment is needed to ensure that those interventions selected are in fact carried out and in the way that was intended. This is referred to as *treatment integrity* or *treatment fidelity*. This can apply to quite different interventions in different ways. For example, training lay people to carry out an intervention to reach many in need must ensure that in fact lay counselors execute the treatment in ways that are likely to make it effective. If changes in policy or law are the intervention (e.g., bans on smoking, bans on advertising near schools), some effort is needed to ensure that in fact the policies or laws were carried out, implemented, or enforced. Evaluating execution and implementation of the intervention are not methodological luxuries. We know from scores of examples that interventions that were planned were either not implemented correctly or not implemented at all (e.g., Sechrest, White, & Brown, 1979). We mistakenly thought that many such programs were ineffective when in fact they were not implemented at all or quite poorly. In short, to address a challenge, execution or implementation of any intervention must be evaluated, sampled, or tested in some way. And this applies to whether the intervention is an EBPI or social policy.

Second, in the case of the burdens of mental illness, it would be important to evaluate penetration or receipt of interventions. There are such enormous mental (and physical) health care disparities in the United States. I have noted that most people (~70 percent) in need of mental health services in the United States receive nothing. Yet this is even worse (higher percentages) for ethnic and minority group members, children, older adults, and other subpopulations. In terms of assessment, we want some index of whether we are penetrating the full set of groups in need of services. In the context of treatment for cigarette smoking (quitlines), research has devised an index called *Reach Ratio* (Baskerville et al., 2015; Campbell et al., 2014). The index calculates the proportion of individuals in a given subgroup (e.g., men, women; but any subgrouping) who receive or are reached by the intervention in proportion to the distribution of that group in the overall population with the problem. Thus a ratio of 1.0 would mean that the intervention is reaching that subgroup in proportion to the extent to which that group shows the problem in the population (prevalence). Disparities in delivery of the intervention would be below that number and show that the reach of treatment is much less than the proportion of individuals overall with the problem. In relation to assessment, we would want much more attention to indices of reach. In discussing novel models of delivering interventions, I mentioned that we want models to scale up the interventions (to reach large numbers) but also to have reach (to get to the groups usually neglected). Critical to measurement would be objective indices that in fact disparities are being reduced and eliminated.

Finally, and most obviously, we need assessment of intervention outcomes. Are there changes in the domains we are focusing on? We can intervene but is there progress or any change in outcomes? Those outcomes could be many (e.g., DALYs, QALYs, prevalence of disorders), and not all measures would correspond and reflect the same pattern. Fundamental to a goal of reducing the burden of mental illness is assessment to monitor mental illness and impairment nationally (i.e., some measure of the mental health of the nation). This would provide a steady stream of information for tracking changes in mental illness and its burden over time across cohorts and across possible social influences that might affect that baseline. There is a need for a national database on mental illness that allows comparisons over time—a point others have articulated well (e.g., Bickman, 2008; Chorpita et al., 2008). There are all sorts of challenges related to feasibility, legal, and ethical issues, of course, but these are not new. We have precedence in addressing large-scale assessment issues. That experience is not an excuse for complacency, but neither is it a reason not to move forward.

Surveillance in Public Health

In public health, surveillance (large-scale assessment) is a critical part of health care. The goals of surveillance usually include measuring and characterizing the extent to which there is a burden (e.g., of disease), identifying emerging conditions that might have an impact on public health, setting priorities based on burdens, evaluating risk and prevalence, and assessing the impact of efforts to improve particular conditions (see Groseclose & Buckeridge, 2017; Institute of Medicine, 2015, 2017b). Surveys typically are population based, select individuals in such a way as to represent the population (or subpopulation) of interest, and often are conducted at regular intervals (e.g., annually). The study, development, and evaluation of surveillance measures, apart from the substantive findings in relation to a particular survey, are core areas in the study of public health.

I mention the topic of surveillance, even if only in passing, for several reasons. First, surveys have been used extensively to elaborate a variety of health problems, including mental health. Large-scale surveys have evaluated the scope of psychiatric disorders in the population, the burdens these disorders cause (e.g., cost, DALYs), the paucity of treatment services for individuals in need, and the nature of the services received (e.g., Reeves et al., 2011; Strine et al., 2015).

Second, the development of EBPIs in the dominant model of delivering treatment generally does not connect with or draw on these surveys and the information they provide. Evaluations of treatment rarely include measures of burdens of mental illness or quality of life relatively standard in public health. This has helped keep treatment evaluation with the dominant model of delivery and research isolated from critical issues about impact. Related, the penetration of treatment among those people (i.e., closing the treatment gap) has not been of interest in the treatment research on EBPIs as it has been in surveillance of mental health needs in public health.

Finally, and also related, many of the models of treatment delivery discussed in this book (e.g., task shifting, extensions of treatment via technology, taxing policies, entertainment-education), unlike the dominant model in use, were selected precisely because they can be scaled and have an impact on the burdens of mental illness. Now more than ever before we have multiple opportunities to address mental illness at the level of large-scale, public health interventions. It naturally follows to integrate surveillance on a large scale and to evaluate impact at that level. There are already examples of this, as I note below.

There are many models that focus both on providing interventions for mental health on a large scale and monitoring the impact over time. Arguably the most comprehensive is Healthy People 2020 in light of the range of measures (Leading Health Indicators) used to evaluate progress. With fewer foci, the Winnable Battles program mentioned previously evaluates diverse areas of focus (e.g., tobacco use, nutrition) on a state-by-state basis annually. For example, for tobacco use, the National Health Interview Survey (www.cdc.gov/nchs/nhis/about_nhis.htm) was used to assess adult cigarette smoking; and the Youth Risk Behavior Surveillance

System (www.cdc.gov/healthyYouth) evaluated youth smoking. Another system of tracking was used (CDC State Tobacco Activities Tracking and Evaluation [STATE] System; www.cdc.gov/statesystem/smokefreeindoorair.html) to evaluate the extent to which states had laws in place to ban smoking in the workplace, bars, and restaurants.

The National Health Interview Survey has been used to monitor the health of the US population for a period spanning six decades and with a focus on many domains beyond the use of tobacco discussed as an example here (see USDHHS, 2010). This is the main means of monitoring the health of the nation. The data for the measure are collected through personal household interviews (35,000 to 40,000 and encompassing 75,000 to 100,000 individuals). The US Census Bureau serves as the agency that collects data for this measure and tracks health status, access to health care, and the extent to which health objectives are achieved. The measure includes a wide range of problem domains and is revised as needed to address new foci of interest. I mentioned tobacco use was one of the Winnable Battles, but large-scale surveillance was used to evaluate progress on each of the "battles" and across each of the states and territories in the United States.

Another large-scale surveillance measure in place is the National Survey on Drug Use and Health. This survey is administered nationwide in the United States and samples approximately 70,000 individuals (12 years and older) (USDHHS, 2017; https://nsduhwebesn.rti.org/respweb/homepage.cfm). The survey provides data on the level and patterns of alcohol, tobacco, and illegal substance use and abuse; tracks trends in use and abuse, assesses the consequences, and identifies groups at high risk. In addition to substance use and abuse, psychopathology (e.g., depression), impairment, and service use are assessed. The interview has had different formats over the course of its use (it began in 1988), including personal interviews, computer-assisted personal interviews, and audio computer-assisted self-interviews. The measure is relied on heavily by diverse federal and state government agencies to make decisions and track trends in various groups (e.g., youth) or specific domains of use and abuse (e.g., alcohol).

There are many other large-scale assessments that provide means of obtaining data over time and in relation to mental and substantive use disorders and related psychological conditions. Here are four of many examples:

- The National Comorbidity Study, which samples the mental health status of thousands of adults and youths, provides data on incidence and prevalence, and encompasses several countries in conjunction with the World Health Organization (www.hcp.med.harvard.edu/ncs/);
- The Monitoring the Future Study, which assesses behaviors, attitudes, and values of school students (http://monitoringthefuture.org/). The project began in 1975 and has provided data on drug, alcohol, and cigarette use nationwide and involves approximately 50,000 students (8th, 10th, and 12th grade) annually;
- The survey of Midlife Development in the US (MIDUS) has been ongoing since the mid-1990s (http://midus.wisc.edu/scopeofstudy.

php). This is an evaluation of age-related variations in health and well-being in the United States and assesses many psychological factors (e.g., personality traits, well-being, affect, sense of control, goal commitments), which are then linked to marital status, family structure, social support, health status, and health care utilization; and
- The Institute for Health Metrics and Evaluation (University of Washington; www.healthdata.org/) focuses specifically on evaluating data on health indicators, including prevalence of major diseases and effectiveness of health programs (Murray & Frenk, 2008). Mental health and major psychological sources of impairment (e.g., substance use, obesity) are included, and pervasive mental disorders (e.g., depression, anxiety) would be natural extensions.

My selective sampling of many assessment options shows that large-scale surveys of the status of mental health of a nation have many models, and many are in place. In terms of challenges, implementation of treatment on a large scale at this point in time might be more of a challenge than measures to evaluate whether we are having an impact. Both are essential, and I wanted to add to the discussion the point that merely deploying novel models of intervention delivery that are scalable and have reach will also require that we show we are achieving these goals and thus reducing the burdens of mental illness. Programs in place, as noted by three illustrations, provide both assessment and interventions. Even so, much more could be accomplished at the level of interventions. The novel models I outlined in Chapters 7 & 8, could be adopted and added on scale and along with a stepped-care model to build on the many programs in place.

SUMMARY AND CONCLUSIONS

In this chapter I have tried to conceptualize the challenge of reducing the burdens of mental illness to place it into broader contexts. The notion of a wicked problem conveys the interconnections of multiple challenges and other features that prepare us for what we can expect as we try to reduce those burdens. Thus we can expect our "one" challenge to be embedded with many others, that there will be no simple or single solution to the challenge that is our focus, that we will not have sufficient data to satisfy ourselves and others to act, but still must act, and that different perspectives on the problem will mean different perspectives on the solutions as well.

Grand challenges more concretely focus on a specific, often multifaceted problem (e.g., global health). Grand challenges promote progress by establishing a specific priority, bringing together resources and multiple partners (e.g., in organizations and others such as scientists, business communities), and identifying the specific barriers or key questions that need to be solved. A grand challenge can be broken down into even more specific and focused questions—subchallenges, so to speak.

The challenge of reducing the burdens of mental illness is included in many initiatives. Assuming that all mental disorders cannot be the focus, the matter is then one of setting priorities and delineating the criteria for selecting among the many disorders. Assessing the burdens of a given disorder and estimating the prospects of having an impact are no doubt among the critical criteria. And final goal selection is often an iterative process involving several experts and constituencies, revisions, reconsideration, and so on before action. All that said, a direct and more concerted focus on depression and anxiety would be very well placed as a national (and international) effort to reduce the burdens of mental illness. Of the 400+ disorders that can be identified, depression and anxiety are most prevalent, have effective interventions on their behalf, and already have in various venues among clinicians and lay individuals evidence that we can have an impact. Also, when coupled with novel models of delivery, there are very feasible ways of scaling up interventions and reaching people in need. A complementary goal to address mental illness and its burdens would be to focus on a particular social change (e.g., exercise, physical activity) that would be likely to have a variety of benefits (e.g., National Physical Activity Plan Alliance, 2016). Here, a disorder (e.g., depression) is not the focus but instead is some broader lifestyle change that could have multiple and diverse benefits.

Currently, the development of psychosocial interventions has not connected well with large-scale surveys of psychological disorders or their indices of impact, in two ways: First, the dependent measures of studies of EBPIs rarely reflect burden of mental illness, but that could be altered. Second, when novel models are used to scale-up interventions, the available systems of surveillance could be integrated to show whether we are having an impact. We have key means to have an impact: interventions, delivery models, and surveillance methods. That these are available is opportune at this point in time. And, for the first time, this is integrated with solid data showing a huge need (e.g., prevalence of disorders) that, despite our current efforts, remains largely unmet.

11

Closing Comments

Key Steps to Reduce the Burdens of Mental Illness

The extreme challenge of reducing the burdens of mental illness is based on the complexity of the problem and on the enormous unmet need for services. I have discussed components that could form the basis for solutions, including the availability of interventions with evidence that could make a difference, the availability of truly novel models of delivering interventions that could reach people in need, and unexplored lines of research and clinical practice in relation to interventions (e.g., weak interventions and low-cost evidence-based psychosocial interventions [EBPIs] would be helpful, targeting possible transmechanisms, developing sequences of stepped-care interventions). This is an opportune time because the components available to meet the challenge would allow us to have the needed impact now. In this closing chapter, I bring together many of the issues and challenges, discuss steps that would help us move forward, and place mental illness in the context of other health issues. These other health issues heighten the importance of and need to change health care significantly.

WHERE ARE WE NOW?

Here is a summary of many of the findings that convey both the challenge of reducing the burdens of mental illness and why now is an opportune time to address that challenge.

- We now have sound evidence that the scope (prevalence, incidence) of mental disorders worldwide is enormous. The data usually focus on clinical disorders (meeting criteria for a psychiatric disorder), which provides a hugely conservative estimate of the problem. Subclinical dysfunction can reflect and portend problems, and many other domains (e.g., loneliness, stress) can still impair functioning in daily life;
- The impact and cost of mental disorders are also enormous by quantifiable indices such as disability and premature death (e.g., disability-adjusted life years [DALYs] and years of life lost [YLLs], respectively). Direct monetary costs, another quantifiable measure, for any given disorder (depression) or set of disorders (e.g., substance use and abuse disorders), run into billions of dollars in the United States in a given year;
- In focusing on populations and large-scale analyses, it is important not to lose sight of the personal burdens that mental illness represents. Suffering, unhappiness, and difficulties in negotiating everyday life are experienced by individuals with mental disorders and families who take care of them early, throughout, or later in life, depending on the type of dysfunction, degree of impairment, and options for care;
- We now have evidence that the vast majority of people in need of treatment for their psychological problems receive nothing systematic at all from a trained or untrained health care worker. Among that small group that does receive something, often it is merely a single check-in session with a doctor or some kind of care taker (healer, religious leader) and not one of the EBPIs or even necessarily a formal regimen of treatment;
- We now have evidence that some interventions are effective and can be considered evidence based. Not all interventions are equally strong in their evidence base, but for many clinical problems, including those with great prevalence, disability, and cost (e.g., depression, anxiety, substance use), we have intervention techniques that could make a difference;
- We have many models of delivery available that can be scaled up to reach individuals in need of services (e.g., task shifting, best buy). Some of these models have been well tested in physical health care, and some have been extended to mental health care. As part of these models, the breakneck pace of technological developments portends disruptive innovations for helping people with physical and mental health problems. I refer to many Web- and app-based self-help techniques with an evidence base, omitting all sorts of cutting-edge innovations yet to emerge and be evaluated (many more apps connected in real-time assessment, widespread use of clothing with sensors to evaluate physical and emotional states, social robots, Internet of Things connected in ways that pertain to our physical and mental health). Yet the available options

for delivering treatment on scale extend well beyond technological advances; and

- There are major efforts in the United States to address grand challenges to promote health and well-being as well as specific domains of mental and physical disorder. I have sampled some of these (e.g., Healthy People 2020, Winnable Battles) and the national surveillance on which they draw to evaluate progress. We need to build on these by uniting often separate efforts toward similar ends (e.g., suicide and tobacco use are covered by multiple initiatives). Also, we need to integrate these remarkable efforts with treatment models on the ground to handle individuals in need of services. Perhaps a way to unify disparate efforts would be to focus on prevalent and costly disorders (e.g., depression and anxiety) and at levels that include federal, state, and local agencies—but more than that, clinical practice and interventions on the ground in a way that is scalable and has reach to those likely to be unserved. The top-down (agency) approach is absolutely essential because of scope of impact, funding, and collaborations that can be brought together; we also need some bottom-up approaches (from clinical care at the level of individuals in need) to have the maximize impact.

The above points rely heavily on sound science. Two reflections follow from that. First, empirical evidence and sound science mean that there are many things to quibble about! Scientists are wont to disagree about findings and their interpretation. Indeed, progress depends on competing views followed by empirical tests, revisions of the views, and debates about what we "really" know. And findings are not always clear or unequivocal. As discussed in Chapter 10 (in the context of wicked problems), we will not necessarily have the full evidence we would want to act. Second, when findings accumulate and there is some consensus, that does not automatically get translated into policy or social change. The leap from findings to policy is enormous because of how policy is formed, the multiple influences and nonlinear process, and the many constituencies involved, often with quite competing goals and agenda (see Malakoff, 2017). Even so, we are in a position in light of what we do know to act, to make a difference, and to reduce the burdens of mental illness. Indeed, programs I have mentioned (e.g., Healthy People 2020, Winnable Battles) are directed to that.

KEY QUESTIONS AS STEPS TOWARD THE GOAL

When summarizing where we are in reducing the burdens of mental illness, it is useful to pose key questions that must be answered to move forward. These are not intended to oversimplify but rather to help summarize steps leading to action. I have identified five such questions, which are listed in Box 11.1 for easy reference but also discussed more fully here.

Box 11.1

Questions That Summarize Our Challenges

1. Can we have an impact?
2. Should we act and do something?
3. Will we move forward and take action?
4. If we were to take action, what are the initial steps?
5. How will we know whether we have had an impact?

Can We Have an Impact?

The first question raises the matter of whether we actually can influence mental illness and related sources of psychological impairment, whether they meet diagnostic criteria or not. By that I mean do we have interventions that could actually make a difference? There are now many EBPIs. One can quibble about measures and indices of change (e.g., effect size) that are used to draw conclusions about the treatments, and I did. Yet, based on the weight of evidence, there are many forms of mental illness in their clinical and subclinical levels that can be treated effectively. Admittedly, the vast majority of demonstrations are in controlled settings and may or may not reflect the impact in real-world settings. Yet some of the evidence is quite strong and has been applied in clinic, as opposed to just laboratory-like settings. The treatment of depression is one example, discussed in large-scale applications previously.

For the moment, let us consider if we focused "only" on major depression, which as noted previously is predicted to be the greatest cause of disability in the world by 2030, among a range of medical and psychiatric disorders and calamities (e.g., cardiovascular disease, traffic accidents, chronic pulmonary disease, and HIV/AIDS) (WHO, 2008b). We have many available interventions, and already efforts in at least one country have increased the workforce to have an impact on depression and on a larger scale than what is normally accomplished (e.g., Clark, 2016). Depression is a single example (but with multiple variants, across the full age spectrum, and with many different samples). But there are many disorders we can now treat (e.g., Nathan & Gorman, 2015; Weisz & Kazdin, 2017), and these are reflected in guidelines for practice that review and update what we know (e.g., National Institute for Health and Care Excellence [NICE], www.nice.org.uk/).

In relation to this first question, I believe we can say that, yes, we can have an impact on mental illness. The now thousands of treatment outcome studies of EBPIs show change on a variety of psychological measures, but rarely connect with measures of burden beyond that (e.g., DALYs, quality-adjusted life years [QALYs], quality of life). Yet some studies do connect with these measures and convey that these, too, reflect change. Another reason we can expect an impact has to do with the base from which we are working—most people receive no special care for their psychological problems. Making things better amounts to surmounting this low bar.

Should We Act and Do Something?

The second question is whether we ought to intervene to reduce the burdens of mental illness. The question might seem silly; surely "of course" is the only answer. Yet I include the question here in part because of long-standing discussion of the relation "ought implies can," as underscored by the philosopher Immanuel Kant (1724–1804). The issue in that context is that if we ought to do something (e.g., on moral grounds), the implication is that in fact we can do something, that is, ought to implies can (Kant, 1793).[1] Certainly, the reverse is not necessarily true (can does not necessarily imply ought). That is, there are many things we can do in life, but ought not to. Yet it is useful to consider whether we should (ought to) reduce the burden in its own right because this discussion will help with other questions (see Box 11.1).

As a philosophical principle, "ought implies can" is certainly a matter of debate (e.g., Graham, 2011). Yet this level of abstraction ignores pressing realities of people suffering from mental disorders, dying earlier than expected for their age, and contracting a variety of other mental and physical disorders along the way. On humane and moral grounds, we ought to focus on reducing the burdens of mental illness. Indeed, to withhold effective interventions from those who are suffering casts the priority more clearly. If the vast majority of people in need receive no services and those rates are even higher for special groups (e.g., minorities, children, older adults), it seems that we are not only withholding intervention in general but also doing so in a discriminatory fashion.

Even if we omitted humane reasons and moral principles, we still ought to intervene to help the majority because doing so would reduce the enormous monetary costs to society from the expense of managing the consequences of mental illness for individuals, for business and industry, and government. And untreated or ineffectively treated mental illness has costs associated with other systems of "care" or interventions (e.g., criminal justice and prison, homeless care, medical care). So, few might argue in the abstract about whether we ought to reduce the burden of mental illness. It is a lose-lose enterprise (for individuals and society) not to.

Will We Move Forward and Take Action?

The third question is, will we in fact make an effort to reduce the burdens of mental illness and try to reach the majority of people in need? We have so many of the key components needed to exert impact. Will we make an effort to intervene and deploy resources? Here "can" and "ought" run into issues related to setting priorities. In any given society and government, resources are inherently constrained. By that I mean, the number of problems and worthy causes that are in need of attention greatly exceeds the number of resources in money, personnel, and often knowledge in being able to address them.

Depending on one's personal view, it is fairly easy for a citizen in any country to ask oneself, "Why is our country focusing so much on *that* (insert here any challenge from Box 10.2 of Chapter 10 or some other issue of which you mildly or vehemently disapprove as a major focus), when we are neglecting or giving so little attention to *this* (insert here any other challenge from Box 10.2 or some other issue that you consider to be a very high priority and even high moral ground)? It is easy to look at a given country and raise the question about priorities and in that evaluation feel that they are misplaced.

For example, depending on the country, resources (monetary, people, and planning) might focus on developing infrastructure (plumbing, availability of electricity), providing clean and disease-free water, promoting sustainable supplies of food and energy, providing prenatal care to reduce medical and psychiatric disabilities, vaccinating all children to prevent diseases, and mounting a space program so as not be left out of the space exploration and colonization race. Even though a country would elect to devote resources to a problem (reducing the burdens of mental illness), in fact those in positions of setting priorities might well argue that we cannot do that or do that very seriously in light of many other priorities. In principle we ought to reduce the burdens of mental illness, but this can be seen in the context of a long list of "ought tos," and for sure all of the ought tos cannot be addressed and funded. So, in fact, "can" is a challenge because we cannot address all the worthwhile ought tos or at least at a given point in time. Stated another way, "can" in one sense challenges whether we have the requisite knowledge to accomplish something. I suggested that we do in relation to reducing the burdens of mental illness on a large scale. But in another sense, "can" challenges whether we are able to in light of multiple other priorities. In this latter context, we cannot unless there is a sharp shift in priorities.

Some funds or resources are allocated to many different priorities, and then the quibbling pertains to the percentage of resources and whether that percentage can have the needed impact. This is still a priority issue. Needless to say, in the United States, resources are provided to treat mental illness, but we are in a bind because we may not be utilizing them in a way that makes much of a difference (e.g., dominant model of delivery), and funds probably are needed for changing the infrastructure of service delivery (e.g., lay people could change the landscape if we did not have professional constraints).

In the scheme of many challenges, it is not clear that reducing the burden of mental illness is very high, and equally it is not clear how to bump the problem up a bit on the priority list. An expression of this frustration was noted in an article about suicide (Lytle, Silenzio, & Caine, 2016) entitled, "Are There Still Too Few Suicides to Generate Public Outrage?" The article begins by noting the astounding data: Suicide is the 10th leading cause of death in the United States, is on the rise, and already surpasses deaths from traffic accidents and homicides. In a prior article by a different set of authors, suicide also was the topic (Rockett & Caine, 2015), and the authors' frustration with the general neglect of the problem was convened with the article's subheading, " 'It Is Time to Pay Attention." One can readily sympathize, but alarming rates alone might not be a very strong incentive in moving us to any action or to action that makes a difference. Information can contribute to shifting priorities, but much more is needed for there to be palpable change.

Consider another example in which alarming information might well be expected to move us to action. A major plane crash was attributed to the depression and suicide of one of the pilots (2015 Germawings Flight in the French Alps). Follow-up research surveying large numbers of pilots found that 12.6 percent meet criteria for depression and 4.1 percent reported having suicidal thoughts (Wu et al., 2016). They do not seek treatment for fear of losing their jobs. Would information like this move the public? It might, but what can the public then do to have an impact? Also, what major changes have been brought about by this tragedy, which enraged many of us?

For some social priorities there are constraints (e.g., laws) and huge sources of influence (e.g., lobbyists) that are in place to ensure that some action is or is not taken (e.g., gun control, banning of cigarettes, placing calorie counts on menus, placing health warnings on many "fast foods"). Also, in prioritizing all the ought-to-do noteworthy causes, segments of the population vary greatly as a function of ethnicity, culture, socioeconomic status, political views, and geography—to mention some influences. In addition, setting policy, making laws, and making decisions about what people can and cannot do, in the United States, invariably clashes with individual rights. Some taxes for the general good (e.g., taxing "junk foods") can readily be seen as too much government control and restriction of individual freedom. In any case, the question about whether we will intervene is not so simple and represents a path obscured by roadblocks, challenges, and points of inertia.

In relation to the present discussion, we begin with a reasonable view that we can intervene to reduce the burden of mental illness, at least as measured by available intervention techniques. And we might for the moment say that we ought to. Perhaps we can agree on that. But whether we will intervene is far less certain and depends on priorities of society and those who make policy and develop laws. These individuals have to juggle multiple priorities and are constantly being lobbied to make a decision that may or may not be in the public interest.

If We Were to Take Action, What Would Be the Initial Steps?

The fourth question I raise is where to begin, assuming that reducing the burdens of mental illness has moved up as a critical priority and will be attended to and with resources. The answer may well depend on the model or models used to administer interventions (e.g., task shifting versus use of technology) and local conditions (e.g., in the country, state, and city). Perhaps some general points can still be made. To begin, one might introduce the novel models or a subset on a small scale as an initial point of departure. Perhaps a state, city, or region would be a place to begin (e.g., https://thrivenyc.cityofnewyork.us/; www.communitypartnersincare.org/). From lessons learned, the implementation could be scaled up. Invariably, each application will introduce new issues. In this approach, an effort is made to have broad impact (e.g., multiple disorders) but on a restricted geographical scale. The restricted scale, such as a given region or state, is only on a temporary basis because the goal is to scale up much more broadly.

Another way to introduce interventions on a small scale is to select just one or two disorders and perhaps one or two interventions and expand gradually from there. This was the approach discussed previously in the treatment dissemination examples from the United Kingdom to make available EBPIs for depression and anxiety and also in the United States in extending treatment to veterans, which began primarily with posttraumatic stress disorder. In the UK example, an extensive effort was made to train existing clinicians and to recruit new ones, and to fold an increasing percentage of clinical services into the program. Over time, more clinical services and more patients were recruited and provided treatment, and the project continues to expand. Critical to this exemplary effort was a central government commitment to the priority of reducing the burdens of mental illness.

Another way to begin reducing the burden would be to piggyback a couple of worthwhile efforts (challenges) where one or two interventions or policy changes would be expected to have multiple benefits. If multiple outcomes (e.g., physical and mental health) might be achieved, then the political and public coalitions that are involved in policy might come together for this priority. There are now a few interventions (e.g., exercise, meditation, mindfulness) that, if extended more to the public, might well have an impact on mental and physical health. Insurance might be structured to reimburse participation in such activities, the workplace might provide incentives and means to do that as well, and of course schools (in the United States) could revert to those olden days (e.g., 50 years ago) in which physical activities (e.g., referred to as physical education or "gym" period) were routine. Many colleges and universities also have intramural athletic activities for individuals not part of intercollegiate competitive sports, and that could be restructured as well to promote greater involvement.

I am suggesting a stepped approach to scaling up interventions and reaching people in need. The range of options and concrete details might be guided by calculating impact, cost, affordability, feasibility, and local conditions (e.g., special groups in the population, regions of the country). It is equally possible that a larger scale application would be a place to begin if, for example, there were some widely available app or self-help program or some best-buy legislation that promoted mental health. There are many disciplines likely to inform the options for proceeding, and I have to defer to others with that special expertise. But we can begin, and there are many options and examples available.

How Will We Know Whether We Have Had an Impact?

Absolutely pivotal to the goal of reducing the burdens of mental illness is to have some indices of how we are doing. As discussed in Chapter 10, assessment in a systematic way is essential in order to more carefully assess the burdens of mental illness over time. I also mentioned that there already are excellent assessments in place to measure health and psychiatric disorders and as part of national services (e.g., National Health Interview Survey, National Survey on Drug Use and Health). These measures are administered at periodic intervals, examine a range of health issues, and can be revised as needed to incorporate new health-related issues. These measures or the model of their administration could readily provide the information we seek and could be supplemented with other measures as needed to evaluate the scalability, reach, and impact of the interventions. I illustrated models of the integration of assessment and intervention on a large scale (e.g., Zero Suicide, Winnable Battles, and Healthy People 2020). In short, we have the mechanisms in place and the measures to obtain the data we would need to evaluate the extent to which we are altering (hopefully reducing) the burdens of mental illness. No doubt there will be discussions about the best assessment format, what new scales or items within the scale will reflect key indices of the burdens, and so on. These are readily addressed given the assessment progress already evident at a national level.

BARRIERS, MOBILIZING THE COST, AND HEALTH CARE ISSUES

Barriers to Providing and Receiving Treatment

The steps I have outlined for expanding how we deliver mental health services may seem reasonable but ignore huge impediments to providing care that were outlined early in the book, namely, the many barriers to participation in and receiving treatment. Moving forward definitely requires addressing these, but "addressing" can be accomplished in different ways. Consider two key types of barriers to represent system factors and attitudinal factors that interfere with providing and obtaining interventions for persons in need of services.

Allocation of Resources and Costs of Treating Mental Illness

System barriers were reviewed previously, and these include high cost of mental health services, policy and legal constraints, and too few professionals to administer treatment, all in the context of assuming the use of the dominant model of delivering treatment. Certainly, a key issue nationally (and worldwide) is the allocation of resources for mental illness. I have mentioned that federal and state budget cuts in the United States often trim services for those in great need, including individuals with mental illness.

Resources for mental illness occasionally are in the public spotlight, especially when there is a local disaster such as seemingly random violent acts that lead to death and injury. Invariably, one might find mental illness in the past of the perpetrator or family member, and the media often conclude that the person slipped through the cracks because of inadequacies in mental health services. Politicians may seize the stage, genuinely lament the tragedy, say this (whatever horrible event happened) cannot go on and advocate for more funds for mental health services. This is not very helpful because the funds, if provided at all, are usually temporary, and even worse, the provided funds just do more of the (ineffective) same. More of the same is nonevaluated, non–evidence-based interventions that cannot reach most of the people in need of mental health services and that have no new ways of picking up (detecting) individuals at risk for dangerous behavior. Again, one does not want to turn down resources, but more funds in response to a crisis gives illusory palliative action. The impact is not likely to be evident and actually could be detract from changes that are needed that could have an impact. We have not made the point to legislators that more of something that has not been shown to work is not a great investment. Perhaps there is mental health illiteracy among those in positions of decision making because we as professionals have not made clear that the existing model of providing services is not very helpful and that typically there is no accountability (assessment, evaluation) to attest the benefits of the services. In any case, one issue to address is costs of services and resources that are needed to have an impact, along with the impact on the clients themselves.

Relevant costs have been allocated to improve access to services. In many countries, this comes from access to physical and mental health care that are provided by the government and draw on the tax base to fund that care. In the United States, there has been an effort to provide health insurance for more of the population. Making insurance available to all and including coverage of mental health services are a plus, and one must be pleased about that in relation to the goals of this book. Yet having insurance for mental health services is not addressing the limitations I have identified here. Insurance in relation to mental health services is encouraging but of small use given the model of service delivery and the lack of access to these services for most people. This is not an argument against insurance—it is "against" the status quo as an ineffective way of reaching people in need of services. The services and model of delivery will need to change to be scaled up and to reach special groups.

A critical cost issue mentioned previously is that cost analyses and cost-benefit analyses need to be routinely included in the delivery of mental health services and evaluations of interventions. The case has been made about how the costs of providing effective treatment of mental illness are recovered by savings in other areas (e.g., DALYs, providing disability payments, lost taxes from workers) (Layard, 2013; Layard et al., 2007). That something will have little or no net cost invariably sounds excellent, but will this actually occur? I noted in the discussion of dissemination of treatment in the United Kingdom that evaluations in fact showed that effective treatment of depression provided a net gain; that is, the government saved more money than it cost to scale up treatment. The critical lesson is that increasing mental health services to reach more people in need is not necessarily expensive. The costs could be neutral (cancelled by savings), or negative (more money is recovered than was spent), or slight to medium (cost is greater than what is recovered). These can be modeled, weighed, and tested but in any case should not serve as a basis for delaying action. Of course, sometimes the issue and debates surround who pays for a given treatment or service, including what government agency (province, state, federal) and what system (mental health, physical health, justice system, social services).

Cost of treatment is a weighty and important issue and central to moving forward to implement what we have available to have an impact. One could move slowly (e.g., one disorder, one region of the country, one age group in need) in a stepped fashion to evaluate benefits, scalability, and net costs. It would help if the many treatment outcome studies would routinely measure cost as well as cost savings. My point is that cost need not necessarily be an impediment to progress. The cost would vary tremendously as a function of what models were adopted to deliver treatments. Arguably, we might well be using the most ineffective model now (aside from doing nothing), namely, individual psychotherapy. The only feature that hides cost is that so few people are treated (so it may not look too costly in absolute dollars) and the costs the untreated incur (e.g., in prisons, homelessness, emergency room visits, unemployment) are too diffuse to easily be attributed to untreated mental disorders.

Stigma as an Impediment to Seeking but Also to Providing Treatment

I have discussed the well-known and more obvious parts of stigma, namely, reticence to seek out mental health services in light of all sorts perceived and real negative consequences. The stigma associated with mental illness in our culture, but in other cultures as well, may be related to the neglect or weak efforts to make a change in providing adequate services and care. There is stigma and rejection of people with mental illness and enduring attributions that are misguided (e.g., mental illness is a weakness of character, mentally ill individuals are dangerous and more violent than others). Worth repeating from Chapter 3, the stigma about mental illness is even evident among mental and physical health care professionals, where this might be least expected. It is not a far leap to consider that those in a position to set policy or legislate may also harbor some of the stigma, and that could be a detriment to action. It was not so long ago that having mental illness was attributed to being possessed by evil spirits and the devil, and as I noted previously, exorcism is still used now to treat mental illness with that causal model in mind. Other challenges (wicked problems) that might be addressed, such as climate change or prenatal care, have their own obstacles but probably do not begin with those leading to rejection of the victims involved.

A hope has been that the stigma and rejection and discriminatory practices associated with mental disorder would change when we clarify that many "mental" disorders (e.g., schizophrenia, autism spectrum disorder) are actually "physical" disorders. Yet, in previous years, trying to convince the public that a given "mental disorder" is actually a physical disorder has not helped in reducing stigma. The most prominent example was trying to convey to the public that alcoholism is a disease (Morse et al., 1992), a view associated with controversy and outright rejection (e.g., Albrecht, 2014; Szasz, 1972). This was an effort to remove the association with vice, moral weakness, and sin, which were long associated with excessive drinking. This has not changed people's views in ways that has altered policy, sympathy, or tolerance toward individuals who drink, or sensitivity to the use of public funds to address the problem (e.g., Crandall & Moriarty, 1995; Crawford & Heather, 1987). For whatever reason, there may not be great public attraction to helping people with mental illness.

Addressing stigma and discrimination associated with mental illness is obviously worthwhile, but reducing those does not necessarily help us to move forward or quickly implement effective interventions and reduce the burdens of mental illness. The reason is that changing attitudes alone is not a very effective way of changing behavior, and reducing stigma (e.g., as reflected in measures such as questionnaires, interviews, and hypothetical situations) may not have an impact on moving large numbers to seek treatment (e.g., follow-through with the requisite behaviors). Indeed, if it did, that would be a disaster because our current model of care cannot handle many people. I am not arguing against attending to and trying to reduce stigma—not at all. Stigma warrants attention and ought to be addressed. However, it is not necessarily the case that reducing stigma (and self-stigma) is a sufficient or even necessary condition to have enormous impact on mental illness.

Stigma is not the only attitudinal barrier, and I have mentioned previously that others, such as mental health literacy and cultural and ethnic beliefs about treatment, play a critical role. We cannot just gloss over them. I also mentioned previously that we can work directly on the barriers (e.g., trying to reduce stigma), or we can try to side-step them. Many models of delivery (e.g., use of technology, use of lay counselors, use of disruptive innovations, providing interventions in everyday setting, setting government policy, entertainment-education) do not require resolving key barriers to get treatments to people and people to treatment. The novel models covered are needed precisely because they have different capacities to reach people and to surmount or sidestep one or more of the barriers that are so salient with the current model of providing treatment. Each model will not surmount all the barriers, but with multiple models of treatment delivery, we will be able to have an impact with a vastly larger swath of the population in need of services.

Mobilizing Different Constituencies to Exert Change

Many different constituencies can be involved in changing and making the reduction of the burdens of mental illness a priority. Those involved in policy making (allocating funds, devising regulations and laws) obviously are key to having an impact on setting the goal as a priority. There often is a reticence of scientists to move into policy, but the health of a nation may well depend on that, that is, scientists leaving their usual domains and stepping into policy to influence public health and societal goals more generally (Press, 2015; Sacher, 2000). How to change policy and the scope of organizations and the professions involved are well beyond the goals of the present book, but their role is critical to mention.

Mobilizing the opinions and actions of mental health professionals, the organizations that represent them, and legislation for which they advocate that restricts the services could have influence on changing the priority of and attention to reducing the burdens of mental illness. In the United States, the dominant model of delivering psychosocial interventions is locked in by required credentials, state laws, and professional organizations protecting clinical practice from intrusions. Much of the rationale is based on protecting the public from people who are not trained in methods, science, and ethical issues that clinical practice requires. Yet this now has neglected the burgeoning literature that supervised lay people can deliver treatment just as effectively and can reach many more people in need. Thus many of the regulations directly interfere with reaching the majority of those in need. Morals demand that we shift the emphasis from protecting clinical services to helping the public or devising solutions in which the benefit of one of these (e.g., the public) is not at the expense or detriment of the other (e.g., professionals who need to earn a living). Right now, in the United States, the public is on the unfortunate side of this—"no treatment" as the most common "intervention" for mental health problems. We have the means to change this (e.g., task shifting) and the science behind it to convey we can have impact. Of course, none of this by itself is very persuasive in mobilizing public opinion and change.

We have seen successful strategies in which public opinion and priorities to change the status quo regarding a public health issue have worked in varying degrees. Some of the more prominent examples include bans on cigarette smoking (e.g., taxes, restricted access to smoking settings, images of smokers as being uncool, fewer examples of people starring in films who smoke cigarettes) and efforts to limit fast-food sales (by promoting lists of calories and contents, by restricting sales in school cafeterias, by pressuring vendors to offer more healthful alternatives from their standard fare). These are promising examples as possible models of effecting change but may be limited in generality to the situation in relation to mental illness and its care.

In the cigarette smoking and fast-food examples, industry was identified as an enemy and served as the basis for mobilizing both public opinion and litigation (e.g., against cigarette manufacturing). There have been massive and enduring class action suits against tobacco companies and an endless stream of cases of individuals who provide real-life and poignant examples of the impact of cigarette smoking. There is no equivalent industry that promotes mental illness in little packages that are dispensed to adolescents or sold to adults. So, we cannot sue a particular company or industry for promoting mental illness behind our backs and producing key products to do that. There are exceptions here—low levels of lead promote attention-deficit disorder and low IQ among children, and that is one domain where there have been litigation and international standards for lead in the air, water, and automobile fuel. But for the 400 or so recognized psychiatric disorders, there is no single source or set of sources that cause the problems in general. It would help to have a visible, common enemy that the media could run with, as they often do, to convey in a dichotomous (evil and good) fashion whom is to blame. This way of thinking invariably is oversimplistic but is helpful and sometimes effective.

Perhaps we can piggyback or attach the goal of reducing mental illness onto other priorities that are more popular and already have some support. Initiatives to reduce air pollution, to better understand the brain, or to make medicine more individualized (personalized medicine) are some of the priorities already in place in the United States, even if not universally supported. We could connect with those priorities by conveying their mental illness implications and by providing evaluative tools to assess the impact or lines of research that support those connections.

Yet it might be better to face directly the challenges of mental illness and its care and to devote resources to this. The significance of the problem might be addressed from the top down, that is, leadership of the nations backed up with specific initiatives drawing on many of the options raised in this book. An excellent illustration of just this was in a speech by the Prime Minister of the United Kingdom (May, 2017), who noted:

> For too long mental illness has been something of a hidden injustice in our country [UK], shrouded in a completely unacceptable stigma and dangerously disregarded as a secondary issue to physical health. Yet left unaddressed, it destroys lives, separates people from each other and deepens the divisions within our society. Changing this goes right to the heart of our humanity; to the heart of the kind of country we are, the attitudes we hold and the values we share." (para. 97)

This same speech was accompanied by concrete proposals to change mental health services to focus on many of the people who are otherwise largely neglected (e.g., youth), problems that are largely neglected (e.g., suicidality), and settings (e.g., the workplace) where problems can be detected and treated. But perhaps more noteworthy, May noted that as Prime Minister she wanted to use "the power of government as a force for good to transform the way we deal with mental health problems right across society, and at every stage of life" (May, 2017, para 72). It is likely we would need that type of commitment and centralized support to have the impact we need.

CHANGING HEALTH CARE: IT IS NOT JUST ABOUT MENTAL ILLNESS

Interestingly, many of the challenges, concerns, and failings of our ability to reach people are not at all unique to mental illness. To convey the point, consider three health domains that seemingly have little relation as challenges: mental illness (the focus of this book), hearing loss, and eye and vision problems. Mental illness, hearing loss, and vision problems of course are quite distinct areas involving very different professions, treatment and preventive interventions, and so on. Indeed, it might be somewhat of a surprise to even take up these latter topics. Yet it is helpful to do so and perhaps especially at the end of the book.

Mental illness, hearing, and vision problems have uncanny commonalities. I have culled the most salient common features for Box 11.2. Consider the scope

Box 11.2

Health Care Challenges: Commonalities Among Three Domains of Disorders: Mental Illness, Hearing Loss, and Vision Problems

Scope of the Problem

The dysfunctions in each domain are a public health problem in light of the high prevalence rates.

Disability (e.g., disability-adjust life years), quality of life, and mortality are related to the dysfunction (e.g., through accidents or other comorbid conditions).

There are physical and mental health comorbidities (for hearing and vision problems) associated with the disability.

Treatment Gap

Most people in need of services for treatment or prevention do not receive them.

There are huge disparities so that some groups (especially minorities) are even less likely to receive care.

There is a need for improved national assessment (surveillance) to evaluate scope of the problem and progress in providing needed care.

Barriers

There are delays in individuals recognizing the problem and then further delays in seeking and obtaining care.

For large numbers of individuals, treatment is not affordable.

There is stigma associated with the problem and seeking help.

Improvements in literacy in relation to each domain are greatly needed so that people have a better understanding of the signs, interventions, and so on.

More attention is needed to convey the connections between general overall health and the onset and course of the disorder.

Intervention Needs to Change

The approach to treatment should include integrated care (personalized care and patient-centered medical home model).

More work is needed to ensure that evidence-based practices are those provided to people in need.

A population approach to intervention is also needed (e.g., social policy, regulations that facilitate screening and intervention).

Note: Prior chapters in this book document these characteristics in relation to mental illness. These same characteristics are evident in relation to treatment and care of hearing (e.g., National Academies of Science, Engineering, and Medicine) ([NASEM], 2016; Pratt, 2010) and vision (e.g., Lam & Leat, 2015; NASEM, 2017).

of the commonalities—high prevalence, most individuals in need of care not receiving treatment, illiteracy in the domain, delays in getting to treatment, health care disparities, stigma, disability, reduced quality of life, and early death! I have focused on these disorders somewhat arbitrarily to make the point. Similar points might be readily raised in relation to other health domains. For example, oral health shares many of the characteristics (see Box 11.2) as well (e.g., most people in need do not receive treatment, access to care is riddled with barriers, there are huge disparities in care, and the domain relates to overall health not just dental health) (Office of the Surgeon General, 2000).

I mention the commonalities not merely because they might be interesting. Rather, the commonalities suggest that our health care system and the ways in which we provide interventions need a major overhaul that goes beyond any one area. One seeming solution recommended in each area is integrated care, certainly part of strategies needed but by far from routinely adopted at this point in time in the United States. Similarly, technology as a way of providing information and leading individuals to services is yet another opportunity.

The book suggested novel models to deliver interventions to reduce the burdens of mental illness. Although it is important to make domain-specific changes (e.g., for mental illness, hearing), it is equally important to look at the much larger system issues that are relevant. I have noted the data showing that most individuals in need of mental health services receive nothing. The broader point is one to which we ought to attend as well: Most people who need all sorts of services (my examples were "only" mental illness, hearing, vision) are not getting them, and these deficiencies relate directly to quality of life, comorbid conditions from another domain, and mortality. There is a need for marked change in health care (see Dzau et al., 2017; Institute of Medicine, 2017a).

FINAL WORDS

The options and opportunities to have an impact on the burdens of mental illness are enormous, in part because of remarkable advances at this point in time in developing effective treatments, models of delivery, better understanding of the nature of disorders, and the ability to monitor health nationally and internationally. Also, repeated cost analyses show more clearly than ever before that neglecting the treatment of mental and substance use disorders is enormously costly—trillions of dollars annually worldwide. Add to those analyses clarity that there is return on investment so that it is likely to be less expensive to treat than not to treat mental illness. These rationales are essential to make the case, but they so often are insufficient to carry the day.

Progress is needed on policy and public will. We need to convey the deeply lamentable consequences of continuing what we are doing at this time. Mental illness is a life-and-death matter, but even apart from that, the scale of day-to-day suffering is enormous. Cost makes the financial case compelling. And that stands on its own. But the human suffering—pain in daily life, unhappiness, comorbid mental and physical diseases, and early death—ought to be front and center. Even if treating mental illness did not "pay" (i.e., cost more than the return on investment), we ought to do it any way. Yet treatment looks like it will pay, so all the more reason for us to act.

The bar is low now in terms of what we accomplish and what we try to accomplish in caring for individuals with a mental disorder. Again, a refrain throughout this book: The most common intervention for mental illness in the United States is no treatment. We can do better than that. Actually, it would be hard to do worse. The goal of this book is to move forward on the many options we now have. Interestingly, we not only "ought" to do this, but actually "can" through many of the means outlined here.

NOTES

Chapter 1

1. The term *mental health professional* can include a range of individuals who work with clients or patients experiencing problems with mental illness. These professionals include individuals trained in clinical psychology, psychiatry, and social work, but many others are involved as well, including psychiatric nurses, mental health counselors, family therapists, and pastoral (as in church) counselors. Also, spiritual leaders and elders in a given culture often explicitly are charged with health care, including psychological health.
2. Complementary and alternative treatments usually are included together. The distinction can be made in which complementary interventions are used along with mainstream interventions (e.g., diet as a complement to chemotherapy for cancer). Alternative interventions are those that are used instead of a more established and well-investigated intervention. Here, the distinction is based on how the intervention is used rather than what the intervention is. The term *integrative health* is sometimes used to draw attention to a combination of complementary and mainstream interventions. In the United States, the National Center for Complementary and Integrative Health serves as a clearing house and source of research on complementary and alternative treatments (see https://nccih.nih.gov/).
3. Multiple terms are introduced throughout the book. They are defined when first presented but also included in the Glossary at the end of the book.
4. The psychiatric disorders are often considered as syndromes, wherein a *syndrome* refers to a group of symptoms that consistently occur together. So *subsyndrome* usually means the person did not quite meet the criteria for the full syndrome. For this book, the terms *subclinical* and *subsyndrome* will be used interchangeably. Each term has problems. Subclinical suggests that something may not be a real problem or enough of a problem to receive help, and that is not necessarily true. Subsyndrome is not a great term because the diagnoses are often in question, and what symptoms should or should not be included in a syndrome and for what duration and whether syndromes (different disorders) are distinguishable all are topics of debate and research.
5. The terms *client* and *patient* are occasionally distinguished in discussions of psychotherapy. The differences reflect varying approaches and views of the entire enterprise of therapy—are we treating mental "illnesses," in which case the term *patient* seems reasonable, or are we working with individuals to help them cope better with

debilitating conditions that affect their everyday lives, in which case some non-patient term such as *client* seems more appropriate? For the present book, I will use *client* when a term is needed. A key reason is that this book moves away from emphasizing one-to-one "treatment" and identifying individuals as *patients*.

Chapter 2

1. The two dominant diagnostic systems are the *International Statistical Classification of Diseases and Related Health Problems* (ICD-10; WHO, 2010) and the *Diagnostic and Statistical Manual of Mental Disorders* (DSM-5; American Psychiatric Association, 2013). Both diagnostic systems list formally recognized psychiatric diagnoses of mental disorders. Each is revised periodically based on evidence about specific disorders as well as consensus among experts. The names of these documents convey their overlapping but also different purposes. The ICD is designed to classify and to track medical and psychiatric diagnoses. The goal is to monitor the incidence and prevalence of diseases, causes of death over time, and trends and changes among diseases within and among countries. Most countries use the ICD to report diseases and causes of death, and of course for that goal the full range of medical conditions is included in the document. Thus the ICD has broader use well beyond mental health professions. Psychiatric diagnoses are covered by a section of that broader focus. In contrast, the DSM is restricted to psychiatric disorders. Many psychiatric conditions of the ICD and the DSM are quite similar, but there are also differences in criteria and recognition of some of the disorders. In the United States, the DSM has dominated both research and clinical practice for decades. Requirements in the United States shifted near the end of 2015 so that the ICD rather than DSM must be used for documentation and reimbursement in clinical application. That shift brought the United States to conformity with many other countries where the ICD has been in use for some time.
2. The term *mental disorders* encompasses substance use and abuse disorders in diagnostic systems. For example, in the ICD-10, multiple diagnoses are included in the category "mental and behavioural disorders due to psychoactive substance use," with separate diagnostic categories based on the specific substance (e.g., alcohol, cannabinoids, cocaine, other stimulants such as caffeine, tobacco, and others) (http://apps.who.int/classifications/icd10/browse/2016/en#/F10-F19). For the present discussion, mental disorders will be used to encompass substance use and abuse disorders. However, epidemiological research occasionally makes the distinction and will be mentioned separately when studies do so.
3. Many different interviews are available and are designed to match the symptoms that need to be assessed for a particular diagnosis. Thus the interviews tend to change as the diagnostic systems (ICD, DSM) are revised. An example is the *Composite International Diagnostic Interview* (CIDI) that includes symptoms of dysfunction but also items related to severity of the symptoms, impairment, and distress (Kessler & Ustun, 2004; WHO, 2004a). A brief description of the instrument, its revisions, and use is available www.hcp.med.harvard.edu/wmhcidi/about-the-who-wmh-cidi/. The use of systematic interviews with established reliability (e.g., different interviewers would obtain the same diagnosis for a given patient) rather than informal clinical observation (winging it) was a breakthrough in mental health research because it meant that patients given a label in one study using

a standardized interview were likely to be very similar to other patients with that same label in other studies. This would better permit the accumulation of many studies on a given disorder.

4. As one might expect, stress is an enormous area of research in part because of the pervasiveness of stressors as a part of life and the impact of diverse domains in mental and physical health. Distinctions I note here among stressors, stress, and distress are generally correct, but these are not uniformly used in research. Even so, the three concepts of stressors, stress, and distress help to go beyond the more generic all-encompassing stress in everyday life. The term *hassles* is sometimes used to refer to the more mundane annoyances of everyday life (e.g., lost items, temporary and minor crises at work), and stressors are more major.
5. We have been delinquent in our interpretation of Juvenal (i.e., many of us are Juvenal delinquents). The reason is that his phrase is misinterpreted and taken out of context. The original statement, "... *orandum est ut sit mens sana in corpore sano*" translates into English as, "It is to be prayed that the mind be sound in a sound body," or "you might pray for a sound mind in a healthy body" (Juvenal—*The Satires*, Satire 10; Rudd, 1991; also see https://en.wikipedia.org/wiki/Satires_(Juvenal)#Satire_X:_Wrong_Desire_is_the_Source_of_Suffering).
6. For example, the National Comorbidity Survey (NCS) and National Comorbidity Survey Replication (NCS-R) are large-scale evaluations of psychopathology, course, risk, and protective factors that have generated scores of publications that have greatly added to our knowledge about disorders over the course of life among adolescents and adults (www.hcp.med.harvard.edu/ncs/). Data sets and measures used in the surveys are available to the public, and research can be accessed for use. Related, the National Institute of Mental Health Collaborative Psychiatric Epidemiology Surveys make available data on the distribution, risk factor, and other characteristics with emphasis on minority groups (www.icpsr.umich.edu/icpsrweb/CPES/). This project brings together three national databases: the NCS-R, the National Survey of American Life (NSAL), and the National Latino and Asian American Study (NLAAS). The project permits the in-depth study of cultural and ethnic influences on mental health. Data, code books, and descriptions of procedures are available for use.
7. Throughout the book references will be made to developed and developing countries. Developed and developing countries are delineated based on economics (e.g., per capita income, gross domestic product) and differ in a variety of other characteristics (e.g., infrastructure and a better environment in terms of health and safety. See other sources for further details of the classification (http://keydifferences.com/difference-between-developed-countries-and-developing-countries.html#ixzz4W2GJ1nfU). Another way of grouping countries has been devised by the WHO and World Bank and also refers to income level. High-income countries are separated from low- and middle-income countries, based on the gross national income and gross domestic product (see other sources for further details of classification; https://datahelpdesk.worldbank.org/knowledgebase/articles/906519-world-bank-country-and-lending-groups). I will refer to developed and developing countries as needed.
8. The WHODAS is a measure developed to reflect impairments associated with diseases and disability and has been elaborated by WHO in a document (and checklist)

referred to as the International Classification of Functioning, Disability, and Health (ICF; WHO, 2001a). This is framework was adopted by WHO member nations (191 countries) in 2001 to serve as the international standard to describe and measure health and disability. The ICF has been extended to cover children and youth as well as adults (www.who.int/classifications/icf/en/).

9. DALY might appear to be straightforward, but there are nuances to its computation (see WHO, 2013). As a brief illustration of these, DALY for a disease or injury is calculated based on the total number of years of life lost (YLL) because of premature mortality in the population and the years lost to disability (YLD) for cases of the disease or injury. The nuances include how severity of the disease is evaluated, with different weights given to early versus later years in life (see WHO, 2004b). The critical point is to be aware of the measure, its international use to measure burden of mental and physical health, and having a common metric (see Gold, Stevenson, & Fryback, 2002, for a fascinating discussion of various metrics and their use). DALYs, YLL, and YLD. Related measures noteworthy in passing include other indices: health adjusted life expectancy (HALE), which takes into account mortality and morbidity; HALE, which refers to the average number of years that a person can expect to live in "full health"; and quality-adjusted life year (QALY), which considers both the quality and quantity of life lived. (All terms noted here are defined in the Glossary at the end of the book.) (For a sample reference that includes many of the indices I have mentioned, see Murray et al., 2014.)

Chapter 3

1. In passing, let me note the well-known consequences associated with cutting mental health budgets by government agencies. Many individuals in need of mental health care often end up in other systems (e.g., homeless shelters, jails and prisons, medical hospital services) or in no systems at all (e.g., the streets) and use other services more frequently (e.g., emergency department visits for psychiatric and neglected physical health problems, social services for homeless care). Rather than saving states and communities money, these cuts to mental health services simply shift financial responsibility and costs to other services, agencies, or settings. The funding insight in any program is to be concerned not only with the cost of providing services but also with the cost of not providing them. Sometimes it is costlier to ignore or undertreat a problem than to provide adequate services.
2. Delays in seeking treatment are not at all unique to mental illness. For example, people with hearing loss take approximately 10 years before they seek assessment and intervention (Davis et al., 2007). This is an interesting example because hearing loss shares some features with mental illness, including the stigma many people experience with the loss and the fact that far more individuals are in need of services than there are professionals and facilities to serve them. Also, hearing loss often leads to social isolation and has been associated with serious psychological problems, including depression, anxiety, and, dementia (Battey, 2016).
3. Knowing what the treatment options are is part of mental health literacy and might be out of reach for all of us. For example, there are hundreds of forms of psychotherapy and all sorts of other psychosocial programs and interventions advocated for mental disorders and substance use and abuse disorders (e.g., Bellack & Hersen,

1985; Kazdin, 2000; Substance Abuse and Mental Health Service Administration, 2017b; https://en.wikipedia.org/wiki/List_of_psychotherapies). It is unlikely that trained mental health professionals (e.g., me) could identify any more than a very small percentage of the treatments in these categories. This is not the same challenge in relation to mental health literacy for the public, which is identifying that treatment is needed and what a viable treatment would be in general terms, and then engaging in the actions necessary to obtain a form of that treatment. Even so, it does not help literacy to have a baffling array of options without any clear way to sort through them.

4. I have designated this in a separate category of barriers as "other factors." It might well fit into system barriers because it is the system rather than attitudinal facets that serves as a barrier. Yet this is worth distinguishing because it is not usually included in lists of barriers and will emerge later in the book with the discussion of novel models that address barriers.
5. When an individual commits a heinous crime, invariably there is interest in going back into the person's history to identify if there was mental disorder or subclinical symptoms. If such a past is found, an implication is that the crime was related to that prior history. There might well be a connection. However, the usual accounts in the media are not a suitable way to find these connections. Among the reasons is that the base rate of mental disorder (ignoring subclinical) in the general population is fairly high (25 percent of individuals in the United States, as elaborated previously). So, we do not know whether the rate of the disorders among individuals who committed the type of crime in question exceeds that rate in the general population and among people who did not commit that type of crime. Also, on the same day of the horrible crime, there were many individuals who helped older adults through the crosswalks, who gave money to charity, and who volunteered at homeless shelters to help individuals in need. For individuals who did such laudable acts, we do not know their rate of mental disorder to help discern if the violent crime perpetrators have a higher rate of disorder. Perhaps more pertinent than abstract argument are the data. Most of the public (approximately 75 percent) considers people with mental illness as dangerous (Link et al., 1999). Actually, individuals with mental disorder are not any more dangerous than others in the general population. An exception is when individuals have both a mental disorder and substance abuse disorder; then the risk for engaging in violent behavior is much higher (Elbogen & Johnson, 2009). However, people with mental illness are much more likely to be victims than perpetrators of a dangerous crime (Hinshaw & Stier, 2008).
6. In the United States, a law was passed referred to as the Plain Writing Act of 2010 (H.R. 946/Public Law 111-274). The law requires that federal agencies use "clear Government communication that the public can understand and use." In 2011, a new Executive Order, "Improving Regulation and Regulatory Review" (E.O. 13563) was issued, which stated that "[our regulatory system] must ensure that regulations are accessible, consistent, written in plain language, and easy to understand" (www.plainlanguage.gov/plLaw/index.cfm). Guidelines are provided and periodically revised (www.plainlanguage.gov/index.cfm) and serve as a critical effort to improve literacy in health care more generally.

Chapter 4

1. The term *metasynthesis* is more often used to refer to analyses of qualitative studies in which multiple qualitative studies are evaluated to examine themes and findings that emerge across many individual studies (e.g., Gale & Schröder, 2014; Gask, Macdonald, & Bower, 2011).
2. There are many measures of the magnitude of an effect and strength of a relation (e.g., r, r^2, R, R^2, omega^2, eta, epsilon^2). Effect size, as measured by Cohen's d, remains the most frequently used. This index refers to the magnitude of the difference between two (or more) conditions or groups and is expressed in standard deviation units. As an admittedly arbitrary but widely used standard of d = .2, .5, and .8 as small, medium, and large effect sizes, respectively (Cohen, 1988).
3. Years ago (2008), a US Congressional Act and subsequent Institute of Medicine Report (2009) gave a high priority to Comparative Effectiveness Research in health care more generally. There are many comparative studies in psychotherapy research, and more often than not, no differences among active treatments are found (e.g., Barth et al., 2013; Olatunji, Cisler, & Deacon, 2010; Smith & Glass, 1977). One interpretation of no differences is that in fact treatment technique makes relatively little difference in comparison to common factors (e.g., alliance) and characteristics of the patient (e.g., Wampold & Imel, 2015). Another interpretation is that the way research is conducted (e.g., usually way underpowered) makes it extremely difficult to show treatment differences even if there truly are differences (Kazdin, 2017b; Kazdin & Bass, 1989). Overall, we know that some treatments have very strong evidence in their behalf. The evidence showing that one of these treatments is better than another is less clear.
4. Statistical significance has several sources of criticism, but key among them is that it leads one to make binary decisions (yes/no) about whether a hypothesis or group difference occurred. Effect size complements this by providing an estimate of the strength of a relation. A relation can vary in strength whether or not the finding was statistically significant (for a detailed discussion, see Kazdin, 2017b).
5. BDNF is a protein dispersed and secreted throughout the body. As a neurotrophin, BDNF stimulates growth and differentiation of new neurons and synapses (neurogenesis) in the brain and is active especially in the hippocampus, cortex, and basal forebrain other areas central to learning, memory, and higher order thinking (see Duman & Aghajanian, 2012).

Chapter 5

1. Other treatments recommended for depression include interpersonal psychotherapy and behavioral activation. Yet cognitive behavioral therapy was the first recommendation and was made across a range of depression and anxiety disorders (NICE, 2009; see Clark, 2011).
2. There are many different terms that are used for integrated care or that overlap with the care. An early effort to codify these identified 52 terms that are used, and that was more than two decades ago (Leathard, 1994). Sample terms to describe the approach to care include *interprofessional, interdisciplinary, multidisciplinary, interagency, cross agency, partnerships,* and many more. *Patient-centered medical homes* is frequently used as a term in contemporary work (e.g., Kazak et al., 2017). Not all terms are interchangeable, and even when the same term is used (e.g., *integrated*

care), there are many versions and variations, in part based on precisely what services are offered and for what population. The distinctions are not central to the present chapter.

3. Transdiagnostic research extends beyond psychiatric disorders. For example, in various cancers and in cancers in relation to other diseases, research has identified core or common pathways and transdiagnostic factors that underlie diverse diseases (e.g., Li, Ishdorj, & Gibson, 2012; Morris, Veeriah, & Chan, 2010; Wong, Engelman, & Cantley, 2010). Here, too, the goal is not only to better understand the disorders but also to develop common or more generic treatment targets that could have broad impact.
4. Many terms are used to refer to the use of technology in the context of treatment delivery (e.g., *telemedicine, telehealth, telecare, eHealth*). The terms have slightly different meanings (see Glossary) and are not used consistently. For this chapter, the term *telehealth* will be used to reflect the broad applications of technology to include health outcomes. Our focus in the chapter is on mental health.
5. The Internet of Things (abbreviated as IoT) refers to the interconnection through the Internet of computing devices embedded in everyday objects, enabling them to send and receive data. The data are transferred from machine to machine without requiring human-to-human or human-to-computer interaction. Connected communication among home appliance, cars, lights, and so on are examples. Health care applications for both physical and mental health care are on the horizon but have not been developed to the extent of other technologies mentioned in this chapter (Metcalf et al., 2016; Stankovic, 2014).

Chapter 6

1. From the 1880s, Anna O arguably is among the most famous and influential case studies in the history of psychotherapy. Anna was a 21-year-old woman who showed several symptoms, including paralysis and loss of sensitivity of the limbs, lapses in awareness, distortions of sight and speech, headaches, and a persistent nervous cough. These symptoms were attributed to anxiety rather than to medical or physical problems. Joseph Breuer (1842–1925), a Viennese physician and collaborator of Sigmund Freud (1856–1939), treated Anna O and wrote up a summary of the case (Breuer & Freud, 1957). Breuer visited Anna regularly to provide treatment. This included talking with Anna and hypnosis. Anna recalled early events in her past and discussed the circumstances associated with the onset of each symptom. As these recollections were made, the symptoms disappeared. This case has had an enormous impact on clinical practice and research and is credited with marking the beginning of the "talking cure" and cathartic method of psychotherapy. This is a historical oddity and at least partial fiction because the therapy was not just talk and included hypnosis and heavy doses of medication (a sleep-inducing agent, chloral hydrate). When talk did not seem to work, the medication was used (see Dawes, 1994)—the "cure" part of the "talking cure" might be readily challenged as well in view of Anna O's subsequent hospitalization and clinical dysfunctions.
2. The *physical Internet* refers to a way of transforming how physical objects (e.g., manufactured goods) are transported, stored, supplied, and used to achieve greater efficiency as well as sustainability. Achieving this transformation requires collaboration and standardization of manufacturing, shipping, retailing, regulating, and the

movement of goods across many boundaries (e.g., geographical, industry, proprietary). This is referred to metaphorically as an Internet to emphasize the standardization and communication that characterizes the more familiar digital Internet. In manufacturing, there are enormous differences among industries, companies, countries, and so on that limit efficiencies, and these influence not only costs but also sustainability of resources and utilization of the workforce (see Montreuil, 2011).

Chapter 7

1. Several such initiatives that focused on mental health include Grand Challenges in Global Mental Health Millennium Villages Program, Integrated Innovations for Global Mental Health, Collaborative Hubs for International Research on Mental Health in Low- and Middle-Income Countries, and Program for Improving Mental Health Care, among others (see Belkin et al., 2011; Patel, Chowdhary et al., 2011). Grand challenges will be discussed further in Chapter 10.
2. The concept behind the frequently used quote is attributed to Brock Chisolm, MD (1896–1971), the first Director-General of the World Health Organization (WHO), who is credited with stating, "without mental health there can be no true physical health" (no date; see Kolappa, Henderson, & Kishore, 2013).
3. Many of the same considerations were part of the rationale for placing physical health, mental health, and substance use and abuse services together as part of integrated care. Integrated care is not task shifting but rather is a collaboration of different services and professionals. Yet they both reflected the zeitgeist of major changes in needed services.
4. Smart tattoos and digital tattoos are implanted in the skin and can be used to control other devices. They are currently used to monitor biological states (e.g., glucose in the case of diabetes; Visweswara & Hua Gan, 2015). These are relatively new, and their potential has yet to be exploited, certainly in the contexts related to markers and indices of psychological states and psychiatric disorder. Here, too, these have not penetrated into everyday life like smartphones and smartwatches. (I expect many people are like me and are waiting the availability of smart butterfly tattoos.)
5. The author has no personal, professional, or financial involvement in or connection to the commercial projects noted as examples here.
6. Although health care–related interventions have been applied in beauty salons for several ethnic groups, several of the applications have focused on African Americans in light of the unique and important role that salons have played in the African American community (e.g., Gill, 2010). Historically, salons have been centers of economic, social, and political change, and beauticians were catalysts for social activism. For example, during the early Civil Rights Movement, beauticians registered their customers to vote and spread information about political rallies and demonstrations. This rich historical context has left the African American beautician or stylist in a valued leadership role and as an ideal messenger of critical information about a variety of topics, including health (Linnan & Ferguson, 2007).

Chapter 8

1. DALY is a measure of overall disease burden, expressed as the number of years lost due to ill health, disability, or early death. This was discussed in more detail in

Chapter 2. The Glossary at the end of the book elaborates this measure and QALY, also referred to in the present chapter.

2. A blog is a shortened version of the term *Web log* and is a medium for posting essays and statements in various lengths. These can also include images, videos, slides, and interactive content.
3. This is distinct from virtual reality and virtual reality exposure therapy, which use a variety of sensory cues and specialized equipment, such as head-mounted displays, to create a believable simulation of reality and a personalized setting for therapy (e.g., Bohil, Alicea, & Biocca, 2011). Much of the work in virtual reality–based interventions has focused on anxiety and traumatic experiences (e.g., Riva, 2005; Rizzo et al., 2010). Because many of these treatments include a therapist (to assist in creating personalized experiences and to help patients process those experiences), these forms of virtual therapy are not elaborated here.
4. Paro is a robot modeled after a harp seal (for photos and more detail see www.parorobots.com/). Through interacting with people, Paro responds as if alive and imitates the voice of a real baby harp seal. Apart from making sounds, Paro responds to petting by moving its tail and opening and closing its eyes and learns a new name given by the person with whom it is interacting. Microprocessors, microphones, tactile sensor, touch-sensitive whiskers, and various motors and actuators that move the limbs make up the inner workings. As a disclosure of any potential source of conflict, as I write this chapter, I am currently funded for social robotics research, and part of that has included use of Paro robots for experimentation.
5. For purposes of conveying the model in broad strokes, I have eliminated the terminology and ways in which facets of the network are identified and their multiple components. Other sources are readily available for more in-depth coverage of networks (Christakis & Fowler, 2009; Rogers, 2003; Valente, 2010).

Chapter 9

1. The most commonly used metric to operationalize "strength" of a treatment in psychotherapy research is one of the many effect size measures. I already discussed in detail why effect size measures have no necessary or clear relation to improvement in ways that make a difference in the lives of clients. Consequently, I do not include those measures here to operationalize strong effect.
2. The number of efforts to raise awareness by government and nongovernment agencies and professional organizations is huge. These are efforts to raise awareness, provide resources available to the public, and devote a day, week, or month to individual problems. Here is a sample for a variety of mental and substance use and abuse disorders: Great American Smokeout (www.cancer.org/healthy/stayawayfromtobacco/greatamericansmokeout/); Children's Mental Health Awareness Day (www.samhsa.gov/children/national-childrens-awareness-day-events/awareness-day-2016); World Bipolar Day (http://www.worldbipolarday.org/); National Posttraumatic Stress Disorder Awareness Day (www.nctsn.org/resources/public-awareness/national-ptsd-awareness-day); National Anxiety and Depression Awareness Week (www.freedomfromfear.org/NationalAnxietyandDepressionAwarenessWeek.en.html); National Autism Awareness Month (www.autism-society.org/get-involved/national-autism-awareness-month/); Schizophrenia Awareness Week (www.rethink.org/news-views/2015/09/schizophrenia-awareness-week-is-coming); National Eating Disorders

Awareness Week (http://nedawareness.org/); Tourette Syndrome Association Advocacy Day (https://www.tourette.org/media/Tourette-Association-National-Advocacy-Day.pdf); National Drug and Alcohol Facts Week (https://teens.drugabuse.gov/national-drug-alcohol-facts-week); and Developmental Disabilities Month (www.specialneedsalliance.org/march-is-developmental-disabilities-awareness-month/). Worth noting that there is also interest in fostering the positive side of mental health, as illustrated by the International Day of Happiness, fostered by the United Nations and its member countries (http://www.un.org/en/events/happinessday/). My listing is quite selective and is restricted to mental health. From the extraordinarily long list of awareness months, weeks, and days, one wonders if any particular cause stands out against a tsunami of genuinely great causes. (I am thinking of proposing a Great Awareness of Nothing Day, in which we have an entire day when we do not have to be aware and we go through consciousness lowering rather than consciousness raising.)

3. The rule has several names in addition to the more commonly used names *(80/20 rule, Pareto's principle)*, including the *law of the vital few* and the *principle of factor sparcity*. This is an informal rule or a rule of thumb, but it also based on mathematical derivations (Chen, Chong, & Tong, 1994). And, of course, the rule is an approximation of 80 and 20, rather than a rigid 80 and 20 in all contexts to which the rule applies.
4. Two researchers warrant special mention: Hideyo Noguchi (1876–1928), a bacteriologist who in 1911 discovered the bacteria of syphilis that caused the progression to the disease; and Julius Wagner-Jauregg (1857–1940), an Austrian physician who discovered that inoculation with malaria was an effective treatment. He received the Nobel Prize in Physiology or Medicine (1927) for this discovery. The work of these investigators, but others, too, firmly established the biological bases for what was considered by many a mental disorder.
5. The notion of pathway is useful to mention to convey the point. The concept of "final common path" was originally developed by Sir Charles Sherrington (1857–1952), a neurophysiologist and pathologist and Nobel laureate (Nobel Prize in Physiology and Medicine in 1932). Sherrington studied how inputs into neural circuits are integrated and join through a final common path to generate muscle/motor movement (see Burke, 2007). The notion has been extended, and "final common pathway" has been used in many different contexts to note how separate factors may converge into a final path leading to an outcome. In the present discussion, I raise a complementary notion that would be equivalent to an initial common origin. In this case, the origin may be common but actually lead to many different outcomes. By transmechanisms, I am suggesting a common initial origin.
6. There is no one "immune system" or single type of response, and my reference to "the" immune system is only to draw attention to the overall topic. The complexities and nuances among various immune responses may well be important for various types of psychiatric symptoms and dysfunction, as they are for physical disorders (e.g., autoimmune diseases). These details are well beyond the scope of the present section. For an overview of the immune system, the reader is referred elsewhere (https://www.niaid.nih.gov/research/immune-system-research; and www.imgt.org/IMGTeducation/Tutorials/ImmuneSystem/UK/the_immune_system.pdf).

7. Actually, with emergency department visits, physical health care correlates of untreated mental illness, and the consequences of mental illness (DALYs, earlier than expected death), providing "no treatment" is probably very expensive. Indeed, one wonders if not providing needed treatment is a "worst buy" (in the spirit of best-buy thinking), leaving aside the inhumanity of it.

Chapter 10

1. The ODPHP is part of the US Department of the Health and Human Services and provides enormous resources that include guidance for consumers on physical and mental conditions, injuries and violence, and well-being in relation to a variety of topics (e.g., material, child, and infant health; reproductive and sexual health; nutrition, activity, and obesity; oral health; injury prevention) (see https://health.gov/). Information and training opportunities are provided in many different formats (e.g., quizzes, blogs, newsletters, and webinars) to promote healthy living. My discussion can provide only an overview of Healthy People 2020. There are many agencies involved and an array of helpful materials to become involved (see the progress that has been made at https://www.healthypeople.gov/2020/about/How-To-Use-HealthyPeople.gov).
2. My mention of diet as a potential place to intervene in relation to mental health is a useful case of how a wicked problem alerts us to cautions. For example, not all agree that the data show a causal relation between improvements in diet and mental illness and whether diet is the issue or a carefully comprised formula of micronutrients, which is a bit different from how we usually think about diet (e.g., see Kaplan et al., 2015; Rucklidge & Kaplan, 2013). There would be a group, maybe a large group, of scientists saying there are insufficient data to act on providing nutrients or micronutrients on a large scale. A wicked problem characteristic is that invariably there will be insufficient data to act, even though some action is needed toward a solution. This is not a rationale for acting on poor data or ignoring data and dissent in interpretation of those data. The challenge is: When is enough inadequate or insufficient data sufficient to act? "Never" is not really feasible because many of the challenges have life and death consequences and academic hedging is a luxury enjoyed only by those not in the line of fire. We need guidelines for when to act when things are not all that clear. My own preference is to act, do so on a small scale at first if that luxury is allowed, and obtain ongoing evidence to be sure some help has been provided and no harm has been incurred. Part of the rationale is that we have to act and cannot delay; but for some of the challenges (e.g., climate change, salvage fisheries in the oceans), a small scale may be too little to expect an impact.

Chapter 11

1. In social policy and science, "ought and can" may have a very different relation from the one considered from a purely philosophical or moral perspective. What we "ought" to do might be used to select a focus or priority or identify a grand challenge (e.g., climate change), and that may foster greater efforts so that the priority "can" be accomplished. For example, policy might say we "ought" to travel to Mars or we "ought" to clean up the oceans, but at this time we cannot, that is, do not have that capacity at present. In this context, ought mobilizes efforts and innovation so that someday in fact we can and will.

ABBREVIATIONS AND GLOSSARY

ABBREVIATION	FULL TERM
BDNF	Brain-derived neurotrophic factor
CDC	Centers for Disease Control and Prevention
DALY	Disability-adjusted life year
DSM	*Diagnostic and Statistical Manual of Mental Disorders*
EBPI	Evidence-based psychosocial intervention
ICD	*International Statistical Classification of Diseases and Related Health Problems*
IOM	Institute of Medicine
NAS	National Academy of Sciences
NASEM	National Academies of Sciences, Engineering, and Medicine
NICE	National Institute for Health and Care Excellence
PTSD	Posttraumatic Stress Disorder
QALY	Quality-adjusted life year
RCT	Randomized controlled trial
SAMHSA	Substance Abuse and Mental Health Services Administration
SARs	Socially assistive robots
TAU	Treatment as usual
WHO	World Health Organization
YLD	Years lived with disability
YLL	Years of life lost to premature mortality

Notes: In 2015, the National Academy of Sciences changed the name of one of components, the Institute of Medicine, to the National Academy of Medicine. The purpose was to better integrate the three different facets of the larger organization, now called the National Academies of Science, Engineering, and Medicine (see www.nationalacademies.org/about/whoweare/index.html).

GLOSSARY

Acceptability: In the context of psychosocial intervention research, acceptability refers to judgments by laypersons, clients, and others about whether the intervention procedures are appropriate, fair, and reasonable for the problem that is to be treated. The extension for this book is that the model of delivery must be acceptable if we are to have large-scale application of the intervention. Acceptability of treatment can be conceived separately from the acceptability of the model of delivering treatment.

Active placebo: A placebo that is inert with respect to direct biological effects on the clinical problem or focus but mimics side effects that the nonplacebo medication has. The presence of side effects makes the placebo more plausible as a "real" medication.

Alternative interventions: See *Complementary and alternative interventions.*

Barriers to treatment: These refer to a variety of obstacles or impediments to obtaining treatment. The barriers can vary in their source (system and attitudinal factors). There are scores of barriers, and a posterchild for these might be the most familiar one, namely, stigma about being labeled as having a mental condition, and the related but less familiar one, namely, self-stigma, in which one's own views interfere with labeling one's symptoms and seeking mental health care.

Benchmarking: A method discussed in the book in the context of evaluating treatments in which the effectiveness of a given intervention is evaluated outside of the context of controlled trials. The effects of that treatment are compared to (i.e., benchmarked against) the magnitude of the effects of treatments that are evaluated in controlled trials and established as evidence based.

Best-buy interventions: Interventions selected based on their cost-effectiveness, affordability, feasibility for the setting (e.g., country, city), and other criteria. Conceived as an economic tool to help countries select among evidence-based strategies to have an impact, where the impact is quantified (estimated) for different strategies. Math models are used to identify likely best buys, and these are followed by empirical tests to evaluate the extent to the model predictions. See *Good-buy interventions.*

Burden: Refers in the context of physical and mental illness to reflect the range of impacts that a particular condition has on measurable outcomes. Commonly used outcomes relate to days or years of functioning that are lost as a result of or associated with the condition and to financial costs. There are many metrics that are used and applied widely to allow comparison of the burdens of different conditions. (For examples of measures to reflect burden, see *DALY, HALE, QALY, YLL,* and *YLD.*)

Case identification: Identified as a barrier to providing treatment services and refers to not identifying individuals at risk early in their course toward dysfunction or with a current dysfunction. This is not a person self-identifying as in need of care or attention but rather the system and public resources (e.g., schools, doctors' offices) that have no systematic way of identifying individuals in need of services.

Client: The term used in this book interchangeably with *patient.* This refers to the individual who is seen for and treated with an intervention. Client is especially useful in the present book because many of the interventions are applied outside of the context of traditional "treatment," and a term outside of the medical reference of "patients" and "treatment" is more appropriate.

Clinical significance: Clinical significance refers to the practical value or importance of the effect of an intervention, that is, whether it makes any "real" difference to the clients or to others in their functioning and everyday life. Researchers have attempted to define and evaluate this to go beyond what statistical significance provides.

Common factors: These are characteristics that are common to many different treatments and considered to be in whole or in part those facets that lead or contribute to or account for the benefits of therapy. These factors include such components as meeting with a therapist, developing and alliance, hearing a credible rationale about one's clinical problem, having hope and expectancies for change mobilized by the treatment, and engaging in some activities or "ritual" designed to be therapeutic.

Comorbidity: The presence of two or more disorders. Many disorders are comorbid so that meeting the criteria for one of them (e.g., depression) increases the likelihood that a person will meet criteria for another disorder (e.g., anxiety) as well.

Complementary and alternative interventions: Procedures in both physical and mental health that are not considered part of mainstream interventions or that have emerged from traditions outside of Western health care. These can include herbs, diet supplements, mind-body exercises, and various therapies like massage and acupuncture. Many of the procedures (e.g., mindfulness, meditation) are part of traditional treatments and main treatments, and hence complementary can blur into mainstream. In general, treatments are considered complementary when they are added to (i.e., complement) standard treatments (e.g., adding special diets to complement chemotherapy for cancer). They are considered alternative therapies when used instead of standard treatment.

DALY: This is an abbreviation for *disability-adjusted life year* and is a metric used to evaluate the burden of disease, accident, injury, and mental disorders. This refers specifically to one year of a healthy life that is lost due to some impairment (e.g., cancer, stroke). One DALY = one year of healthy life that is lost based on life expectancy. Stated another way, the measure is the difference or gap between current health status and an ideal situation based on how long one would be likely to live into old age, free of disease and disability. See also *HALE, QALY, YLD,* and *YLL.*

Disparities in health care: Refers to the differences in access to care and services that are not the result of differences in the health status (e.g., prevalence of dysfunction) or preferences of the groups. In the United States, there are huge disparities across ethnic, cultural, and socioeconomic lines in which non-White individuals who are not part of the majority cultural group and have lower income and education are less likely to receive services.

Disruptive innovation: The concept pertains to a change in a product or service that is not a linear, evolutionary, or incremental step. The product or service often provides a disruptive, disjunctive, or qualitative leap and develops or extends a market that is not otherwise being served. The innovation involves taking a product or service that is complicated, expensive, and less affordable and providing something that changes these.

Disruptive technology: See *Disruptive innovation.*

Dissemination of treatment: Efforts to extend treatments that have been developed in research so that are used in clinical work. There are multiple steps in dissemination involving agencies, administrators, and clinicians, training in the new treatments, developing procedures to monitor implementation of treatment correctly, and others.

Distress: A reaction to stressful events or experiences that are maladaptive and may include the emergence of symptoms such as anxiety and depression. Distress reflects a reaction that interferes with functioning in some way.

Dominant model of therapy: The most frequent way that psychosocial interventions (evidence based and non–evidence based) are provided. The model includes three main characteristics: (1) treatment sessions are provided in person and one-to-one with a client (individual, couple, family); (2) treatment is administered by a highly trained (e.g., master's or doctoral level) mental health professional; and (3) sessions are held at a clinic, private office, or health care facility. The model is the one used in clinical practice, graduate school training, clinical program accreditation, predoctoral and postdoctoral internships, and research on psychosocial interventions.

Effect size: A measure of the strength or magnitude of an experimental effect. Also, a way of expressing the difference between conditions (e.g., treatment versus control) in terms of a common metric across measures and studies. The most common method of computing effect size (Cohen's *d*) is based on computing the difference between the means of interest on a particular measure and dividing this by the standard deviation (e.g., pooled standard deviation of the conditions).

eHealth: The use of the Internet as a basis for health care, including providing information, opportunities to interaction, and more broadly extending health information and technology on a larger scale. See www.ncbi.nlm.nih.gov/pmc/articles/PMC1761894/.

Entertainment-education: Use of television or radio to deliver health care messages and to model health-promoting behaviors. A culturally sensitive long-running series (e.g., TV series) is developed in which different characters take on different roles, deal with the challenges related to the focus of the intervention, and model adaptive strategies in relation to the goal of the particular series (e.g., family planning). The series is devised in the context of cultural and ethnic considerations to ensure that characters and their daily lives embrace commonly held values and practices of the culture.

Experience sampling: This is a method of assessment in which participants are asked to stop at various points in time during their everyday lives and in real time to respond to questions about their experience (e.g., how they are feeling, what they are thinking, and what they are doing). When to provide the assessment can be signaled (e.g., beeper, cell phone call, or text message) and randomized over a given time period. The assessment is not necessarily self-report, and increasingly biological indices (and correlates) of psychological states continue to come online. This is a breakthrough in clinical research because of the assessment of daily life in real time and also because interventions can be programmed to be applied as needed in response to the information obtained by that assessment.

Good-buy interventions: In developing interventions using the best-buy model, interventions occasionally are distinguished that do not meet all of the criteria to make them best buys. Even so, they are considered to be "good buys" because they meet some or most of the criteria and could make a difference in expanding the availability of services. See *Best-buy interventions*.

Grand challenge: A major problem area that is identified as an important focus that could be resolved or seriously mitigated if critical barriers were removed. Delineation of a challenge identifies the goal, focuses attention on the barriers and tasks that need to be addressed, and mobilizes many resources and partners to help reach the goal. The implication is that if the barriers were resolved, significant progress could be made. Many of the grand challenges are in the area of health, but also a very many disciplines have identified these to move a given topic forward (e.g., archaeology, engineering, mathematics, nutrition and food science, robotics, and many more).

HALE: This is an abbreviation of *health adjusted life expectancy* and is a metric to measure the burden of illness. The measure considers mortality and morbidity and includes the average number of years that a person can expect to live in "full health." This is expected life expectancy minus the amount of time expected to be hampered by a disabling condition (physical or mental health). See also *DALY, QALY, YLD,* and *YLL*.

Impairment: Refers to interruption or interference with functioning and in meeting role requirements in relation to work, social relations, or other domains of daily activity and responsibility. Also, impairment includes increased risk in suffering in some way (e.g., death, pain, or loss of freedom).

Integrated care: A model of providing health care in which physical health care and mental and substance abuse services and behavioral health (e.g., to address health related lifestyle issues) are in the same setting or closely coordinated if not exactly in the same setting. The goal is to facilitate delivery and receipt of services by coordination and integration of multiple foci in a single setting and to reduce barriers (e.g., stigma, seeking treatment for different problems at different services). Integrated care is person centered, that is, meeting the full set of needs of the patient, rather than specialty care centered. See www.integration.samhsa.gov/about-us/what-is-integrated-care.

Internet of things: Refers to the interconnection via the Internet of computing devices embedded in everyday objects, enabling them to send and receive data. The data are transferred from machine to machine without requiring human-to-human or human-to-computer interaction.

Lifestyle changes: Refers to a range of behaviors in everyday life that individuals can engage in that positively affect health. Diet, exercise, alcohol consumption, and cigarette smoking are familiar practices that relate to health. Others include walks in nature, meditation, and yoga.

Loneliness: Refers to the subjective experience of social isolation. This is not necessarily *being* socially isolated or having few or no social contacts. Rather, loneliness it is how one experiences the world and how one feels, rather than objective information about a person's contacts with others.

Mechanism: The steps or processes through which the intervention (or some independent variable) unfolds and exerts its influence. Mechanism explains more about underlying processes and how they lead change and goes beyond merely a statistical association (mediation) or a conceptual interpretation of what explains change.

Mediator: A construct that shows a statistical relation between an experimental manipulation or intervention and the dependent variable or outcome. This is an intervening construct that suggests processes about why change occurs or on which change depends. Typically, mediators are not causes or mechanisms, but they might point the way to either of those.

Mental disorder: Refers to formally recognized symptom patterns that are delineated in various diagnostic systems in which psychiatric disorders are described. Several specific criteria have to be met to have a designated psychiatric diagnosis. For present purposes, psychiatric disorder and mental disorders will be used interchangeably. The focus of the book includes reducing the burdens of mental disorders but also going beyond formally recognized psychiatric disorders. See *Subclinical disorder.*

Mental health literacy: Identified a barrier to receiving services and refers to information individuals have and what they know about mental disorders, whether they recognize that they have symptoms or a disorder that warrants treatment, what the options are for treatment, and how to pursue those options and obtain treatment.

Meta-analysis: A quantitative method of evaluating a body of research in which effect size is used as the common metric. Studies are combined so that inferences can be drawn across multiple studies and as a function of several of their characteristics (e.g., types of interventions, quality of their methodologies).

mHealth: The use of mobile communications (e.g., smartphones, smartwatch, computer) for health services and information. The emphasis is on mobile or portable devices that can develop, store, deliver, and retrieve health information in real time.

Mindfulness: Mindfulness involves attention to and awareness of the present moment (e.g., focusing on present thoughts, feelings, sensations). This also includes acknowledging and accepting these thoughts, feelings, and sensations.

Nonspecific treatment factors: See *Common factors.*

Pareto's principle: This is commonly referred to as the *80/20 rule* and is based on observations that approximately 80 percent of an outcome is the result of 20 percent of the causes or input. The rule, named after Vilfredo Pareto (1848–1923), has been applied very widely in many contexts (e.g., business, economics, sports, science, and health). An illustration noted is that in the United States, approximately 20 percent of patients use 80 percent of health care resources. The rule has other names used less frequently, including the *law of the vital few* and the *principle of factor sparcity.*

Physician's practice model: A model of providing treatment that grew out of medicine in which the professional (doctor) meets individually with a patient in an office to provide or prescribe the treatment. That model was central in the formal development of various psychosocial therapies (e.g., mesmerism, hypnosis, psychoanalysis) and is continued as the dominant model of psychotherapy.

Placebo: A substance that has no active pharmacological properties that would be expected to produce change in the condition to which it is applied.

Placebo effect: Change in an outcome due to expectancies for improvement on the part of clients or those who are administering a medication or other intervention procedure.

Proportionate universalism: Refers to the means of providing health care services to all (universally) but allocating the proportion of resources and services in relation to the level of disadvantage, burden, or need.

Psychiatric diagnosis: See *Mental disorder*.

Psychological dysfunction: This will be used along with "psychological problems" as a broad term to encompass not only psychiatric disorders but all psychological domains that can interfere with functioning in daily life. Maladaptive thoughts (cognitions) and difficult-to-control emotions (affect) and actions (behaviors) alone and in combination can lead to problems in our individual lives.

Psychosocial intervention: A broad term needed in the book to encompass a variety of interventions that can have an impact on psychological problems and daily functioning. These will include but go well beyond what is traditionally covered by various forms of psychotherapy (e.g., behavior therapy, cognitive therapy, psychodynamic therapy) and treatment. Psychosocial emphasizes that strategies of change are mostly based on psychological rather than medical and biological means of intervention.

QALY: Abbreviation for *quality-adjusted life* years that refers to a measure of burden (e.g., of disease) that integrates both the quality and the quantity of life lived. One QALY refers to one year of life in perfect health. The measure is used as part of cost calculations, namely, what is the cost of interventions using as a measure a gain in one QALY. See also *DALY, HALE, YLD,* and *YLL*.

Quality-adjusted life year: See *QALY*.

Randomized controlled trial: A intervention outcome study in which clients with a particular problem (e.g., depression, cancer) are randomly assigned to various intervention and control conditions. This is usually regarded by many as the "gold standard," that is, the best and most definitive way of demonstrating that an intervention is effective.

Reach of treatment: Capacity of treatment to extend to individuals not usually served or well served by the traditional dominant service delivery model.

Research-practice gap: Refers to the fact that what has been shown to work well in research is not what is being carried out in practice. The gap in integrating findings from research to clinical practice is evident both in physical and mental health care. The research to application gap is common in many fields in which knowledge is used toward applied ends (e.g. agriculture, economics, education, farming, forestry, and many others).

Scalability of treatment: The capacity of the intervention to be applied in a way that reaches a large number (and proportion) of individuals.

Self-stigma: Refers to the view that individuals may hold in relation to their own mental health and reticence and perhaps shame in labeling themselves as having a mental disorder and worthy of seeking treatment. Self-stigma is internalization of the broader view (stigma) one might hold toward others or that others hold toward them.

Socially assistive robots: Robots that interact with humans in some way. They can provide education and feedback, coach clients through activities and tasks, and provide companionship.

Stigma: Refers to negative beliefs and practices by a group about a condition that others may have, such as mental disorder or a disability. Stigma can lead to genuine discriminatory practices and domains of rejection (e.g., employment, promotion, access to other services). This is a barrier because people are less likely to identify themselves as having a mental disorder or seeking treatment because of the stigma. See *Self-stigma*.

Stressor: Refers to those conditions that pose threats, challenges, and demands that exceed the usual regulatory processes of the individual. Stress can also refer to the temporary psychological and biological reactions (e.g., worry, loss of sleep, nausea, anxiety). See *Distress*.

Subclinical disorder: This is a term often used to refer to psychological dysfunctions that miss meeting the criteria for a psychiatric disorder (e.g., major depression). The individual with a subclinical dysfunction may still experience impairment in daily functioning and still benefit from treatment. Subclinical disorders can be important in part because the cutoff for meeting and not meeting criteria is arbitrary. Also, having a subclinical disorder is a risk factor for meeting the criteria for a "full" disorder sometime later. See *Subsyndromal disorder*.

Subsyndromal disorder: Many individuals have sources of impairment and symptoms but do not meet the cutoff and criteria for a formal psychiatric disorder. Because psychiatric disorders can be considered syndromes, not quite meeting the criteria can refer to subsyndrome. The term will be used interchangeably with *subclinical disorder*. See *Syndrome* and *Subclinical disorder*.

Syndrome: A group of symptoms that consistently go together and may have characteristics that go beyond those particular symptoms. These other characteristics may include antecedent factors (e.g., risk factors, family history), other comorbid conditions, and long-term course. Psychiatric disorders reflect groups of symptoms that go together, but in many cases (e.g., schizophrenia, depression) much more is known.

Task sharing: A variant of task shifting in which tasks of delivering services are not completely turned over to nonprofessionals and lay individuals. Rather, both trained lay individuals and professionals work together and *share* in the activities and task. Task sharing and task shifting can be a matter of degree depending on whether, but also the extent to which, professionals are involved in delivering the intervention. See *Task shifting*.

Task shifting: A method of strengthening and expanding the health care workforce by redistributing the tasks of delivering services to a broad range of individuals with less training and fewer qualifications than traditional health care workers (e.g., doctors, nurses). This redistribution allows an increase in the total number of health workers (e.g., nonprofessionals, lay individuals) to scale up the scope of providing services. See *Task sharing*, a related term that is sometimes used interchangeably with, but also occasionally distinguished from, task shifting.

Telehealth: Refers broadly to a model of delivering health care services through information and communication technologies. The focus is on diagnosis, treatment, education, case management, and self-management. This is a broader term that encompasses multiple technologies (e.g., mhealth) and foci (e.g., physical and mental health, occupational therapy, disaster management). Telehealth also encompasses telemedicine, which began with a more restricted focus on diagnosis, assessment, and intervention with medical disorders. See www.cchpca.org/what-is-telehealth.

Telemedicine: The use of telecommunications technologies to provide remote access to assess, diagnosis, and treat patients. The term has been expanded to eHealth as technologies and uses have expanded, but many of the terms (e.g., ehealth, mhealth, telehealth) are not used consistently. See www.amdtelemedicine.com/telemedicine-resources/telemedicine-defined.html.

The 80/20 rule: See *Pareto's principle.*

Therapeutic alliance: Refers to the quality and nature of the client–therapist relationship, the collaborative interaction between them, and the bond or personal attachment that emerges during treatment.

Transdiagnosis: Refers to the study of processes (e.g., risk factors, etiology) that span many different manifestations of clinical dysfunction. Many disorders show several underlying commonalities that include family history, genetic, and psychosocial (e.g., socioeconomic, cultural) factors.

Transtreatment: A broad term that encompasses interventions that are designed to treat many different disorders. This contrasts with the traditional approach of developing individual treatments for specific disorders. Psychosocial transtreatments draw on components of evidence-based interventions that can be applied broadly.

Treatment as usual: The routine treatment that is provided in a given setting for the same clinical problem or intervention focus that is included in the study. This group receives whatever is usually done, that is, usual care.

Treatment gap: Refers to the difference between the proportion of people who have disorders or suffer psychological dysfunction (prevalence) and the proportion of those individuals who receive care. This is a core concept for the book because the vast majority of individuals with psychological dysfunction receive no care for their problems.

Wicked problem: The term is used in policymaking, social planning, and business and captures several special features of such as having no single, definitive, or simple formulation of the problem, the likelihood that the problem is embedded in several other challenges and wicked problems, there is no one solution, and the problem and solution have multiple formulations based on different stakeholders, values, culture, politics, and other features.

Years lived with disability: See *YLD.*

Years of life lost to premature mortality: See *YLL.*

YLD: Abbreviation for *years lived with disability* that is another measure to reflect the burden of disease or dysfunction. This is used less frequently than DALYs but gives separate information. See also *DALY, HALE, QALY,* and *YLL.*

YLL: Abbreviation for *years of life lost to premature mortality* that is a measure to reflect the burden of disease or dysfunction. Used less frequently than DALYs but gives separate information. See also *DALY, HALE, QALY,* and *YLD.*

REFERENCES

Adams, R. (2010). *If you build it will they come? Three steps to test and validate any market opportunity*. Hoboken, NJ: John Wiley & Sons.

Addis, M. E. (2002). Methods for disseminating research products and increasing evidence-based practice: Promises, obstacles, and future directions. *Clinical Psychology: Science and Practice*, *9*(4), 367–378.

Adelborg, K., Schmidt, M., Sundboll, J., Pedersen, L., Videbech, P., Botker, H. E., . . . Sorensen, H. T. (2016). Mortality risk among heart failure patients with depression: A nationwide population-based cohort study. *Journal of the American College of Cardiology*, *67*(13_S), 1318.

Agency for Healthcare Research and Quality (AHRQ). (2017). Patient centered Medical Home Resource Center. Retrieved from https://pcmh.ahrq.gov/page/defining-pcmh

Ahmead, M. K., Rahhal, A. A., & Baker, J. A. (2010). The attitudes of mental health professionals towards patients with mental illness in an inpatient setting in Palestine. *International Journal of Mental Health Nursing*, *19*(5), 356–362.

Alarcón, R. D. (2009). Cultural factors and psychiatric diagnosis: Review and projections. *World Psychiatry*, *8*(3), 131–139.

Albrecht, M. (2014). Alcoholism is not a disease. In N. Ishibashi (Ed.), *Arguing with the DSM-5* (pp. 9–18). Chicago: Nora L. Ishibashi (publisher).

Alderman, H. (Ed.) (2011). *No small matter: The impact of poverty, shocks, and human capital*. Washington, DC: The World Bank.

Alegria, M, Jackson, J. S., Kessler, R. C., & Takeuchi, D. (2003). National Comorbidity Survey Replication (NCS-R), 2001–2003. Ann Arbor: Interuniversity Consortium for Political and Social Research.

Allinder, R. M., & Oats, R. G. (1997). Effects of acceptability on teachers' implementation of curriculum-based measurement and student achievement in mathematics computation. *Remedial and Special Education*, *18*, 113–120.

Allumbaugh, D. L., & Hoyt, W. T. (1999). Effectiveness of grief therapy: A meta-analysis. *Journal of Counseling Psychology*, *46*(3), 370–380.

American College of Lifestyle Medicine. (2009). *Lifestyle medicine: Evidence review*. Retrieved from www.lifestylemedicine.org/

American Psychiatric Association. (2013). *Diagnostic and statistical manual of mental disorders* (5th ed.). Arlington, VA: American Psychiatric Publishing.

American Psychological Association Presidential Task Force on Evidence-Based Practice. (2006). Evidence-based practice in psychology. *American Psychologist*, *61*, 271–285.

American Psychological Association Task Force on Promotion and Dissemination of Psychological Procedures. (1995). Training in and dissemination of empirically-validated psychological procedures: Report and recommendations. *Clinical Psychologist*, *48*(1), 3–23.

American Psychological Association. (2015, February). *Stress in America™: Paying with our health*. Washington, DC: American Psychological Association.

Amini, M. (2016, September). Aetna giving 50,000 Apple Watches to employees, deduction to customers buying them. CNBC News, Health Care. Retrieved from www.cnbc.com/2016/09/28/aetna-giving-50000-apple-watches-to-employees-deduction-to-customers-buying-them.html

Anderson, K. M. (2012). *How far have we come in reducing health disparities? Progress since 2000*. Washington, DC: The National Academies Press.

Anderson, L. A., & Whiston, S. C. (2005). Sexual assault education programs: A meta-analytic examination of their effectiveness. *Psychology of Women Quarterly*, *29*(4), 374–388.

Andersson, G., Cuijpers, P., Carlbring, P., Riper, H., & Hedman, E. (2014). Guided Internet-based vs. face-to-face cognitive behavior therapy for psychiatric and somatic disorders: A systematic review and meta-analysis. *World Psychiatry*, *13*(3), 288–295.

Andrews, G., Cuijpers, P., Craske, M. G., McEvoy, P., & Titov, N. (2010). Computer therapy for the anxiety and depressive disorders is effective, acceptable and practical health care: A meta-analysis. *PLoS One*, *5*(10), e13196.

Anestis, M. D., Anestis, J. C., Zawilinski, L. L., Hopkins, T. A., & Lilienfeld, S. O. (2014). Equine-related treatments for mental disorders lack empirical support: A systematic review of empirical investigations. *Journal of Clinical Psychology*, *70*(12), 1115–1132.

Ankuta, G. Y., & Abeles, N. (1993). Client satisfaction, clinical significance, and meaningful change in psychotherapy. *Professional Psychology: Research and Practice*, *24*, 70–74.

Ansseau, M., Dierick, M., Buntinkx, F., Cnockaert, P., De Smedt, J., Van Den Haute, M., & Vander Mijnsbrugge, D. (2004). High prevalence of mental disorders in primary care. *Journal of Affective Disorders*, *78*(1), 49–55.

Arnberg, F. K., Linton, S. J., Hultcrantz, M., Heintz, E., & Jonsson, U. (2014). Internet-delivered psychological treatments for mood and anxiety disorders: A systematic review of their efficacy, safety, and cost-effectiveness. *PLoS One*, *9*(5), p.e98118.

Arndorfer, R. E., Allen. K. D., & Aljazireh, L. (1999). Behavioral health needs in pediatric medicine and the acceptability of behavioral solutions: Implications for behavioral psychologists. *Behavior Therapy*, *30*, 137–148.

Asarnow, J. R., Rozenman, M., Wiblin, J., & Zeltzer, L. (2015). Integrated medical-behavioral care compared with usual primary care for child and adolescent behavioral health: A meta-analysis. *JAMA Pediatrics*, *169*(10), 929–937.

Awad, A. G., & Voruganti, L. N. (2012). Measuring quality of life in patients with schizophrenia. *Pharmacoeconomics*, *30*(3), 183–195.

Ayllon T., & Michael, J. (1959). The psychiatric nurse as a behavioral engineer. *Journal of the Experimental Analysis of Behavior*, *2*, 323–334.

Babyak, M., Blumenthal, J. A., Herman, S., Khatri, P., Doraiswamy, M., Moore, K., . . . Krishnan, K. R. (2000). Exercise treatment for major depression: Maintenance of therapeutic benefit at 10 months. *Psychosomatic Medicine*, *62*, 633–638.

Backhaus, A., Agha, Z., Maglione, M. L., Repp, A., Ross, B., Zuest, D., . . . Thorp, S. R. (2012). Videoconferencing psychotherapy: A systematic review. *Psychological Services*, *9*(2), 111.

Bailey, D. G., Dresser, G., & Arnold, J. M. O. (2013). Grapefruit–medication interactions: Forbidden fruit or avoidable consequences? *Canadian Medical Association Journal, 185*(4), 309–316.

Bair, M. J., Robinson, R. L., Katon, W., & Kroenke, K. (2003). Depression and pain comorbidity: A literature review. *Archives of Internal Medicine, 163*(20), 2433–2445.

Baker, J. R., & Moore, S. M. (2008). Blogging as a social tool: A psychosocial examination of the effects of blogging. *Cyberpsychology & Behavior, 11*, 747–749.

Balaji, M., Chatterjee, S., Koschorke, M., Rangaswamy, T., Chavan, A., Dabholkar, H., . . . Patel, V. (2012). The development of a lay health worker delivered collaborative community based intervention for people with schizophrenia in India. *BioMed Central Health Services Research, 12*. Retrieved from http://www.biomedcentral.com/1472-6963/12/42/

Bandura, A. (1969). *Principles of behavior modification.* New York: Holt, Rinehart & Winston.

Bang, A. T., Reddy, H. M., Deshmukh, M. D., Baitule, S. B., & Bang, R. A. (2005). Neonatal and infant mortality in the 10 years (1993–2003) of the Gadchiroli field trial: Effect of home-based neonatal care. *Journal of Perinatology, 25*, 92–107.

Banks, M. R., Willoughby, L. M., & Banks, W. A. (2008). Animal-assisted therapy and loneliness in nursing homes: Use of robotic versus living dogs. *Journal of the American Medical Directors Association, 9*, 173–177.

Barak, A., Hen, L., Boniel-Nissim, M., & Shapira, N. A. (2008). A comprehensive review and a meta-analysis of the effectiveness of internet-based psychotherapeutic interventions. *Journal of Technology in Human Services, 26*(2-4), 109–160.

Bardo, M. T., & Pentz, M. A. (2012). Translational research. In H. Cooper (Ed.), *APA handbook of research methods in psychology* (Vol. 3, pp. 553–568). Washington, DC: American Psychological Association.

Barlow, D. H., Bullis, J. R., Comer, J. S., & Ametaj, A. A. (2013). Evidence-based psychological treatments: An update and a way forward. *Annual Review of Clinical Psychology, 9*, 1–27.

Barlow, D. H., Ellard, K. K., Fairholme, C., Farchione, T. J., Boisseau, C., Allen, L., & Ehrenreich-May, J. (2011). *Unified protocol for the transdiagnostic treatment of emotional disorders.* New York, NY: Oxford University Press.

Barlow, D. H., Farchione, T. J., Fairholme, C. P., Ellard, K. K., Boisseau, C. L., Allen, L. B., & Ehrenreich-May, J. (2011). *The unified protocol for transdiagnostic treatment of emotional disorders: Therapist guide.* New York, NY: Oxford University Press.

Barlow, D. H., Sauer-Zavala, S., Carl, J. R., Bullis, J. R., & Ellard, K. K. (2014). The nature, diagnosis, and treatment of neuroticism: Back to the future. *Clinical Psychological Science, 2*(3), 344–365.

Barnett, J., & Adger, W. N. (2007). Climate change, human security and violent conflict. *Political Geography, 26*(6), 639–655.

Barth, J., Munder, T., Gerger, H., Nüesch, E., Trelle, S., Znoj, H., . . . Cuijpers, P. (2013). Comparative efficacy of seven psychotherapeutic interventions for patients with depression: A network meta-analysis. *PLoS Medicine, 10*(5), e1001454.

Baskerville, N. B., Hayward, L., Brown, K. S., Hammond, D., Kennedy, R. D., & Campbell, H. S. (2015). Impact of Canadian tobacco packaging policy on quitline reach and reach equity. *Preventive Medicine, 81*, 243–250.

Baskin, T. W., Tierney, S. C., Minami, T., & Wampold, B. E. (2003). Establishing specificity in psychotherapy: A meta-analysis of structural equivalence of placebo controls. *Journal of Consulting and Clinical Psychology, 71*, 973–979.

Bastiampillai, T., Sharfstein, S. S., & Allison, S. (2016). Increase in US suicide rates and the critical decline in psychiatric beds. *JAMA*, *316*(24), 2591–2592.

Batsis, M., Dagalakis, U., Stratakis, C. A., Prodanov, T., Papadakis, G. Z., Adams, K., . . . Pacak, K. (2016). Attention deficit hyperactivity disorder in pediatric patients with pheochromocytoma and paraganglioma. *Hormone and Metabolic Research*, *48*, 509–513.

Battey, J. F. Jr., (2016, June 2). Statement on National Academies' Hearing Health Care Report by NIDCD Director National Institute of Deafness and Other Communication Disorders, US Department of Health and Human Services. Retrieved from www.nidcd.nih.gov/director-statement-on-AAHHC

Bauer, I. E., Gálvez, J. F., Hamilton, J. E., Balanzá-Martínez, V., Zunta-Soares, G. B., Soares, J. C., & Meyer, T. D. (2016). Lifestyle interventions targeting dietary habits and exercise in bipolar disorder: A systematic review. *Journal of Psychiatric Research*, *74*, 1–7.

Becker, A. E., & Kleinman, A. (2013). Mental health and the global agenda. *New England Journal of Medicine*, *369*(1), 66–73.

Belkin, G. S., Unutzer, J., Kessler, R. C., Verdeli, H., Raviola, G. J., Sachs, K., . . . Eustache, E. (2011). Scaling up for the "bottom billion": "5 × 5" implementation of community mental health care in low-income regions. *Psychiatric Services*, *62*, 1494–1502.

Bellack, A. S., & Hersen, M. (Eds.) (1985). *Dictionary of behavior therapy techniques*. New York: Pergamon.

Bemelmans, R., Gelderblom, G. J., Jonker, P., & De Witte, L. (2012). Socially assistive robots in elderly care: A systematic review into effects and effectiveness. *Journal of the American Medical Directors Association*, *13*(2), 114–120.

Benach, J., Malmusi, D., Yasui, Y., & Matinez, J. M. (2013). A new typology of policies to tackle health inequalities and scenarios of impact based on Rose's population approach. *Journal of Epidemiology and Community Health*, *67*, 286–291.

Bender, J. L., Jimenez-Marroquin, M. C., & Jadad, A. R. (2011). Seeking support on Facebook: A content analysis of breast cancer groups. *Journal of Medical Internet Research*, *13*, e16.

Benedetti, F. (2009). *Placebo effects: Understanding the mechanisms in health and disease*. New York: Oxford University Press.

Bennett-Levy, J., Richards, D. A., Farrand, P., Christensen, H., Griffiths, K. M., Kavanagh, D. J., . . . Williams, C. (Eds.). (2010). *Oxford guide to low intensity CBT interventions*. Oxford, UK: Oxford University Press.

Ben-Zeev, D., Davis, K. E., Kaiser, S., Krzsos, I., & Drake, R. E. (2013). Mobile technologies among people with serious mental illness: Opportunities for future services. *Administration and Policy in Mental Health and Mental Health Services Research*, *40*(4), 340–343.

Bergin, A. E., & Garfield, S. L. (Eds.) (1994). *Handbook of psychotherapy and behavior change* (4th ed.). New York: John Wiley & Sons.

Berk, M., Dean, O., Drexhage, H., McNeil, J. J., Moylan, S., O'Neil, A., . . . Maes, M. (2013). Aspirin: A review of its neurobiological properties and therapeutic potential for mental illness. *BMC Medicine*, *11*, 74.

Berman, M. G., Kross, E., Krpan, K. M., Askren, M. K., Burson, A., Deldin, P. J., . . . Jonides, J. (2012). Interacting with nature improves cognition and affect for individuals with depression. *Journal of Affective Disorders*, *140*(3), 300–305.

Berntsen, D., Johannessen, K. B., Thomsen, Y. D., Bertelsen, M., Hoyle, R. H., & Rubin, D. C. (2012). Peace and war trajectories of posttraumatic stress disorder symptoms before, during, and after military deployment in Afghanistan. *Psychological Science*, *23*(12), 1557–1565.

Bertolote, J. M., & Fleischmann, A. (2015). A global perspective in the epidemiology of suicide. *Suicidologi*, *7*(2). Retrieved from www.iasp.info/pdf/papers/Bertolote.pdf

Bethony, J., Brooker, S., Albonico, M., Geiger, S. M., Loukas, A., Diemert, D., & Hotez, P. J. (2006). Soil-transmitted helminth infections: Ascariasis, trichuriasis, and hookworm. *Lancet*, *367*(9521), 1521–1532.

Bettmann, J. E., Gillis, H. L., Speelman, E. A., Parry, K. J., & Case, J. M. (2016). A Meta-analysis of wilderness therapy outcomes for private pay clients. *Journal of Child and Family Studies*, *25*(9), 2659–2673.

Bickman, L. (2008). A measurement feedback system (MFS) is necessary to improve mental health outcomes. *Journal of the American Academy of Child and Adolescent Psychiatry*, *47*, 1114–1119.

Birken, S. A., Powell, B. J., Presseau, J., Kirk, M. A., Lorencatto, F., Gould, N. J., . . . Haines, E. (2017). Combined use of the Consolidated Framework for Implementation Research (CFIR) and the Theoretical Domains Framework (TDF): A systematic review. *Implementation Science*, *12*(1), 2.

Birks, M., Bodak, M., Barlas, J., Harwood, J., & Pether, M. (2016). Robotic seals as therapeutic tools in an aged care facility: A qualitative study. *Journal of Aging Research*. Retrieved from www.hindawi.com/journals/jar/2016/8569602/abs/

Blanton, H., & Jaccard, J. (2006). Arbitrary metrics in psychology. *American Psychologist*, *61*, 27–41.

Bleich, A., Gelkopf, M., & Solomon, Z. (2003). Exposure to terrorism, stress-related mental health symptoms, and coping behaviors among a nationally representative sample in Israel. *JAMA*, *290*(5), 612–620.

Blendon, R. J., Steel Fisher, G. K., Weldon, K. J., Benson, J., Brule, M., Mann, F., . . . Kramer, A. (2014). The burden of stress in America. *NPR/Robert Wood Johnson Foundation Harvard School of Public Health*, 1–12. Retrieved from https://media.npr.org/documents/2014/july/npr_rwfj_harvard_stress_poll.pdf

Bloom, D. E., Cafiero, E. T., Jané-Llopis, E., Abrahams-Gessel, S., Bloom, L. R., Fathima, S., . . . Weinstein, C. (2011). *The global economic burden of noncommunicable diseases*. Geneva: World Economic Forum.

Boehm, J. K., & Kubzansky, L. D. (2012). The heart's content: The association between positive psychological well-being and cardiovascular health. *Psychological Bulletin*, *138*(4), 655–691.

Bohil, C. J., Alicea, B., & Biocca, F. A. (2011). Virtual reality in neuroscience research and therapy. *Nature Reviews Neuroscience*, *12*, 752–762.

Bolton, P., Lee, C., Haroz, E. E., Murray, L., Dorsey, S., Robinson, C., . . . Bass, J. (2014). A transdiagnostic community-based mental health treatment for comorbid disorders: Development and outcomes of a randomized controlled trial among Burmese refugees in Thailand. *PLoS Medicine*, *11*(11), e1001757.

Bond, R. M., Fariss, C. J., Jones, J. J., Kramer, A. D., Marlow, C., Settle, J. E., & Fowler, J. H. (2012). A 61-million-person experiment in social influence and political mobilization. *Nature*, *489*(7415), 295–298.

Boniel-Nissim, M., & Barak, A. (2013). The therapeutic value of adolescents' blogging about social–emotional difficulties. *Psychological Services*, *10*(3), 333–341.

Boot, W. R., Simons, D. J., Stothart, C., & Stutts, C. (2013). The pervasive problem with placebos in psychology why active control groups are not sufficient to rule out placebo effects. *Perspectives on Psychological Science*, *8*(4), 445–454.

Boothe, J., Borrego, J., Jr., Hill, C., & Anhalt, K. (2005). Treatment acceptability and treatment compliance in ethnic minority populations. In C. L. Frisby & C. R. Reynolds (Eds.), *Comprehensive handbook of multicultural school psychology* (pp. 945–972). Hoboken, NJ: John Wiley & Sons.

Borkovec, T., & Rachman, S. (1979). The utility of analogue research. *Behaviour Research and Therapy, 17*, 253–261.

Boulos, M. N. K., Hetherington, L., & Wheeler, S. (2007). Second Life: An overview of the potential of 3-D virtual worlds in medical and health education. *Health Information & Libraries Journal, 24*(4), 233–245.

Bouma, G., Admiraal, J. M., de Vries, E. G., Schröder, C. P., Walenkamp, A. M., & Reyners, A. K. (2015). Internet-based support programs to alleviate psychosocial and physical symptoms in cancer patients: A literature analysis. *Critical Reviews in Oncology/Hematology*. Retrieved from www.croh-online.com/article/S1040-8428(15)00014-1/pdf

Bourque, F., & Cunsolo Willox, A. (2014). Climate change: The next challenge for public mental health? *International Review of Psychiatry, 26*(4), 415–422.

Bowen, D. J., & Neill, J. T. (2013). A meta-analysis of adventure therapy outcomes and moderators. *Open Psychology Journal, 6*(1), 28–53.

Bower, J. L., & Christensen, C. M. (1995). Disruptive technologies: Catching the wave. *Harvard Business Review, 73*(1), 43–53.

Bradley, E. H., Canavan, M., Rogan, E., Talbert-Slagle, K., Ndumele, C., Taylor, L., & Curry, L. A. (2016). Variation in health outcomes: The role of spending on social services, public health, and health care, 2000–09. *Health Affairs, 35*(5), 760–768.

Bradley, E. H., & Taylor, L. (2013). *The American health care paradox: Why spending more is getting us less*. New York: Public Affairs.

Bradley, R. H., & Corwyn, R. F. (2002). Socioeconomic status and child development. *Annual Review of Psychology, 53*(1), 371–399.

Brady, K. T., & Sinha, R. (2005). Co-occurring mental and substance use disorders: The neurobiological effects of chronic stress. *American Journal of Psychiatry, 162*(8), 1483–1493.

Bratman, G. N., Hamilton, J. P., Hahn, K. S., Daily, G. C., & Gross, J. J. (2015). Nature experience reduces rumination and subgenual prefrontal cortex activation. *Proceedings of the National Academy of Sciences, 112*(28), 8567–8572.

Breazeal, C. (2003). Emotion and sociable humanoid robots. *International Journal of Human-Computer Studies, 59*(1), 119–155.

Breuer, J., & Freud, S. (1957). *Studies in hysteria*. New York: Basic Books.

Brinkman, H. J., & Hendrix, C. S. (2011). *Food insecurity and violent conflict: Causes. consequences, and addressing the challenges*. Rome, Italy: *World Food Programme*. Retrieved from https://ucanr.edu/blogs/food2025/blogfiles/14415.pdf

Broadbent, E. (2017). Interactions with robots: The truths we reveal about ourselves. *Annual Review of Psychology, 68*, 627–652.

Brown, R. A., Abrantes, A. M., Read, J. P., Marcus, B. H., Jakicic, J., Strong, J. R., . . . Gordon, A. A. (2010). A pilot study of aerobic exercise as an adjunctive treatment for drug dependence. *Mental Health and Physical Activity, 1*, 27–34.

Brown, C. A., & Weisman de Mamani, A. (2017). A comparison of psychiatric symptom severity in individuals assessed in their mother tongue versus an acquired language: A two-sample study of individuals with schizophrenia and a normative population. *Professional Psychology: Research and Practice, 48*(1), 1–10.

Brownell, K. D., & Frieden, T. R. (2009). Ounces of prevention—the public policy case for taxes on sugared beverages. *New England Journal of Medicine*, *360*(18), 1805–1808.

Brownson, R. C., Colditz, G. A., & Proctor, E. K. (Eds.). (2012). *Dissemination and implementation research in health: Translating science to practice.* Oxford, UK: Oxford University Press.

Bruce, T. J., &. Sanderson, W. C. (2005). Evidence-based psychosocial practices: Past, present, and future. In C. E. Stout & R. A. Hayes (Eds.), *The evidence-based practice: Methods, models, and tools for mental health professionals* (pp. 220–243). New York: John Wiley & Sons.

Bruckner, T. A., Scheffler, R. M., Shen, G., Yoon, J., Chisholm, D., Morris, J., . . . Saxena, S. (2011). The mental health workforce gap in low-and middle-income countries: A needs-based approach. *Bulletin of the World Health Organization*, *89*(3), 184–194.

Buche, J., Singer, P. M., King, E., Maniere, E., & Beck, A. J. (2016). Primary care and behavioral health workforce integration: Barriers and best practices. Behavioral Health Workforce Resource Center, University of Michigan. Retrieved from http://www.behavioralhealthworkforce.org/wp-content/uploads/2017/02/FA2P3_Team-based-Care-Case-Studies_Full-Report.pdf

Buck, J., Manges, K., & Kaboli, P. (2016). Asynchronous teleneurology: A systematic review of electronic provider-to-provider communications (P3. 400). *Neurology*, *86*(16 Suppl.), P3–400.

Buckland, M. K. (1975). *Book availability and the library user*. New York: Pergamon.

Bullock, J. G., Green, D. P., & Ha, S. E. (2010). Yes, but what's the mechanisms? Don't expect an easy answer. *Journal of Personality and Social Psychology*, *98*, 550–558.

Burke, R. E. (2007). Sir Charles Sherrington's The integrative action of the nervous system: A centenary appreciation. *Brain*, *130*(4), 887–894.

Bush, D. E., Ziegelstein, R. C., Patel, U. V., Thombs, B. D., Ford, D. E., Fauerbach, J. S., . . . Patel, A. L. 2005. *Post-myocardial infarction depression: Summary*. Agency for Healthcare Research and Quality (AHRQ) Pub. No. 05-E018-1. Evidence reports/technology assessment number 123. Rockville, MD: AHRQ.

Butler, A. C., Chapman, J. E., Forman, E. M., & Beck, A. T. (2006). The empirical status of cognitive-behavioral therapy: A review of meta-analyses. *Clinical Psychology Review*, *26*(1), 17–31.

Cacioppo, J. T., Cacioppo, S., Cole, S. W., Capitanio, J. P., Goossens, L., & Boomsma, D. I. (2015). Loneliness across phylogeny and a call for comparative studies and animal models. *Perspectives on Psychological Science*, *10*(2), 202–212.

Cacioppo, J. T., & Patrick, W. (2008). *Loneliness: Human nature and the need for social connection*. New York: W. W. Norton & Company.

Cacioppo, S., Capitanio, J. P., & Cacioppo, J. T. (2014). Toward a neurology of loneliness. *Psychological Bulletin*, 140(6), 1464–1504.

Cahill, J., Barkham, M., & Stiles, W. B. (2010), Systematic review of practice-based research on psychological therapies in routine clinic settings. *British Journal of Clinical Psychology*, *49*, 421–453.

Calderón-Garcidueñas, L., Calderón-Garcidueñas, A., Torres-Jardón, R., Avila-Ramírez, J., Kulesza, R. J., & Angiulli, A. D. (2015). Air pollution and your brain: What do you need to know right now. *Primary Health Care Research & Development*, *16*(04), 329–345.

Campbell, H. S., Baskerville, N. B., Hayward, L. M., Brown, K. S., & Ossip, D. J. (2014). The reach ratio: A new indicator for comparing quitline reach into smoking subgroups. *Nicotine & Tobacco Research*, *16*(4), 491–495.

Campbell, S. W., & Park, Y. J. (2008). Social implications of mobile telephony: The rise of personal communication society. *Sociology Compass, 2*, 371–387.

Canetti, D., Russ, E., Luborsky, J., Gerhart, J. I., & Hobfoll, S. E. (2014). Inflamed by the flames? The impact of terrorism and war on immunity. *Journal of Traumatic Stress, 27*(3), 345–352.

Cannon, T. D. (2015). How schizophrenia develops: Cognitive and brain mechanisms underlying onset of psychosis. *Trends in Cognitive Sciences, 19*(12), 744–756.

Capezza, N. M., Zlotnick, C., Kohn, R., Vicente, B., & Saldivia, S. (2012). Perceived discrimination is a potential contributing factor to substance use and mental health problems among primary care patients in Chile. *Journal of Addiction Medicine, 6*(4), 297–303.

Carrington, P. J., Scott, J., & Wasserman, S. (Eds.). (2005). *Models and methods in social network analysis* (Vol. 28). New York: Cambridge University Press.

Carroll, L. (1865). *Alice's adventures in wonderland.* New York, NY: MacMillan.

Carter, S. L. (2007). Review of recent treatment acceptability research. *Education and Training in Developmental Disabilities, 42*(3), 301–316.

Carvalho, C., Caetano, J. M., Cunha, L., Rebouta, P., Kaptchuk, T. J., & Kirsch, I. (2016). Open-label placebo treatment in chronic low back pain: A randomized controlled trial. *Pain, 157*(12), 2766–2772.

Caspi, A., Houts, R. M., Belsky, D. W., Goldman-Mellor, S., Harrington, H., Israel, S., . . . Moffitt, T. E. (2014). The "p factor": One general psychopathology factor in the structure of psychiatric disorders? *Clinical Psychological Science, 2*, 119–137.

Castonguay, L. G., Constantino, M. J., Boswell, J. F., & Kraus, D. R. (2011). The therapeutic alliance: Research and theory. In L. M. Horowitz & S. Strack (Eds.), *Handbook of interpersonal psychology: Theory, research, assessment and therapeutic interventions* (pp. 509–518). Hoboken, NJ: John Wiley & Sons.

Cazalé, A., Sant, W., Ginot, F., Launay, J. C., Savourey, G., Revol-Cavalier, F., . . . Temple-Boyer, P. (2016). Physiological stress monitoring using sodium ion potentiometric microsensors for sweat analysis. *Sensors and Actuators B: Chemical, 225*, 1–9.

Centers for Disease Control and Prevention. (2009, October 15). *2009 H1N1 vaccination recommendations.* Retrieved from www.cdc.gov/h1n1flu/vaccination/acip.htm

Center for Disease Control and Prevention. (2015). Suicide: Facts at a glance: 2015. Retrieved from www.cdc.gov/violenceprevention/pdf/suicide-datasheet-a.pdf

Centers for Disease Control and Prevention (2016a). *Plain language.* Atlanta, GA: CDC Retrieved from www.cdc.gov/healthliteracy/developmaterials/plainlanguage.html

Centers for Disease Control and Prevention (2016b). *Winnable Battles: Final report.* Washington, DC: US Department of Health and Human Services.

Charles, D. (2009). Soap operas to save energy. *Science, 325*, 807.

Chisholm, D., & Saxena, S. (2012). Cost effectiveness of strategies to combat neuropsychiatric conditions in sub-Saharan Africa and South East Asia: Mathematical modelling study. *British Medical Journal, 344*, e609.

Ciesla, J. A., & Roberts, J. E. (2014). Meta-analysis of the relationship between HIV infection and risk for depressive disorders. *American Journal of Psychiatry, 158*, 725–730.

Clark, D. M. (2011). Implementing NICE guidelines for the psychological treatment of depression and anxiety disorders: The IAPT experience. *International Review of Psychiatry, 23*(4), 318–327.

Clark, D. M. (2012). The English Improving Access to Psychological Therapies (IAPT) program. In R. K. McHugh & D. H. Barlow (Eds.). *Dissemination and implementation of evidence-based psychological interventions* (pp. 61–77). New York: Oxford University Press.

Clark, D. M. (2016, May). Developing and disseminating effective psychological therapies: Science, economics, and politics. Keynote Addresses presented at the 28th annual meeting of the Association for Psychological Science, Chicago, IL.

Clayton, S., Manning, C. M., Krygsman, K., & Speiser, M. (2017). Mental health and our changing climate: Impacts, implications, and guidance. Washington, DC: American Psychological Association.

Clement, S., Schauman, O., Graham, T., Maggioni, F., Evans-Lacko, S., Bezborodovs, N., . . . Thornicroft, G. (2015). What is the impact of mental health-related stigma on help-seeking? A systematic review of quantitative and qualitative studies. *Psychological Medicine, 45*(01), 11–27.

Coeckelbergh, M., Pop, C., Simut, R., Peca, A., Pintea, S., David, D., & Vanderborght, B. (2016). A survey of expectations about the role of robots in robot-assisted therapy for children with ASD: Ethical acceptability, trust, sociability, appearance, and attachment. *Science and Engineering Ethics, 22*(1), 47–65.

Cohen, J. (1988). *Statistical power analysis in the behavioral sciences.* (2nd ed.). Hillsdale, NJ: Lawrence Erlbaum.

Cohen, J. (2015a). HIV/AIDS care for all—on a budget. *Science, 350*(6266), 1305.

Cohen, J. (2015b). Means to an end. *Science, 349*(6245), 226–231.

Cohen, S., & Janicki-Deverts, D. (2009). Can we improve our physical health by altering our social networks? *Perspectives on Psychological Science, 4*(4), 375–378.

Cohn, D., & Taylor, P. (2010). Baby boomers approach 65—glumly. *Pew Research Social & Demographic Trends.* Washington, DC: Pew Research Center.

Coker, A. L., Davis, K. E., Arias, I., Desai, S., Sanderson, M., Brandt, H. M., & Smith, P. H. (2002). Physical and mental health effects of intimate partner violence for men and women. *American Journal of Preventive Medicine, 23*(4), 260–268.

Collins, P. Y., Insel, T. R., Chockalingam, A., Daar, A., & Maddox, Y. T. (2013). Grand challenges in global mental health: Integration in research, policy, and practice. *PLoS Medicine, 10*(4), e1001434.

Commission on Ethnic Minority Recruitment, Retention, and Training. (2008). *Progress report.* Washington, DC: American Psychological Association.

Conklin, J. (2006). *Dialogue mapping: Building shared understanding of wicked problems.* West Sussex, UK: John Wiley & Sons.

Conrad, C. D. (Ed.). (2011). *The handbook of stress: Neuropsychological effects on the brain*, Oxford, UK: John Wiley & Sons.

Constantine, M. G., & Sue, D. W. (Eds.). (2005). *Strategies for building multicultural competence in mental health and educational settings.* New York: John Wiley & Sons.

Consumers Union. (1995, November). Mental health: Does therapy help? *Consumer Reports, 60*, 734–739.

Cooney, G. M., Dwan, K., Greig, C. A., Lawlor, D. A., Rimer, J., Waugh, F. R., . . . Mead, G. E. (2013). Exercise for depression. *Cochrane Library.* Retrieved from http://onlinelibrary.wiley.com/doi/10.1002/14651858.CD004366.pub6/abstract?TB_iframe=true&width=288&height=432

Cooper, Z., & Scott-Morton, F. (2016). Out-of-network emergency-physician bills: An unwelcome surprise. *New England Journal of Medicine, 375*, 1915–1918.

Corrigan, P. (2004). How stigma interferes with mental health care. *American Psychologist, 59*, 614–625.

Corrigan, P. W., Morris, S. B., Michaels, P. J., Rafacz, J. D., & Rüsch, N. (2012). Challenging the public stigma of mental illness: A meta-analysis of outcome studies. *Psychiatric Services, 63*(10), 963–973.

Cotton, R., Wilkins, A., Irwin, J., & Young, C. (2014). *The future's digital: Mental health and technology*. Mental Health Network, National Health Service Confederation, United Kingdom. Retrieved from www.nhsconfed.org/resources/2014/09/the-future-s-digital-mental-health-and-technology

Countryside Recreation Network. (2006). *A countryside for health and wellbeing: The Physical and mental health benefits of green exercise*. Retrieved from www.thehealthwell.info/node/3900

Coventry, P., Lovell, K., Dickens, C., Bower, P., Chew-Graham, C., McElvenny, D., . . . Baguley, C. (2015). Integrated primary care for patients with mental and physical multimorbidity: Cluster randomised controlled trial of collaborative care for patients with depression comorbid with diabetes or cardiovascular disease. *BMJ, 350*, h638.

Coviello, L., Sohn, Y., Kramer, A. D., Marlow, C., Franceschetti, M., Christakis, N. A., & Fowler, J. H. (2014). Detecting emotional contagion in massive social networks. *PLoS One, 9*(3), e90315.

Cowen, E. L., Gesten, E. L., Boike, M., Norton, P. L., Wilson, A., & DeStafano, M. (1979). Hairdressers as caregivers: A descriptive profile of interpersonal help-giving involvement. *American Journal of Community Psychology, 7*, 633–648.

Crabtree, A. (1993). *From Mesmer to Freud: Magnetic sleep and the roots of psychological healing*. New Haven, CT: Yale University Press.

Cragun, D., Cragun, R. T., Nathan, B., Sumerau, J. E., & Nowakowski, A. C. (2016). Do religiosity and spirituality really matter for social, mental, and physical health? A tale of two samples. *Sociological Spectrum, 36*(6), 359–377.

Crandall, C. S., & Moriarty, D. (1995). Physical illness stigma and social rejection. *British Journal of Social Psychology, 34*(1), 67–83.

Crawford, J., & Heather, N. (1987). Public attitudes to the disease concept of alcoholism. *International Journal of the Addictions, 22*(11), 1129–1138.

Crawford, M. J., Thana, L., Farquharson, L., Palmer, L., Hancock, E., Bassett, P., . . . Parry, G. D. (2016). Patient experience of negative effects of psychological treatment: Results of a national survey. *British Journal of Psychiatry, 208*, 260–265.

Creswell, J. D. (2017). Mindfulness interventions. *Annual Review of Psychology, 68*, 491–516.

Crits-Christoph, P., Gibbons, M. B. C., & Mukherjee, D. (2013). Psychotherapy process outcome research. In M. J. Lambert (Ed.), *Bergin and Garfield's handbook of psychotherapy and behavior change* (6th ed., pp. 298–339). New York: John Wiley & Sons.

Cross-Disorder Group of the Psychiatric Genomics Consortium. (2013). Genetic relationship between five psychiatric disorders estimated from genome-wide SNPs. *Nature Genetics, 45*(9), 984–994.

Crowley, R. A., & Kirschner, N. (2015). The integration of care for mental health, substance abuse, and other behavioral health conditions into primary care: Executive summary of an American College of Physicians Position Paper. Integration of behavioral health into primary care. *Annals of Internal Medicine, 163*(4), 298–299.

Cubic, B., Neumann, C., Kearney, L., McGrath, R., Ruddy, N., Rybarczyk, B., & Zamudio, A. (2012). Report of the Primary Care Training Task Force to the APA Board of Educational Affairs. Washington, DC: American Psychological Association. Retrieved from www.apa.org/ed/graduate/task-force-report.pdf

Cuijpers, P., Driessen, E., Hollon, S. D., van Oppen, P., Barth, J., & Andersson, G. (2012). The efficacy of non-directive supportive therapy for adult depression: A meta-analysis. *Clinical Psychology Review, 32*(4), 280–291.

Cuijpers, P., Koole, S. L., van Dijke, A., Roca, M., Li, J., & Reynolds, C. F. (2014). Psychotherapy for subclinical depression: Meta-analysis. *British Journal of Psychiatry, 205*(4), 268–274.

Cummins, S. E., Bailey, L., Campbell, S., Koon-Kirby, C., & Zhu, S. (2007). Tobacco quitlines in North America: A descriptive study. *Tobacco Control, 16*, i9 –i15

Curtin, S. C., Warner, M., & Hedegaard, H. (2016). Increase in suicide in the United States, 1999–2014. NCHS data brief, no 241. Hyattsville, MD: National Center for Health Statistics.

Cuthbert, B. N., & Insel, T. R. (2013). Toward the future of psychiatric diagnosis: The seven pillars of RDoC. *BMC Medicine, 11*(1), 126. Retrieved from www.biomedcentral.com/1741-7015/11/126

Chakrabarti, S. (2015). Usefulness of telepsychiatry: A critical evaluation of videoconferencing-based approaches. *World Journal of Psychiatry, 5*(3), 286–304.

Chaloupka, F. J., & Davidson, P. A. (2010). *Applying tobacco control lessons to obesity: Taxes and other pricing strategies to reduce consumption.* Saint Paul, MN: Tobacco Control Legal Consortium.

Chambless, D. L., Baker, M. J., Baucom, D. H., Beutler, L. E., Calhoun, K. S., Crits-Christoph, P., . . . Johnson, S. B. (1998). Update on empirically validated therapies, II. *Clinical Psychologist, 51*(1), 3–6.

Chambless, D. L., & Hollon, S. D. (1998). Defining empirically supported therapies. *Journal of Consulting and Clinical Psychology, 66*, 1–18.

Chambless, D. L., & Ollendick, T. H. (2001). Empirically supported psychological interventions: Controversies and evidence. *Annual Review of Psychology, 52*, 685–716.

Chand, P. K., & Murthy, P. (2008). Climate change and mental health. *Regional Health Forum, 12* (1), 43–48.

Charman, D., & Barkham, M. (2005). Psychological treatments: Evidence-based practice and practice-based evidence. *InPsych*. Retrieved from www.psychology.org.au/publications/inpsych/highlights2005/

Chen, L. M., Farwell, W. R., & Jha, A. K. (2009). Primary care visit duration and quality: Does good care take longer? *Archives of Internal Medicine, 169*(20), 1866–1872.

Chen, M., Ma, Y., Song, J., Lai, C. F., & Hu, B. (2016). Smart clothing: Connecting human with clouds and big data for sustainable health monitoring. *Mobile Networks and Applications, 21*(5), 825–845.

Chen, Y. S., Chong, P. P., & Tong, M. Y. (1994). Mathematical and computer modelling of the Pareto principle. *Mathematical and Computer Modelling, 19*(9), 61–80.

Cheok, A. D., Levy, D., Karunanayaka, K., & Morisawa, Y. (2017). Love and sex with robots. In R. Nakatsu, M. Rauterberg, & P. Ciancarini (Eds.), *Handbook of digital games and entertainment technologies* (pp. 833–858). Singapore: Springer.

Chiang, W., Cheng, P., Su, M., Chen, H., Wu, S., & Lin, J. (2011, June). *Socio-health with personal mental health records: Suicidal-tendency observation system on Facebook*. Paper presented at the International Conference on e-Health Networking, Applications, and Services, Columbia, MO.

Chisholm, D., Lund, C., & Saxena, S. (2007). Cost of scaling up mental healthcare in low- and middle-income countries. *British Journal of Psychiatry, 191*, 528–535.

Chisholm, D., Sweeny, K., Sheehan, P., Rasmussen, B., Smit, F., Cuijpers, P., & Saxena, S. (2016). Scaling-up treatment of depression and anxiety: a global return on investment analysis. *Lancet Psychiatry*, *3*(5), 415–424.

Chorpita, B. F., Bernstein, A. D., Daleiden, E. L., & The Research Network on Youth Mental Health. (2008). Driving with roadmaps and dashboards: Using information resources to structure the decision models in service organizations. *Administration and Policy in Mental Health and Mental Health Services Research*, *35*, 114–123.

Chorpita, B. F., & Weisz, J. R. (2009). Modular Approach to Therapy for Children with Anxiety, Depression, Trauma, or Conduct problems *(MATCH-ADTC) PracticeWise LLC: Satellite Beach.*

Christakis, N. A., & Fowler, J. H. (2007). The spread of obesity in a large social network over 32 years. *New England Journal of Medicine*, *357*(4), 370–379.

Christakis, N. A., & Fowler, J. H. (2009). *Connected: The surprising power of our social networks and how they shape our lives*. New York: Little, Brown.

Christakis, N. A., & Fowler, J. H. (2013). Social contagion theory: Examining dynamic social networks and human behavior. *Statistics in Medicine*, *32*(4), 556–577.

Christensen, A., Miller, W. R., & Muñoz, R. F. (1978). Paraprofessionals, partners, peers, paraphernalia, and print: Expanding mental health service delivery. *Professional Psychology*, *9*, 249–270.

Christensen, C. M. (2003). *The innovator's solution: Creating and sustaining successful growth*. Boston: Harvard Business School.

Christensen, C. M., Grossman, J. H., & Hwang, J. (2009). *The innovator's prescription: A disruptive solution for health care*. New York: McGraw-Hill.

Chua, S. E., & McKenna, P. J. (1995). Schizophrenia—a brain disease? A critical review of structural and functional cerebral abnormality in the disorder. *British Journal of Psychiatry*, *166*(5), 563–582.

Chwastiak, L. (2015). Making evidence-based lifestyle modification programs available in community mental health centers: Why so slow? *Journal of Clinical Psychiatry*, *76*(4), e519.

D'Amato, G., Bergmann, K. C., Cecchi, L., Annesi-Maesano, I., Sanduzzi, A., Gennaro Liccardi, G., . . . D'Amato, M. (2014). Climate change and air pollution. *Allergo Journal International*, *23*(1), 17–23.

Dale, R. (2016). The return of the chatbots. *Natural Language Engineering*, *22*(5), 811–817.

Danese, A., & Baldwin, J. R. (2017). Hidden wounds? Inflammatory links between childhood trauma and psychopathology, *Annual Review of Psychology*, *68*, 517–544.

David, D., Matu, S. A., & David, O. A. (2014). Robot-based psychotherapy: Concepts development, state of the art, and new directions. *International Journal of Cognitive Therapy*,*7*(2), 192–210.

Davis, A., Smith, P., Ferguson, M., Stephens, D., & Gianopoulos, I. (2007). Acceptability, benefit and costs of early screening for hearing disability: A study of potential screening tests and models. *Health Technology Assessment-Southampton, 11*(42).

Davis, G. (2012). The most deadly disease of asylumdom: general paralysis of the insane and Scottish psychiatry, c. 1840–1940. *JR College of Physicians Edinburgh*, *42*, 266–273.

Dawes, R. M. (1994). *House of cards: Psychology and psychotherapy built on myth*. New York: Free Press.

de Girolamo, G., Dagani, J., Purcell, R., Cocchi, A., & McGorry, P. D. (2012). Age of onset of mental disorders and use of mental health services: needs, opportunities and obstacles. *Epidemiology and Psychiatric Sciences*, *21*(01), 47–57.

De la Torre-Díez, I., Díaz-Pernas, F. J., & Antón-Rodríguez, M. (2012). A content analysis of chronic diseases social groups on Facebook and Twitter. *Telemedicine and e-Health*, *18*, 1–5.

De Los Reyes, A., Aldao, A., & Augenstein, T. M. (2017). Assessment issues in child and adolescent psychotherapy. In J. R. Weisz & A. E. Kazdin (Eds.), *Evidence-based psychotherapies for children and adolescents* (3rd ed.). New York: Guilford Press.

De Los Reyes, A., & Kazdin, A. E. (2006). Conceptualizing changes in behavior in intervention research: The Range of Possible Changes Model. *Psychological Review*, *113*, 554–583.

Delgadillo, J., McMillan, D., Leach, C., Lucock, M., Gilbody, S., & Wood, N. (2014). Benchmarking routine psychological services: A discussion of challenges and methods. *Behavioural and Cognitive Psychotherapy*, *42*(01), 16–30.

Demyttenaere, K., Bruffaerts, R., Lee, S., Posada-Villa, J., Kovess, V., Angermeyer, M. C., . . . Von Korff, M. (2007). Mental disorders among persons with chronic back or neck pain: Results from the World Mental Health Surveys. *Pain*, *129*(3), 332–342.

Denissenko, M. F., Pao, A., Tang, M., & Pfeifer, G. P. (1996). Preferential formation of benzo[*a*]pyrene adducts at lung cancer mutational hotspots in *P53*. *Science*, *274*, 430–432.

Depp, C. A., Mausbach, B., Granholm, E., Cardenas, V., Ben-Zeev, D., Patterson, T. L., . . . Jeste, D. V. (2010). Mobile interventions for severe mental illness: Design and preliminary data from three approaches. *Journal of Nervous and Mental Disease*, *198*(10), 715–721.

Deslandes, A., Moraes, H., Ferreira, C., Veiga, H., Silveira, H., Mouta, R., . . . Laks, J. (2009). Exercise and mental health: Many reasons to move. *Neuropsychobiology*, *59*, 191–198.

DeVault, D., Artstein, R., Benn, G., Dey, T., Fast, E., Gainer, A., . . . Lucas, G. (2014, May). SimSensei Kiosk: A virtual human interviewer for healthcare decision support. In *Proceedings of the 2014 international conference on Autonomous agents and multi-agent systems* (pp. 1061–1068). Paris, France: International Foundation for Autonomous Agents and Multiagent Systems.

Dew, S. E., & Bickman, L. (2005). Client expectancies about therapy. *Mental Health Services Research*, *7*(1), 21–33.

Dieleman, J. L., Baral, R., Birger, M., Bui, A. L., Bulchis, A., Chapin, A., . . . & Lavado, R. (2016). US spending on personal health care and public health, 1996–2013. *JAMA*, *316*(24), 2627–2646.

Diener, E., & Chan, M. Y. (2011). Happy people live longer: Subjective well-being contributes to health and longevity. *Applied Psychology: Health and Well-Being*, *3*, 1–43.

DiMatteo, M. R., Lepper, H. S., & Croghan, T. W. (2000). Depression is a risk factor for noncompliance with medical treatment: Meta-analysis of the effects of anxiety and depression on patient adherence. *Archives of Internal Medicine*, *160*(14), 2101–2107.

Dimidijian, S., Hollon, S. D., Dobson, K. S., Schmaling, K. B., Kohlenberg, R. J., Addis, M. E., . . . Jacobson, N. S. (2006). Randomized trial of behavioral activation, cognitive therapy, and antidepressant medication in the acute treatment of adults with major depression. *Journal of Consulting and Clinical Psychology*, *74*, 658–670.

Diniz, B. S., Reynolds, C. F., Butters, M. A., Dew, M. A., Firmo, J. O., Lima-Costa, M. F., & Castro-Costa, E. (2014). The effect of gender, age, and symptom severity in late-life depression on the risk of all-cause mortality: The Bambuí cohort study of aging. *Depression and Anxiety, 31*(9), 787–795.

Doherty, T. J., & Clayton, S. (2011). The psychological impacts of global climate change. *American Psychologist, 66*(4), 265–276.

Doman, L. C., & Le Roux, A. (2012). The relationship between loneliness and psychological well-being among third-year students: A cross-cultural investigation. *International Journal of Culture and Mental Health, 5*(3), 153–168.

Dombeck, M., & Wells-Moran, J. (2006). *Dealing with avoidance-motivated behavior: Exposure*. Retrieved from www.mentalhelp.net/poc/view_doc.php?type=doc&id=9738

Donker, T., Petrie, K., Proudfoot, J., Clarke, J., Birch, M. R., & Christensen, H. (2013). Smartphones for smarter delivery of mental health programs: A systematic review. *Journal of Medical Internet Research, 15*(11), e247.

Draper, C., & O'Donohue, W. (Eds.) (2011). *Stepped care and e-health: Practical applications to behavioral disorders*. New York: Springer Science + Business Media, LLC.

Drapkin, M. L., Wilbourne, P., Manuel, J. K., Baer, J., Karlin, B., & Raffa, S. (2016). National dissemination of motivation enhancement therapy in the Veterans health administration: Training program design and initial outcomes. *Journal of Substance Abuse Treatment, 65*, 83–87.

Druss, B. G., & Rosenheck, R. A. (2014). Patterns of health care costs associated with depression and substance abuse in a national sample. *Psychiatric Services, 50*(2), 214–218.

Druss, B. G., Hwang, I., Petukhova, M., Sampson, N. A., Wang, P. S., & Kessler, R. C. (2009). Impairment in role functioning in mental and chronic medical disorders in the United States: results from the National Comorbidity Survey Replication. *Molecular Psychiatry, 14*, 728–737.

Duman, C. H., Schlesinger, L., Russell, D. S., & Duman, R. S. (2008). Voluntary exercise produces antidepressant and anxiolytic behavioral effects in mice. *Brain Research, 1199*, 148–158.

Duman, R. S., & Aghajanian, G. K. (2012). Synaptic dysfunction in depression: Potential therapeutic targets. *Science, 338*, 68–72.

Dunbar-Jacob, J., & Mortimer-Stephens, M. (2001). Treatment adherence in chronic disease. *Journal of Clinical Epidemiology, 54*(12), S57–S60.

Duncan, B. L., Miller, S. D., Wampold, B. E., & Hubble, M. A. (Eds.). (2010). *The heart and soul of change: Delivering what works in therapy* (2nd ed.). Washington, DC: American Psychological Association.

Dunn, A. L., Trivedi, M. H., Kampert, J. B., Clark, C. G., & Cham-bliss, H. O. (2005). Exercise treatment for depression: Efficacy and dose response. *American Journal of Preventative Medicine, 28*, 1–8.

Dzau, V. J., McClellan, M. B., McGinnis, J. M., Burke, S. P., Coye, M. J., Diaz, A., . . . Henney, J. E. (2017). Vital directions for health and health care: Priorities from a National Academy of Medicine Initiative. *JAMA, 317*(14), 1461–1470.

Eaton, N. R., Rodriguez-Seijas, C., Carragher, N., & Krueger, R. F. (2015). Transdiagnostic factors of psychopathology and substance use disorders: A review. *Social Psychiatry and Psychiatric Epidemiology, 50*, 171–182.

Edlund, M. J., Wang, P. S., Berglund, P. A., Katz, S. J., Lin, E., & Kessler, R. C. (2002). Dropping out of mental health treatment: Patterns and predictors among epidemiological survey respondents in the United States and Ontario. *American Journal of Psychiatry, 159*(5), 845–851.

Eftekhari, A., Ruzek, J. I., Crowley, J. J., Rosen, C. S., Greenbaum, M. A., & Karlin, B. E. (2013). Effectiveness of national implementation of prolonged exposure therapy in Veterans Affairs care. *JAMA Psychiatry, 70*(9), 949–955.

Egan, M., Kearns, A., Katikireddi, S. V., Curl, A., Lawson, K., & Tannahill, C. (2016). Proportionate universalism in practice? A quasi-experimental study (GoWell) of a UK neighbourhood renewal programme's impact on health inequalities. *Social Science and Medicine, 152*, 41–49.

Egan, S. J., Wade, T. D., & Shafran, R. (2011). Perfectionism as a transdiagnostic process: A clinical review. *Clinical Psychology Review, 31*, 203–212.

Egger, G., Binns, A., & Rossner, S. (2008). *Lifestyle medicine*. New York: McGraw-Hill.

Eisenberger, N. I., & Cole, S. W. (2012). Social neuroscience and health: Neurophysiological mechanisms linking social ties with physical health. *Nature Neuroscience, 15*(5), 669–674.

Elbogen, E. B., & Johnson, S. C. (2009). The intricate link between violence and mental disorder: Results from the National Epidemiologic Survey on Alcohol and Related Conditions. *Archives of General Psychiatry, 66*(2), 152–161.

Elliot, R. (1998). Editor's introduction: A guide to the empirically supported treatments controversy. *Psychotherapy Research, 8*(2), 115–125.

Elliott, R. (2002). The effectiveness of humanistic therapies: A meta-analysis. In D. J. Cain (Ed.), *Humanistic psychotherapies: Handbook of research and practice* (pp. 57–81). Washington, DC: American Psychological Association.

Ellis, A. (1957). Outcome of employing three techniques of psychotherapy. *Journal of Clinical Psychology, 13*, 344–350.

El-Sayed, A. M., & Galea, S. (2015). Climate change and population mental health. In G. Luber & J. Lemery (Eds.), *Global climate change and human health: From science to practice* (pp. 311–332). San Francisco, CA: John Wiley & Sons.

England, M. J., Butler, A. S., & Gonzalez, M. L. (Eds.). (2015). *Psychosocial interventions for mental and substance use disorders: A framework for establishing evidence-based standards*. Washington, DC: National Academies Press.

Erlangsen, A., Runeson, B., Bolton, J. M., Wilcox, H. C., Forman, J. L., Krogh, J., . . . Conwell, Y. (2017). Association between spousal suicide and mental, physical, and social health outcomes: A longitudinal and nationwide register-based study. *JAMA Psychiatry, 74*(5), 456–464.

Estes, M. L., & McAllister, A. K. (2016). Maternal immune activation: Implications for neuropsychiatric disorders. *Science, 353*(6301), 772–777.

Evans, B. (2014). *The 80/20 Pareto Principle: Its application in daily life and business.* Success First Publishing Kindle Edition.

Eysenck, H. J. (1952). The effects of psychotherapy: An evaluation. *Journal of Consulting Psychology, 16*, 319–324.

Eysenck, H. J. (1966). *The effects of psychotherapy* (with commentaries). New York: International Science Press.

Eysenck, H. J. (1995). The outcome problem in psychotherapy: What have we learned? *Behaviour Research and Therapy, 32*, 477–495.

Fabiano, G. A., Schatz, N. K., Aloe, A. M., Chacko, A., & Chronis-Tuscano, A. (2015). A systematic review of meta-analyses of psychosocial treatment for attention-deficit/hyperactivity disorder. *Clinical Child and Family Psychology Review, 18*(1), 77–97.

Fairburn, C. G., Cooper, Z., & Shafran, R. (2003). Cognitive behaviour therapy for eating disorders: A "transdiagnostic" theory and treatment. *Behaviour Research and Therapy, 41*(5), 509–528.

Fairburn, C. G., & Patel, V. (2014). The global dissemination of psychological treatments: A road map for research and practice. *American Journal of Psychiatry, 171*(5), 495–498.

Fasola, J., & Matarić, M. J. (2010). Robot exercise instructor: A socially assistive. *9th International Symposium in Robot and Human Interactive Communication*, Viareggio. Published in RO-MAN, 2010 IEEE, 416–421.

Fazel, M., Wheeler, J., & Danesh, J. (2005). Prevalence of serious mental disorder in 7000 refugees resettled in Western countries: A systematic review. *Lancet, 365*(9467), 1309–1314.

Feil-Seifer, D., & Matarić, M. J. (2011). Socially assistive robotics. *IEEE Robotics and Automation Magazine, 18*(1), 24–31.

Ferrari, A. J., Charlson, F. J., Norman, R. E., Patten, S. B., Freedman, G., Murray, C. J., . . . Whiteford, H. A. (2013). Burden of depressive disorders by country, sex, age, and year: Findings from the Global Burden of Disease Study 2010. *PLoS Medicine, 10*(11), e1001547.

Fine, A. (Ed.). (2015). *Handbook on animal-assisted therapy: Theoretical foundations and guidelines for practice* (4th ed.). New York: Elsevier.

Finniss, D. G., Kaptchuk, T. J., Miller, F., & Benedetti, F. (2010). Biological, clinical, and ethical advances of placebo effects. *Lancet, 375*(9715), 686–695.

Fixsen, D. L., Blase, K. A., Naoom, S. F., & Wallace, F. (2009). Core implementation components. *Research on Social Work Practice, 19*(5), 531–540.

Fixsen, D. L., Naoom, S. F., Blase, K. A., Friedman, R. M., & Wallace, F. (2005). Implementation research: A synthesis of the literature. Tampa, FL: University of South Florida, Louis de la Parte Florida Mental Health Institute.

Forman-Hoffman, V. L., Muhuri, P. K., Novak, S. P., Pemberton, M. R., Ault, K. L., & Mannix, D. (2014). Psychological distress and mortality among adults in the US household population. Center for Behavioral Health Statistics and Quality, Rockville, MD: SAMHSA.

Fornito, A., & Bullmore, E. T. (2015). Connectomics: A new paradigm for understanding brain disease. *European Neuropsychopharmacology, 25*(5), 733–748.

Frank, J. D. (1961). *Persuasion and healing: A comparative study of psychopathology.* Baltimore: Johns Hopkins University Press.

Frank, J. D., & Frank, J. B. (1991). *Persuasion and healing* (3rd ed.). Baltimore, MD: Johns Hopkins University Press.

Franzese, R. J., Covey, H. C., Tucker, A. S., McCoy, L., & Menard, S. (2014). Adolescent exposure to violence and adult physical and mental health problems. *Child Abuse & Neglect, 38*(12), 1955–1965.

Frattaroli, J. (2006). Experimental disclosure and its moderators: A meta-analysis. *Psychological Bulletin, 132*, 823–865.

Frattaroli, J., Weidner, G., Dnistrian, A. M., Kemp, C., Daubenmier, J. J., Marlin, R. O., . . . Ornish, D. (2008). Clinical events in prostate cancer lifestyle trial: Results from two years of follow-up. *Urology, 72*, 1319–1323.

Frewen, P. A., Dozois, D. J. A., & Lanius, R. A. (2008). Neuroimaging studies of psychological interventions for mood and anxiety disorders: Empirical and methodological review. *Clinical Psychology Review*, *28*, 228–246.

Frisina, P. G., Borod, J. C., & Lepore, S. J. (2004). A meta-analysis of the effects of written emotional disclosure on the health outcomes of clinical populations. *Journal of Nervous and Mental Disease*, *192*(9), 629–634.

Fulton, B. D., Scheffler, R. M., Sparkes, S. P., Auh, E. Y., Vujicic, M., & Soucat, A. (2011). Health workforce skill mix and task shifting in low income countries: A review of recent evidence. *Human Resources for Health*, *9*(1), 1.

Gale, C., & Schröder, T. (2014). Experiences of self-practice/self-reflection in cognitive behavioural therapy: A meta-synthesis of qualitative studies. *Psychology and Psychotherapy: Theory, Research and Practice*, *87*(4), 373–392.

Gallagher, K. M., & Updegraff, J. A. (2012). Health message framing effects on attitudes, intentions, and behavior: A meta-analytic review. *Annals of Behavioral Medicine*, *43*(1), 101–116.

Gallo, K. P., Comer, J. S., & Barlow, D. H. (2013). Direct-to-consumer marketing of psychological treatments for anxiety disorders. *Journal of Anxiety Disorders*, *27*(8), 793–801.

Garfield, S. L. (1980). *Psychotherapy: An eclectic approach.* New York: Wiley & Sons.

Gask, L., Macdonald, W., & Bower, P. (2011). What is the relationship between diabetes and depression? A qualitative meta-synthesis of patient experience of co-morbidity. *Chronic Illness*, *7*(3), 239–252.

Gavin, A. R., Walton, E., Chae, D. H., Alegria, M., Jackson, J. S., & Takeuchi, D. (2010). The associations between socio-economic status and major depressive disorder among Blacks, Latinos, Asians and non-Hispanic Whites: Findings from the Collaborative Psychiatric Epidemiology Studies. *Psychological Medicine*, *40*(01), 51–61.

Gee, B. L., Griffiths, K. M., & Gulliver, A. (2016). Effectiveness of mobile technologies delivering ecological momentary interventions for stress and anxiety: A systematic review. *Journal of the American Medical Informatics Association*, *23*(1), 221–229.

Geffner, R., Igelman, R. S., & Zellner, J. (Eds.). (2014). *The effects of intimate partner violence on children*. New York: Routledge.

Gelo, O., & Pritz, A. (Eds.) (2015). *Psychotherapy research: Foundations, process, and outcome*. Vienna: Springer-Verlag.

Germer, C. (2004). What is mindfulness. *Insight Journal*, *22*, 24–29.

Germer, C. K., Siegel, R. D., & Fulton, P. R. (Eds.). (2013). *Mindfulness and psychotherapy*. New York: Guilford Press.

Gibbons, M. B. C., Rothbard, A., Farris, K. D., Stirman, S. W., Thompson, S. M., Scott, K., . . . Crits-Christoph, P. (2011). Changes in psychotherapy utilization among consumers of services for major depressive disorder in the community mental health system. *Administration and Policy in Mental Health and Mental Health Services Research*, *38*(6), 495–503.

Gill, T. M. (2010). *Beauty shop politics: African American women's activism in the beauty industry*. Champaign, IL: University of Illinois Press.

Gold, M. R., Stevenson, D., & Fryback, D. G. (2002). HALYS and QALYS and DALYS, Oh My: Similarities and differences in summary measures of population health. *Annual Review of Public Health*, *23*(1), 115–134.

Goldman, R. (2012, May 2). *States see instant spike in organ donors following Facebook push.* Retrieved from http://abcnews.go.com/Health/states-instant-spike-organ-donors-facebook-push/story?id=16255979#.UAblFo7R3dk

Goldstein, B. I., Kemp, D. E., Soczynska, J. K., & McIntyre, R. S. (2009). Inflammation and the phenomenology, pathophysiology, comorbidity, and treatment of bipolar disorder: A systematic review of the literature. *Journal of Clinical Psychiatry, 70*(8), 1078–1090.

Gonzalez, J. S., Batchelder, A. W., Psaros, C., & Safren, S. A. (2011). Depression and HIV/AIDS treatment nonadherence: A review and meta-analysis. *Journal of Acquired Immune Deficiency Syndrome, 58*(2), 181–187.

Gonzalez, J. S., Peyrot, M., McCarl, L. A., Collins, E. M., Serpa, L., Mimiaga, M. J., & Safren, S. A. (2008). Depression and diabetes treatment nonadherence: A meta-analysis. *Diabetes Care, 31*(12), 2398–2403.

Good, A., Gnanayutham, P., Sambhanthan, A., & Panjganj, P. (2011, June). *HCI considerations in designing a Second Life virtual therapeutic community for the support and treatment of people with borderline personality disorder.* Paper presented at the Seventh Annual International Conference on Computer Science and Information Systems, Athens, Greece.

Goodell, A., Druss, B. G., & Walker, E. R. (2011). *Mental disorders and medical comorbidity. The synthesis project: Policy brief.* Robert Wood Johnson Foundation. Retrieved from http://www.researchgate.net/profile/Elizabeth_Walker12/publication/51220912_Mental_disorders_and_medical_comorbidity/links/0a85e53c973139cf16000000.pdf

Goodheart, C. D., Kazdin, A. E., & Sternberg, R. J. (Eds.). (2006). *Evidence-based psychotherapy: Where practice and research meet.* Washington, DC: American Psychological Association.

Goodman, S. H., Rouse, M. H., Connell, A. M., Broth, M. R., Hall, C. M., & Heyward, D. (2011). Maternal depression and child psychopathology: A meta-analytic review. *Clinical Child and Family Psychology Review, 14*(1), 1–27.

Gorini, A., Gaggioli, A., & Riva, G. (2008). A second life for eHealth: Prospects for the use of 3-D virtual worlds in clinical psychology. *Journal of Medical Internet Research, 10*(3), e21.

Gorini, A., & Riva, G. (2008). Virtual reality in anxiety disorders: The past and the future. *Expert Review of Neurotherapeutics, 8*, 215–233.

Goschke, T. (2014). Dysfunctions of decision-making and cognitive control as transdiagnostic mechanisms of mental disorders: Advances, gaps, and needs in current research. *International Journal of Methods in Psychiatric Research, 23*(S1), 41–57.

Graham, A. L., Cobb, N. K., Papandonatos, G. D., Moreno, J. L., Kang, H., Tinkelman, D. G., . . . Abrams, D. B. (2011). A randomized trial of Internet and telephone treatment for smoking cessation. *Archives of Internal Medicine, 171*(1), 46–53.

Graham, P. A. (2011). "Ought" and ability. *Philosophical Review, 120*(3), 337–382.

Grajales III, F. J., Sheps, S., Ho, K., Novak-Lauscher, H., & Eysenbach, G. (2014). Social media: A review and tutorial of applications in medicine and health care. *Journal of Medical Internet Research, 16*(2), e13.

Grand Challenges Canada™ (2011, January). *The grand challenges approach.* Grand Challenges Canada. Retrieved from http://www.grandchallenges.ca/

Grandjean, P., & Landrigan, P. J. (2014). Neurobehavioural effects of developmental toxicity. *Lancet Neurology, 13*(3), 330–338.

Grant, B. F., Goldstein, R. B., Saha, T. D., Chou, S. P., Jung, J., Zhang, H., . . . Hasin, D. S. (2015). Epidemiology of DSM-5 alcohol use disorder: Results from the National Epidemiologic Survey on Alcohol and Related Conditions III. *JAMA Psychiatry, 72*(8), 757–766.

Gray, J. J. (2000). *The Hilbert challenge.* Oxford, UK: Oxford University Press.

Green, B., Horel, T., & Papachristos, A. V. (2017). Modeling contagion through social networks to explain and predict gunshot violence in Chicago, 2006 to 2014. *JAMA Internal Medicine*. (Online Jan 3).

Green, J. G., McLaughlin, K. A., Berglund, P. A., Gruber, M. J., Sampson, N. A., Zaslavsky, A. M., & Kessler, R. C. (2010). Childhood adversities and adult psychiatric disorders in the national comorbidity survey replication. I: Associations with first onset of DSM-IV disorders. *Archives of General Psychiatry*, *67*, 113–123.

Green, S. J., Littell, J. H., Hammerstrøm, K. T., Tanner-Smith, E., & Wilen, J. S. (2013). *The therapeutic alliance and psychotherapy outcomes for young adults aged 18 to 34: Protocol for a systematic review*. Graduate School of Social Work and Social Research, Faculty Research and Scholarship. Paper 59. The Campbell Collaboration. http://repository.brynmawr.edu/cgi/viewcontent.cgi?article=1061&context=gsswr_pubs

Greenberg, G. A., & Rosenheck, R. A. (2008). Jail incarceration, homelessness, and mental health: A national study. *Psychiatric Services*, *59*(2), 170–177.

Greenwood, B. M., Greenwood, A. M., Snow, R. W., Byass, P., Bennett, S., & Hatib-N'Jie, A. B. (1989). The effects of malaria chemoprophylaxis given by traditional birth attendants on the course and outcome of pregnancy. *Transactions of the Royal Society of Tropical Medicine and Hygiene Journal*, *83*, 589–594.

Greeson, J., Garland, E. L., & Black, D. (2014). A transtherapeutic approach for transdiagnostic mental processes. In Le, A., Ngnoumen, C. T., & Langer, E. J. (Eds.), *The Wiley Blackwell handbook of mindfulness* (pp. 533–562). New York: John Wiley & Sons.

Griner, D., & Smith, T. B. (2006). Culturally adapted mental health intervention: A meta-analytic review. *Psychotherapy: Theory, Research, Practice, Training*, *43*(4), 531–548.

Grissom, R. J. (1996). The magical number .7 +/- .2: Meta-meta-analysis of the probability of superior outcome in comparisons involving therapy, placebo, and control. *Journal of Consulting and Clinical Psychology*, *64*, 973–982.

Groseclose, S. L., & Buckeridge, D. L. (2017). Public health surveillance systems: Recent advances in their use and evaluation. *Annual Review of Public Health*, *38*(8), 8.1–8.23.

Grunbaum, A. (1985). *The foundations of psychoanalysis: A philosophical critique*. Berkeley, CA: University of California Press.

Haaga, D. A. F. (2000). Introduction to the special section on stepped-care models in psychotherapy. *Journal of Consulting and Clinical Psychology*, *68*, 547–548.

Hair Care Services Industry Profile (2016), First Research, Hoover's Inc. Retrieved from http://www.firstresearch.com/industry-research/Hair-Care-Services.html

Hamer, M., & Chida, Y. (2008). Active commuting and cardiovascular risk: A meta-analytic review. *Preventive Medicine*, *46*, 9–13.

Hanlon, P. (2011, May). Mindstylz: Making personal connections. *New England Psychologist*, *19*(4). Retrieved from www.mindstylz.org/assets/NEPSY_Mindstylz_Making_personal_connections.pdf

Hansen, N. B., Lambert, M. J., & Forman, E. M. (2002). The psychotherapy dose-response effect and its implications for treatment delivery services. *Clinical Psychology: Science and Practice*, *9*(3), 329–343.

Hansen, P. G., Skov, L. R., & Skov, K. L. (2016). Making healthy choices easier: Regulation versus nudging. *Annual Review of Public Health*, *37*, 237–251.

Harvey, A. G., Lee, J., Williams, J., Hollon, S. D., Walker, M. P., Thompson, M. A., & Smith, R. (2014). Improving outcome of psychosocial treatments by enhancing memory and learning. *Perspectives on Psychological Science*, *9*(2), 161–179.

Harvey, A. G., Murray, G., Chandler, R. A., & Soehner, A. (2011). Sleep disturbance as transdiagnostic: Consideration of neurobiological mechanisms. *Clinical Psychology Review, 31*(2), 225–235.

Harvey, A. G., Watkins, E., Mansell, W., & Safran, R. (2004). *Cognitive behavioural processes across psychological disorders: A transdiagnostic approach to research and treatment*. New York: Oxford University Press.

Harwood, T. M., & L'Abate, L. (2010). *Self-help in mental health: A critical review.* New York: Springer.

Hasin, D. S., Goodwin, R. D., Stinson, F. S., & Grant, B. F. (2005). Epidemiology of major depressive disorder: Results from the National Epidemiologic Survey on Alcoholism and Related Conditions. *Archives of General Psychiatry, 62*(10), 1097–1106.

Hatch, O. G. (1982). Psychology, society, and politics. *American Psychologist, 37*, 1031–137.

Health Resources and Services Administration. (2010). *Health professional shortage areas: Mental health designated populations*. Rural Assistance Center. See www.ruralhealthinfo.org/

Heath, B., Wise, R. P., & Reynolds K. A (2013). *Standard framework for levels of integrated healthcare.* Washington, DC: SAMHSA-HRSA Center for Integrated Health Solutions. Retrieved from www.integration.samhsa.gov/integrated-care-models/A_Standard_Framework_for_Levels_of_Integrated_Healthcare.pdf

Hefner, J. L., Wexler, R., & McAlearney, A. S. (2015). Primary care access barriers as reported by nonurgent emergency department users: Implications for the US primary care infrastructure. *American Journal of Medical Quality, 30*(2), 135–140.

Henn, F. A., & Nasrallah, H. A. (1982). *Schizophrenia as a brain disease*. New York: Oxford University Press.

Herbert, J. D. (2003). The science and practice of empirically supported treatments. *Behavior Modification, 27*(3), 412–430.

Hernandez, M. Y., & Organista, K. C. (2013). Entertainment–education? A fotonovela? A new strategy to improve depression literacy and help-seeking behaviors in at-risk immigrant Latinas. *American Journal of Community Psychology, 52*(3-4), 224–235.

Hert, M., Correll, C. U., Bobes, J., Cetkovich-Bakmas, M., Cohen, D., Asai, I., . . . Newcomer, J. W. (2011). Physical illness in patients with severe mental disorders. I. Prevalence, impact of medications and disparities in health care. *World Psychiatry, 10*(1), 52–77.

Hettema, J. M., Prescott, C. A., Myers, J. M., Neale, M. C., & Kendler, K. S. (2005). The structure of genetic and environmental risk factors for anxiety disorders in men and women. *Archives of General Psychiatry, 62*(2), 182–189.

Hill, C. E., Chui, H., & Baumann, E. (2013). Revisiting and re envisioning the outcome problem in psychotherapy: An argument to include individualized and qualitative measurement. *Psychotherapy, 50*, 68–76.

Hinkle, S. N., Louis, G. M. B., Rawal, S., Zhu, Y., Albert, P. S., & Zhang, C. (2016). A longitudinal study of depression and gestational diabetes in pregnancy and the postpartum period. *Diabetologia, 59*(12), 2594–2602.

Hinshaw, S. P., & Stier, A. (2008). Stigma as related to mental disorders. *Annual Review of Clinical Psychology, 4*(1), 367–393.

Hirschberg, D. L., Betts, K., Emanuel, P., & Caples. M. (2014). *Assessment of wearable sensor technologies for biosurveillance*. Aberdeen Proving Ground, MD: Defense Threat Reduction Agency, US Army Edgewood Chemical Biological Center.

Hoagwood, K., Hibbs, E., Brent, D., & Jensen, P. J. (1995). Efficacy and effectiveness in studies of child and adolescent psychotherapy. *Journal of Consulting and Clinical Psychology, 63*, 683–687.

Hoagwood, K. E., Peth-Pierce, R., Glaeser, E. Whitmyre, E., Shorter, P., & Vardanian, M. M. (2017). Implementing evidence-based psychotherapies for children and adolescents within complex mental health systems. In J. R. Weisz & A. E. Kazdin (Eds.), *Evidence-based psychotherapies for children and adolescents* (3rd. ed.). New York: Guilford Press.

Hoeft, T. J., Fortney, J. C., Patel, V., & Unützer, J. (2017). Task-sharing approaches to improve mental health care in rural and other low-resource settings: A systematic review. *Journal of Rural Health*. Retrieved from http://onlinelibrary.wiley.com/doi/10.1111/jrh.12229/full

Hofmann, S. G., Asnaani, A., Vonk, I. J., Sawyer, A. T., & Fang, A. (2012). The efficacy of cognitive behavioral therapy: A review of meta-analyses. *Cognitive Therapy and Research, 36*(5), 427–440.

Hoge, M. A., Morris, J. A., Daniels, A. S., Stuart, G. W., Huey, L. Y., & Adams, N. (2007). *An action plan for behavioral health workforce development*. Washington, DC: Department of Health and Human Services.

Holliday, B. G., Dawes, D. E, Al-Mohamed, D., & Figueroa-Garcia, A. (Eds.). (2009, March). Special Issue: Psychological and behavioral perspectives on health disparities, *Communiqué*. Retrieved from www.apa.org/pi/oema/resources/communique/2009/03/march.pdf

Hollon, S. D., & Beck, A. T. (2004). Cognitive and cognitive behavioral therapies. In M. J. Lambert (Ed.), *Bergin and Garfield's handbook of psychotherapy and behavior change* (5th ed., pp. 447–492). New York: John Wiley & Sons.

Holt, S., Buckley, H., & Whelan, S. (2008). The impact of exposure to domestic violence on children and young people: A review of the literature. *Child Abuse & Neglect, 32*(8), 797–810.

Holt-Lunstad, J., Smith, T. B., Baker, M., Harris, T., & Stephenson, D. (2015). Loneliness and social isolation as risk factors for mortality: A meta-analytic review. *Perspectives on Psychological Science, 10*(2), 227–237.

Honberg, R., Diehl, S., Kimball, A., Gruttadaro, D., & Fitzpatrick, M. (2011). *State mental health cuts: A national crisis*. The National Alliance on Mental Illness.

Horn, R. E., & Weber, R. P. (2007). *New tools for resolving wicked problems: Mess mapping and resolution mapping processes*. Strategy Kinetics LLC. Retrieved from www.strategykinetics.com

Horvath, A. O., & Bedi, R. P. (2002). The alliance. In J. C. Norcross (Ed.). *Psychotherapy relationships that work: Therapist contributions and responsiveness to patients* (pp. 37–69). New York: Oxford University Press.

Horvath, A. O., Del Re, A. C., Flückiger, C., & Symonds, D. (2011). Alliance in individual psychotherapy. *Psychotherapy, 48*, 9–16.

Howell, K. H., Coffey, J. K., Fosco, G. M., Kracke, K., Nelson, S. K., Rothman, E. F., & Grych, J. H. (2016). Seven reasons to invest in well-being. *Psychology of Violence, 6*(1), 8–14.

Howick, J., Bishop, F. L., Heneghan, C., Wolstenholme, J., Stevens, S., Hobbs, F. R., & Lewith, G. (2013). Placebo use in the United Kingdom: Results from a national survey of primary care practitioners. *PLoS One, 8*(3), e58247.

Howren, M. B., & Gonzalez, J. S. (2016). Treatment adherence and illness self-management: introduction to the special issue. *Journal of Behavioral Medicine, 39*(6), 931–934.

Hum, J. D. (1998). *The history of general paralysis of the insane in Britain, 1830 to 1950*: London: University of London. Retrieved from http://discovery.ucl.ac.uk/1349281/1/339949.pdf

Hunsley, J., & Lee, C. M. (2007). Research-informed benchmarks for psychological treatments: Efficacy studies, effectiveness studies, and beyond. *Professional Psychology: Research and Practice, 38*, 21–33.

Hurling, R., Catt, M., De Boni, M., Fairley, B. W., Hurst, T., Murray, P., . . . Sodhi, J. S. (2007). Using Internet and mobile phone technology to deliver an automated physical activity program: Randomized controlled trial. *Journal of Medical Internet Research, 9*(2), e7.

Hvistendahl, M. (2016). Crime forecasters, *Science, 353*(6307), 1484–1487.

Insel, T. R. (2008). Assessing the economic costs of serious mental illness. *American Journal of Psychiatry, 165*(6), 663–665.

Insel, T. R. (2013, November 22). Culture clash. *Director's Blog*. National Institute of Mental Health. Retrieved from www.nimh.nih.gov/about/director/2013/culture-clash.shtml?utm_source=govdelivery&utm_medium=email&utm_campaign=govdelivery

Insel, T. R., & Cuthbert, B. M. (2015). Brain disorders? Precisely. *Science, 348*(6234), 499–500.

Institute of Medicine. (2001). *Crossing the quality chasm: A new health system for the 21st century*. Washington, DC: National Academies Press.

Institute of Medicine. (2006). *Improving the quality of care for mental and substance use conditions*. Washington, DC: National Academies Press.

Institute of Medicine. (2009). *Comparative effectiveness research*. Washington, DC: National Academies Press.

Institute of Medicine. (2010). *Promoting cardiovascular health in the developing world: A critical challenge to achieve global health*. Washington, DC: National Academies Press.

Institute of Medicine. (2011). *Country-level decision making for control of chronic diseases*. Washington, DC: National Academy Press.

Institute of Medicine. (2012). *The mental health and substance use workforce for older adults: In whose hands?* Washington, DC: National Academies Press.

Institute of Medicine. (2015). *Vital signs: Core metrics for health and health care progress*. Washington, DC: National Academies Press.

Institute of Medicine. (2017a). *Best care at lower cost: The path to continuously learning health care in America*. Washington, DC: National Academy Press.

Institute of Medicine. (2017b). *Vital signs: Core metrics for heal and health care progress*. Washington, DC: National Academy Press.

Jackson, D., Roberts, G., Wu, M. L., Ford, R., & Doyle, C. (2016). A systematic review of the effect of telephone, internet or combined support for careers of people living with Alzheimer's, vascular or mixed dementia in the community. *Archives of Gerontology and Geriatrics, 66*, 218–236.

Jacobs, D. (2016). MindKare® Kiosks. Screening for Mental Health, Inc. Retrieved from https://mentalhealthscreening.org/about

Jacobson, N. S., & Truax, P. (1991). Clinical significance: A statistical approach to defining meaningful change in psychotherapy research. *Journal of Consulting and Clinical Psychology, 59*(1), 12–19.

Jasper, K., Weise, C., Conrad, I., Andersson, G., Hiller, W., & Kleinstäuber, M. (2014). The working alliance in a randomized controlled trial comparing Internet-based self-help and face-to-face cognitive behavior therapy for chronic tinnitus. *Internet Interventions, 1*(2), 49–57.

Jayakody, K., Gunadasa, S., & Hosker, C. (2013). Exercise for anxiety disorders: Systematic review. *British Journal of Sports Medicine*. Retrieved from http://bjsm.bmj.com/content/48/3/187

Jim, H. S., Pustejovsky, J. E., Park, C. L., Danhauer, S. C., Sherman, A. C., Fitchett, G., . . . Salsman, J. M. (2015). Religion, spirituality, and physical health in cancer patients: A meta-analysis. *Cancer, 121*(21), 3760–3768.

Johnson, B. T., Scott-Sheldon, L. A. J., & Carey, M. P. (2010). Meta-synthesis of health behavior change meta-analyses. *American Journal of Public Health, 100*(11), 2193–2198.

Johnston, L., Titov, N., Andrews, G., Dear, B. F., & Spence, J. (2013). Comorbidity and Internet-delivered transdiagnostic cognitive behavioural therapy for anxiety disorders. *Cognitive Behaviour Therapy, 42*(3), 180–192.

Johnston-Wilson, N. L., Sims, C. D., Hofmann, J. P., Anderson, L., Shore, A. D., Torrey, E. F., & Yolken, R. H. (2000). Disease-specific alterations in frontal cortex brain proteins in schizophrenia, bipolar disorder, and major depressive disorder. *Molecular Psychiatry, 5*(2), 142–149.

Jonas, S., Khalifeh, H., Bebbington, P. E., McManus, S., Brugha, T., Meltzer, H., & Howard, L. M. (2014). Gender differences in intimate partner violence and psychiatric disorders in England: Results from the 2007 adult psychiatric morbidity survey. *Epidemiology and Psychiatric Sciences, 23*(02), 189–199.

Jørgensen, T. S., Wium-Andersen, I. K., Wium-Andersen, M. K., Jørgensen, M. B., Prescott, E., Maartensson, S., . . . Osler, M. (2016). Incidence of depression after stroke, and associated risk factors and mortality outcomes, in a large cohort of Danish patients. *JAMA Psychiatry, 73*(10), 1032–1040.

Jorm, A. F. (2012). Mental health literacy: Empowering the community to take action for better mental health. *American Psychologist, 67*, 231–243.

Jorm, A. F., Korten, A. E., Jacomb, P. A., Christensen, H., Rodgers, B., & Pollitt, P. (1997). Mental health literacy: A survey of the public's ability to recognise mental disorders and their beliefs about the effectiveness of treatment. *Medical Journal of Australia, 166*(4), 182–186.

Judd, L. L., Paulus, M. P., Wells, K. B., & Rapaport, M. H. (1996). Socioeconomic burden of subsyndromal depressive symptoms and major depression in a sample of the general population. *American Journal of Psychiatry, 153*(11), 1411–1417.

Jürgens, R., Ball, A., & Verster, A. (2009). Interventions to reduce HIV transmission related to injecting drug use in prison. *Lancet Infectious Diseases, 9*, 57–66.

Juvenal, *The Satires* (1991; N. Rudd, Translation). New York: Oxford University Press.

Kalichman, S. C., Ramachandran, B., & Catz, S. (1999). Adherence to combination antiretroviral therapies in HIV patients of low health literacy. *Journal of General Internal Medicine, 14*(5), 267–273.

Kaltenthaler, E., Sutcliffe, P., Parry, G., Beverley, C., Rees, A., & Ferriter, M. (2008). The acceptability to patients of computerized cognitive behaviour therapy for depression: A systematic review. *Psychological Medicine, 38*(11), 1521–1530.

Kam-Hansen, S., Jakubowski, M., Kelley, J. M., Kirsch, I., Hoaglin, D. C., Kaptchuk, T. J., & Burstein, R. (2014). Altered placebo and drug labeling changes the outcome of episodic migraine attacks. *Science Translational Medicine, 6*(218), 218ra5.

Kanamori, M., Suzuki, M., Oshiro, H., Tanaka, M., Inoguchi, T., Takasugi, H., & Yokoyama, T. (2003). Pilot study on improvement of quality of life among elderly using a pet-type robot. *Proceedings of the IEEE International Symposium on Computational Intelligence in Robotics and Automation. 1*, 107–112.

Kang, K. I., Freedman, S., Matarić, M. J., Cunningham, M. J., & Lopez, B. (2005, June). A hands-off physical therapy assistance robot for cardiac patients. 9th International Conference. In *Proceedings of the International Conference on Rehabilitation Robotics, ICORR*, 337–340.

Kant, I. (1793). *Religion within the boundaries of mere reason*. Edited and translated by R. M. Adams, G. Di Giovanni, &. A. Wood (1999). New York: Cambridge University Press.

Kao, H. L. C., Holz, C., Roseway, A., Calvo, A., & Schmandt, C. (2016, September). DuoSkin: Rapidly prototyping on-skin user interfaces using skin-friendly materials. In *Proceedings of the 2016 Association for Computing Machinery (ACM) International Symposium on Wearable Computers* (pp. 16–23). ACM. Retrieved from http://duoskin.media.mit.edu/

Kaplan, B. J. Rucklidge, J. J., Romijn, A., & McLeod, K. (2015). The emerging field of nutritional mental health: Inflammation, the microbiome, oxidative stress, and mitochondrial function. *Clinical Psychological Science*, 3, 964–980.

Kaptchuk, T. J., Friedlander, E., Kelley, J. M., Sanchez, M. N., Kokkotou, E., Singer, J. P., . . . Lembo, A. J. (2010). Placebos without deception: A randomized controlled trial in irritable bowel syndrome. *PLoS One*, *5*(12), e15591.

Karlin, B. E., & Cross, G. (2014). From the laboratory to the therapy room: National dissemination and implementation of evidence-based psychotherapies in the US Department of Veterans Affairs Health Care System. *American Psychologist*, *69*(1), 19–33.

Karlin, B. E., Trockel, M., Taylor, C. B., Gimeno, J., & Manber, R. (2013). National dissemination of cognitive behavioral therapy for insomnia in veterans: Clinician and patient-level outcomes. *Journal of Consulting and Clinical Psychology, 81*(5), 912–917.

Kazak, A. E., Nash, J. M., Hiroto, K., & Kaslow, N. J. (2017). Psychologists in patient-centered medical homes (PCMHs): Roles, evidence, opportunities, and challenges. *American Psychologist*, *72*(1), 1–12.

Kazdin, A. E. (1977). Assessing the clinical or applied significance of behavior change through social validation. *Behavior Modification*, *1*, 427–452.

Kazdin, A. E. (1978a). Evaluating the generality of findings in analogue therapy research. *Journal of Consulting and Clinical Psychology*, *46*, 673–686.

Kazdin, A. E. (1978b). *History of behavior modification: Experimental foundations of contemporary research*. Baltimore: University Park Press. (Sponsored by the National Academy of Sciences.)

Kazdin, A. E. (1999). The meanings and measurement of clinical significance. *Journal of Consulting and Clinical Psychology*, *67*, 332–339.

Kazdin, A. E. (2000). *Psychotherapy for children and adolescents: Directions for research and practice.* New York: Oxford University Press.

Kazdin, A. E. (2013). Evidence-based treatment and usual care: Cautions and qualifications. *JAMA Psychiatry*, *70*, 666–667.

Kazdin, A. E. (2014). Moderators, mediators, and mechanisms of change in psychotherapy. In W. Lutz & S, Knox (Eds.), *Quantitative and qualitative methods in psychotherapy* (pp. 87–101). East Sussex, UK: Routledge.

Kazdin, A. E. (2015). Treatment as usual and routine care in research and clinical practice. *Clinical Psychology Review, 42*, 168–178.

Kazdin, A. E. (2017a). Parent management training and problem-solving skills training for child and adolescent conduct problems. In J. R. Weisz & A. E. Kazdin (Eds.), *Evidence-based psychotherapies for children and adolescents* (3rd ed.). New York: Guilford Press.

Kazdin, A. E. (2017b). *Research design in clinical psychology* (5th ed.). Boston: Pearson.

Kazdin, A. E., & Bass, D. (1989). Power to detect differences between alternative treatments in comparative psychotherapy outcome research. *Journal of Consulting and Clinical Psychology, 57*, 138–147.

Kazdin, A. E., & Blase, S. L. (2011). Rebooting psychotherapy research and practice to reduce the burden of mental illness. *Perspectives on Psychological Science, 6*, 21–37.

Kazdin, A. E., Holland, L., & Crowley, M. (1997). Family experience of barriers to treatment and premature termination from child therapy. *Journal of Consulting and Clinical Psychology, 65*, 453–463.

Kazdin, A. E., & Rabbitt, S. (2013). Novel models for delivering mental health services and reducing the burdens of mental illness. *Clinical Psychological Science, 1*, 170–191.

Kazdin, A. E., & Wilcoxon, L. A. (1976). Systematic desensitization and non-specific treatment effects: A methodological evaluation. *Psychological Bulletin, 83*, 729–758.

Kazdin, A. E., & Wilson, G. T. (1978). *Evaluation of behavior therapy: Issues, evidence, and research strategies*. Cambridge, MA: Ballinger.

Kazrin, A., Durac, J., & Agteros, T. (1979). Meta-meta analysis: A new method for evaluating therapy outcome. *Behaviour Research and Therapy, 17*, 397–399.

Keil, D. (2011). An ounce of prevention is worth a pound of cure: Reframing the debate about law school affirmative action, *Denver Law Review, 88*, 791–806.

Kendall, P. C., & Grove, W. M. (1988). Normative comparisons in therapy outcome. *Behavioral Assessment, 10*, 147–158.

Kendell, R. E. (2001). The distinction between mental and physical illness. *British Journal of Psychiatry, 178*(6), 490–493.

Kendler, K. S., Prescott, C. A., Myers, J., & Neale, M. C. (2003). The structure of genetic and environmental risk factors for common psychiatric and substance use disorders in men and women. *Archives of General Psychiatry, 60*(9), 929–937.

Kessler, R. C., Aguilar-Gaxiola, S., Alonso, J., Chatterji, S., Lee, S., Ormel, J., . . . Wang, P. S. (2009). The global burden of mental disorders: An update from the WHO World Mental Health (WMH) Surveys. *Epidemiologia e Psichiatria Sociale,18*, 23–33.

Kessler, R. C., Angermeyer, M., Anthony, J. C., De Graaf, R., Demyttenaere, K., Gasquet, I., . . . Uestuen, T. B. (2007). Lifetime prevalence and age-of-onset distributions of mental disorders in the World Health Organization's World Mental Health Survey Initiative. *World Psychiatry, 6*(3), 168–176.

Kessler, R. C., Berglund, P., Demler, O., Jin, R., Merikangas, K. R., & Walters, E. E. (2005). Lifetime prevalence and age-of-onset distributions of DSM-IV disorders in the National Comorbidity Survey Replication. *Archives of General Psychiatry, 62*(6), 593–602.

Kessler, R. C., & Bromet, E. J. (2013). The epidemiology of depression across cultures. *Annual Review of Public Health, 34*, 119–138.

Kessler, R. C., Chiu, W. T., Demler, O., & Walters, E. E. (2005). Prevalence, severity, and comorbidity of 12-month DSM-IV disorders in the National Comorbidity Survey Replication. *Archives of General Psychiatry, 62*(6), 617–627.

Kessler, R. C., Heeringa, S., Lakoma, M. D., Petukhova, M., Rupp, A. E., Schoenbaum, M., . . . Zaslavsky, A. M. (2008). Individual and societal effects of mental disorders on earnings in the United States: Results from the national comorbidity survey replication. *American Journal of Psychiatry, 165*(6), 703–711.

Kessler, R. C., McGonagle, K. A., Zhao, S., Nelson, C. B., Hughes, M., Eshleman, S., . . . Kendler, K. S. (1994). Lifetime and 12-month prevalence of DSM-III-R psychiatric disorders in the United States: Results from the National Comorbidity Survey. *Archives of General Psychiatry, 51*, 8–19.

Kessler, R. C., Mickelson, K. D., & Williams, D. R. (1999). The prevalence, distribution, and mental health correlates of perceived discrimination in the United States. *Journal of Health and Social Behavior, 40*(3), 208–230.

Kessler, R. C., & Üstün, T. B. (2004). The World Mental Health (WMH) Survey initiative version of the World Health Organization (WHO) Composite International Diagnostic Interview (CIDI). *International Journal of Methods in Psychiatric Research, 13*(2), 93–121.

Kessler, R. C., & Wang, P. S. (2008). The descriptive epidemiology of commonly occurring mental disorders in the United States. *Annual Review of Public Health, 29*, 115–129.

Khoury, B., Lecomte, T., Fortin, G., Masse, M., Therien, P., Bouchard, V., . . . Hofmann, S. G. (2013). Mindfulness-based therapy: A comprehensive meta-analysis. *Clinical Psychology Review, 33*(6), 763–771.

Killeen, C. (1998). Loneliness: an epidemic in modern society. *Journal of Advanced Nursing, 28*(4), 762–770.

Kilpatrick, D. G., & Acierno, R. (2003). Mental health needs of crime victims: Epidemiology and outcomes. *Journal of Traumatic Stress, 16*(2), 119–132.

Kilpela, L. S., Hill, K., Kelly, M. C., Elmquist, J., Ottoson, P., Keith, D., . . . Becker, C. B. (2014). Reducing eating disorder risk factors: A controlled investigation of a blended task-shifting/train-the-trainer approach to dissemination and implementation. *Behaviour Research and Therapy, 63*, 70–82.

Kim, B. S., Ng, G. F., & Ahn, A. J. (2005). Effects of client expectation for counseling success, client-counselor worldview match, and client adherence to Asian and European American cultural values on counseling process with Asian Americans. *Journal of Counseling Psychology, 52*(1), 67–76.

Kim, C. C., Lee, H. H., Oh, K. H., & Sun, J. Y. (2016). Highly stretchable, transparent ionic touch panel. *Science, 353*(6300), 682–687.

Kim, S. (2015, April). Priceline acknowledges baby as "unusual" purchaser of $516 car rental. ABC News, Good Morning America. Retrieved from https://gma.yahoo.com/priceline-acknowledges-baby-unusual-purchaser-516-car-rental-201043173--abc-news-personal-finance.html

Kim, Y., & Sundar, S. S. (2009). Me, myself, and my avatar. In N. T. Wood & M. R. Solomon (Eds.), *Virtual social identity and consumer behavior* (pp. 141–156). Armonk, NY: M. E. Sharpe, Inc.

Kipper, D. A., & Ritchie, T. D. (2003). The effectiveness of psychodramatic techniques: A meta-analysis. *Group Dynamics: Theory, Research, and Practice, 7*(1), 13–25.

Kirsch, I. (1985). Response expectancy as a determinant of experience and behavior. *American Psychologist, 40*(11), 1189–1202.

Kiume, S. (2013). *Top 10 mental health apps*. Psych Central, World of Psychology Blog. Retrieved from http://psychcentral.com/blog/archives/2013/01/16/top-10-mental-health-apps/

Klauser, P., Baker, S. T., Cropley, V. L., Bousman, C., Fornito, A., Cocchi, L., . . . Michie, P. T. (2017). White matter disruptions in schizophrenia are spatially widespread and topologically converge on brain network hubs. *Schizophrenia Bulletin, 43*(2), 425–435.

Klein, R. G., Mannuzza, S., Olazagasti, M. A. R., Roizen, E., Hutchison, J. A., Lashua, E. C., & Castellanos, F. X. (2012). Clinical and functional outcome of childhood attention-deficit/hyperactivity disorder 33 years later. *Archives of General Psychiatry, 69*(12), 1295–1303.

Kleindorfer, D., Miller, R., Sailor-Smith, S., Moomaw, C., Khoury, J., & Frankel, M. (2008). The challenges of community-based research: The beauty shop stroke education project. *Stroke, 39*, 2331–2335.

Knapp, M., Mangalore, R., & Simon, J. (2004). The global costs of schizophrenia. *Schizophrenia Bulletin, 30*(2), 279–293.

Knapp, M., McDaid, D., & Personage, M. (Eds.). (2011). *Mental health promotion and mental illness prevention: The economic case*. London: Department of Health.

Knuesel, I., Chicha, L., Britschgi, M., Schobel, S. A., Bodmer, M., Hellings, J. A., . . . Prinssen, E. P. (2014). Maternal immune activation and abnormal brain development across CNS disorders. *Nature Reviews Neurology, 10*(11), 643–660.

Koch, R. (2011). *Living the 80/20 way: Work less, worry less, succeed more, enjoy more.* (New ed.). London: Nicholas Brealey Publishing.

Koffel, E., Krebs, E. E., Arbisi, P. A., Erbes, C. R., & Polusny, M. A. (2016). The unhappy triad: Pain, sleep complaints, and internalizing symptoms. *Clinical Psychological Science, 4*(1) 96–106.

Koh, H. K., Piotrowski, J. J., Kumanyika, S., & Fielding, J. E. (2011). Healthy people: A 2020 vision for the social determinants approach. *Health Education & Behavior, 38*(6), 551–557.

Kohn, R., Saxena, S., Levav, I., & Saraceno, B. (2004). The treatment gap in mental health care. *Bulletin of the World Health Organization, 82*(11), 858–866.

Kolappa, K., Henderson, D. C., & Kishore, S. P. (2013). No physical health without mental health: Lessons unlearned? *Bulletin of the World Health Organization, 91*(1), 3–3a.

Korenman, S., Miller, J. E., & Sjaastad, J. E. (1995). Long-term poverty and child development in the United States: Results from the NLSY. *Children and Youth Services Review, 17*(1), 127–155.

Kotov, R., Krueger, R. F., Watson, D., Achenbach, T. M., Althoff, R. R., Bagby, R. M., . . . Eaton, N. R. (2017). The Hierarchical Taxonomy of Psychopathology (HiTOP): A dimensional alternative to traditional nosologies. *Journal of Abnormal Psychology, 126*(4), 454–477.

Kraemer, H. C., Kazdin, A. E., Offord, D. R., Kessler, R. C., Jensen, P. S., & Kupfer, D. J. (1997). Coming to terms with the terms of risk. *Archives of General Psychiatry, 54*, 337–343.

Kring, A. M., & Sloan, D. M. (Eds.). (2009). *Emotion regulation and psychopathology: A transdiagnostic approach to etiology and treatment*. New York: Guilford Press.

Krol, D. M., Redlener, M., Shapiro, A., & Wajnberg, A. (2007). A mobile medical care approach targeting underserved populations in post-Hurricane Katrina Mississippi. *Journal of Health Care for the Poor and Underserved, 18*, 331–340.

Krpan, K. M., Kross, E., Berman, M. G., Deldin, P. J., Askren, M. K., & Jonides, J. (2013). An everyday activity as a treatment for depression: The benefits of expressive writing for people diagnosed with major depressive disorder. *Journal of Affective Disorders, 150*(3), 1148–1151.

Kuchler, F., Tegene, A., & Harris, J. M. (2005). Taxing snack foods: Manipulating diet quality or financing information programs? *Applied Economic Perspectives and Policy, 27*(1), 4–20.

Lam, N., & Leat, S. J. (2015). Barriers to accessing low-vision care: The patient's perspective. *Canadian Journal of Ophthalmology/Journal Canadien d'Ophtalmologie, 50*, S34–S39.

Lamanna, D., Kirst, M., Shapiro, G., Matheson, F., Nakhost, A., & Stergiopoulos, V. (2015). Toronto Mobile Crisis Intervention Team (MCIT): Outcome evaluation report. Toronto, CA.

Lambert, M. J. (Ed.). (2013). *Bergin and Garfield's handbook of psychotherapy and behavior change* (6th ed.). New York: John Wiley & Sons.

Lambert, M. J., & Ogles, B. M. (2013). The efficacy and effectiveness of psychotherapy. In M. J. Lambert (Ed.), *Bergin and Garfield's handbook of psychotherapy and behavior change* (6th ed., pp. 169–218). New York: John Wiley & Sons.

Lambert, W., Salzer, M. S., & Bickman, L. (1998). Clinical outcome, consumer satisfaction, and ad hoc ratings of improvement in children's mental health. *Journal of Consulting and Clinical Psychology, 66*, 270–279.

Lancaster, A. (2016). Evidence for joint police and mental health responses for people in mental health crisis. *Mental Health Practice, 19*(10), 20–26.

Lancet Global Mental Health Group. (2007). Scale up services for mental disorders: A call for action. *Lancet, 370, 1241–1252.*

Lancet Psychiatry. (2015, April). Series on diabetes and psychiatric disorder. *2*(5), 431–476.

Larkin, I., Ang, D., Avorn, J., & Kesselheim, A. S. (2014). Restrictions on pharmaceutical detailing reduced off-label prescribing of antidepressants and antipsychotics in children. *Health Affairs, 33*(6), 1014–1023.

Larun, L., Nordeim, L. V., Ekeland, E., Hagen, K. B., & Heian, F. (2006). Exercise in prevention and treatment of anxiety and depression among children and young people. *Cochrane Database of Systematic Reviews, 19*, 1–49.

Lasgaard, M., Goossens, L., & Elklit, A. (2011). Loneliness, depressive symptomatology, and suicide ideation in adolescence: Cross-sectional and longitudinal analyses. *Journal of Abnormal Child Psychology, 39*(1), 137–150.

Lauber, C., Anthony, M., Ajdacic-Gross, V., & Rössler, W. (2004). What about psychiatrists' attitude to mentally ill people? *European Psychiatry, 19*(7), 423–427.

Layard, R. (2013). Mental health: The new frontier for labour economics. *IZA Journal of Labor Policy, 2*(1), 2. Retrieved from http://izajolp.springeropen.com/articles/10.1186/2193-9004-2-2

Layard, R., & Clark, D. M. (2014). *Thrive: The power of evidence-based psychological therapies*. London: Penguin Books.

Layard, R., Bell, S., Clark, D. M., Knapp. M., Meacher, M., Priebe, S., & Wright, B. (2006). The depression report: A new deal for depression and anxiety disorders. Centre for Economic Performance Report. London: London School of Economics. Retrieved from http://cep.lse.ac.uk

Layard, R., Clark, D. M., Knapp, M., & Mayraz, G. (2007). Cost-benefit analysis of psychological therapy. *National Institute Economic Review, 202*, 90–98.

Lazányi, K. (2016, August). Investing in social support: Robots as perfect partners? *14th International Symposium*. In *Intelligent Systems and Informatics (SISY)*, 25–30. IEEE.

Lazarus, A. A. (1961). Group therapy of phobic disorders by systematic desensitization. *Journal of Abnormal and Social Psychology, 63*, 504–510.

Leahy, R. L., Holland, S. J. F., & McGinn, L. K. (2012). *Treatment plans and interventions for depression and anxiety disorders*. New York: Guilford Press.

Leamy, M., Bird, V., Le Boutillier, C., Williams, J., & Slade, M. (2011). Conceptual framework for personal recovery in mental health: Systematic review and narrative synthesis. *British Journal of Psychiatry, 199*(6), 445–452.

Leathard, A. (Ed.) (1994). *Going Inter-professional: Working together for health and welfare*. London: Routledge.

Leblanc, M., & Ritchie, M. (2001). A meta-analysis of play therapy outcomes. *Counselling Psychology Quarterly, 14*(2), 149–163.

Lee, J., Carvallo, M., & Lee, E. (2015). Feasibility of utilizing ethnic beauty salons for cervical cancer screening education. *Western Journal of Nursing Research, 37*, 1489–1509.

Lehman, A. F., & Dixon, L. (Eds.). (2016). *Double jeopardy: Chronic mental illness and substance use disorders*. London: Routledge.

Leichsenring, F., Rabung, S., & Leibing, E. (2004). The efficacy of short-term psychodynamic psychotherapy in specific psychiatric disorders: A meta-analysis. *Archives of General Psychiatry, 61*(12), 1208–1216.

Lester, R. T., Ritvo, P., Mills, E. J., Kariri, A., Karanja, S., Chung, M. H., . . . Marra, C. A. (2010). Effects of a mobile phone short message service on antiretroviral treatment adherence in Kenya (WelTel Kenya1): A randomised trial. *Lancet, 376*(9755), 1838–1845.

Levack, B. (2013). *The devil within: Possession and exorcism in the Christian West*. New Haven, CT: Yale University Press.

Levitt, E. E. (1957). The results of psychotherapy with children: An evaluation. *Journal of Consulting Psychology, 21*, 189–196.

Levitt, E. E. (1963). Psychotherapy with children: A further evaluation. *Behaviour Research and Therapy, 60*, 326–329.

Lewinsohn, P. M. (1975). The behavioral study and treatment of depression. In M. Hersen, R. M. Eisler, & P. M. Miller (Eds.), *Progress in behavioral modification* (Vol. 1, pp. 19–65). New York: Academic.

Lewis, Y. R., Shain, L., Quinn, S., Turner, K., & Moore, T. (2002). Building community trust: Lessons from a STID/HIV peer educator program with African American barbers and beauticians. *Health Promotion Practice, 3*, 133–143.

Lewis-Fernández, R., & Aggarwal, N. K. (2013). Culture and psychiatric diagnosis. *Advances in Psychosomatic Medicine, 33*, 15–30.

Li, L., Ishdorj, G., & Gibson, S. B. (2012). Reactive oxygen species regulation of autophagy in cancer: implications for cancer treatment. *Free Radical Biology and Medicine, 53*(7), 1399–1410.

Libin, A., & Cohen-Mansfield, J. (2004). Therapeutic robocat for nursing home residents with dementia: Preliminary inquiry. *American Journal of Alzheimer's Disease and Other Dementias, 19*, 111–116.

Lichtenstein, E., Glasgow, R. E., Lando, H. A., Ossip-Klein, D. J., & Boles, S. M. (1996). Telephone counseling for smoking cessation: Rationales and meta-analytic review of evidence. *Health Education Research, 11*(2), 243–257.

Lichtenstein, E., Zhu, S. H., & Tedeschi, G. J. (2010). Smoking cessation quitlines: An underrecognized intervention success story. *American Psychologist, 65*(4), 252–261.

Lichtman, J. H., Froelicher, E. S., Blumenthal, J. A., Carney, R. M., Doering, L. V., Frasure-Smith, N., . . . Wulsin, L. (2014). Depression as a risk factor for poor prognosis among patients with acute coronary syndrome: Systematic review and recommendations a scientific statement from the American Heart Association. *Circulation, 129*(12), 1350–1369.

Lick, J., & Bootzin, R. (1975). Expectancy factors in the treatment of fear: Methodological and theoretical issues. *Psychological Bulletin*, 1975, *82*, 917–931.

Lindert, J., von Ehrenstein, O. S., Grashow, R., Gal, G., Braehler, E., & Weisskopf, M. G. (2014). Sexual and physical abuse in childhood is associated with depression and anxiety over the life course: Systematic review and meta-analysis. *International Journal of Public Health, 59*(2), 359–372.

Ling, R. (2004). *The mobile connection: The cell phone's impact on society*. San Francisco, CA: Morgan Kaufman Publishers.

Link, B. G., Phelan, J. C., Bresnahan, M., Stueve, A., & Pescosolido, B. A. (1999). Public conceptions of mental illness: Labels, causes, dangerousness, and social distance. *American Journal of Public Health, 89*(9), 1328–1333.

Linnan, L. A., D'Angelo, H., & Harrington, C. B. (2014). A literature synthesis of health promotion research in salons and barbershops. *American Journal of Preventive Medicine, 47*(1), 77–85.

Linnan, L. A., & Ferguson, Y. (2007). Beauty salons: A promising health promotion setting for reaching and promoting health among African American women. *Health Education and Behavior, 34*, 517–530.

Litz, B. T., Gray, M. J., Bryant, R. A., & Adler, A. B. (2002). Early intervention for trauma: Current status and future directions. *Clinical Psychology: Science and Practice, 9*(2), 112–134.

Locher, C., Hasler, S., & Gaab, J. (2016). Placebos in der psychotherapieforschung-eine systematische Analyse am beispiel der systematischen desensibilisierung. *Verhaltenstherapie, 26*, 9–20.

Loewenthal, D., & Samuels, A. (2014). *Relational psychotherapy, psychoanalysis and counselling: Appraisals and reappraisals*. East Sussex, UK: Routledge.

Loncar, M., Plasc, I. D., Bunjevac, T., Hrabac, P., Jaksic, N., Kozina, S., & Marcinko, D. (2014). Predicting symptom clusters of posttraumatic stress disorder (PTSD) in Croatian war veterans: the role of socio-demographics, war experiences and subjective quality of life. *Psychiatria Danubina, 26*(3), 231–238.

London, P. (1986). *The modes and morals of psychotherapy* (2nd ed.). Abingdon, UK: Routledge.

Lopresti, A. L., Hood, S. D., & Drummond, P. D. (2013). A review of lifestyle factors that contribute to important pathways associated with major depression: Diet, sleep and exercise. *Journal of Affective* disorders, *148*(1), 12–27.

Lora, A., Kohn, R., Levav, I., McBain, R., Morris, J., & Saxena, S. (2012). Service availability and utilization and treatment gap for schizophrenic disorders: A survey in 50 low-and middle-income countries. *Bulletin of the World Health Organization, 90*(1), 47–54B.

Lorenc, T., Clayton, S., Neary, D., Whitehead, M., Petticrew, M., Thomson, H., . . . Renton, A. (2012). Crime, fear of crime, environment, and mental health and wellbeing: Mapping review of theories and causal pathways. *Health & Place, 18*(4), 757–765.

Luborsky, L., Singer, B., & Luborsky, L. (1975). Comparative studies of psychotherapies: Is it true that "everyone has won and all must have prizes"? *Archives of General Psychiatry, 32*, 995–1008.

Lucas, R. E., & Diener, E. (2009). Personality and subjective well-being. In E. Diener (Ed.), *The science of well-being* (pp. 75–102). Netherlands: Springer.

Lund, C., De Silva, M., Plagerson, S., Cooper, S., Chisholm, D., Das, J., . . . Patel, V. (2011). Poverty and mental disorders: Breaking the cycle in low-income and middle-income countries. *Lancet, 378*(9801), 1502–1514.

Lundahl, B. W., Kunz, C., Brownell, C., Tollefson, D., & Burke, B. L. (2010). A meta-analysis of motivational interviewing: Twenty-five years of empirical studies. *Research on Social Work Practice, 20*(2) 137–160.

Luo, R., Shi, Y., Zhang, L., Liu, C., Rozelle, S., Sharbono, B., . . . Martorell, R. (2011, January). *Nutrition and educational performance in rural China's elementary schools: Results of a randomized con- trolled trial in Shaanxi Province.* Paper presented at the annual meeting of the American Economic Association, Denver, CO.

Luo, Y., Hawkley, L. C., Waite, L. J., & Cacioppo, J. T. (2012). Loneliness, health, and mortality in old age: A national longitudinal study. *Social Science & Medicine, 74*(6), 907–914.

Luque, J. S., Ross, L., & Gwede, C. K., (2014). Qualitative systematic review of barber-administered health education, promotion, screening and outreach programs in African-American communities. *Journal of Community Health, 39*(1), 181–90.

Lutz, W., Stulz, N., & Kock, K. (2009). Patterns of early change and their relationship to outcome and follow-up among patients with major depressive disorders. *Journal of Affective Disorders, 118*, 60–68.

Luxton, D. D., McCann, R. A., Bush, N. E., Mishkind, M. C., & Reger, G. M. (2011). mHealth for mental health: Integrating smartphone technology in behavioral healthcare. *Professional Psychology: Research and Practice, 42*(6), 505–512.

Lydecker, J. A., & Grilo, C. M. (2016). The apple of their eye: Attitudinal and behavioral correlates of parents' perceptions of child obesity. *Obesity, 24*, 1124–1131.

Lyness, J. M., Kim, J., Tu, X., Conwell, Y., King, D. A., & Caine, E. D. (2007). The clinical significance of subsyndromal depression in older primary care patients. *American Journal of Geriatric Psychiatry, 15*(3), 214–223.

Lynn, S. J., O'Donohue, W. T., & Lilienfeld, S. O. (Eds.). (2015). *Health, happiness, and well-being: Better living through psychological science.* Los Angeles, CA: Sage Publications.

Lyon, A. R., & Koerner, K. (2016). User-centered design for psychosocial intervention development and implementation. *Clinical Psychology: Science and Practice, 23*(2), 180–200.

Lytle, M. C., Silenzio, V. M., & Caine, E. D. (2016). Are there still too few suicides to generate public outrage? *JAMA Psychiatry, 73*, 1003–1004.

Macdonald W, Beeston C, & McCullough S. (2014). *Proportionate universalism and health inequalities.* Edinburgh: NHS Health Scotland. Retrieved from www.healthscotland.com/uploads/documents/24296-ProportionateUniversalismBriefing.pdf

Macoveanu, J., Rowe, J. B., Hornboll, B., Elliott, R., Paulson, O. B., Knudsen, G. M., & Siebner, H. R. (2013). Playing it safe but losing anyway: Serotonergic signaling of negative outcomes in dorsomedial prefrontal cortex in the context of risk-aversion. *European Neuropsychopharmacology, 23*(8), 919–930.

Madigan, M. E., Smith-Wheelock, L., & Krein, S. L. (2007). Healthy hair starts with a healthy body: Hair stylists as lay health advisors to prevent chronic kidney disease. *Preventing Chronic Disease, 4*, A64.

Maercker, A., Brewin, C. R., Bryant, R. A., Cloitre, M., van Ommeren, M., Jones, L., & Reed, G. M. (2013). Diagnosis and classification of disorders specifically associated with stress: Proposals for ICD-11. *World Psychiatry, 12*, 198–206.

Maes, M., Kubera, M., Obuchowiczwa, E., Goehler, L., Brzeszcz, J. (2011). Depression's multiple comorbidities explained by (neuro)inflammatory and oxidative and nitrosative stress pathways. *Neuroendocrinology Letters, 32*, 7–24.

Magidson, J. F., Blashill, A. J., Safren, S. A., & Wagner, G. J. (2015). Depressive symptoms, lifestyle structure, and ART adherence among HIV-infected individuals: A longitudinal mediation analysis. *AIDS and Behavior, 19*(1), 34–40.

Maher, C. A., Lewis, L. K., Ferrar, K., Marshall, S., De Bourdeaudhuij, I., & Vandelanotte, C. (2014). Are health behavior change interventions that use online social networks effective? A systematic review. *Journal of Medical Internet Research, 16*(2), e40.

Maher, J. E., Rohde, K., Dent, C. W., Stark, M. J., Pizacani, B., Boysun, M. J., . . . Yepassis-Zembrou, P. L. (2007). Is a statewide tobacco quitline an appropriate service for specific populations? *Tobacco Control, 16*(Suppl 1), i65–i70.

Maier, C. B., & Aiken, L. H. (2016). Task shifting from physicians to nurses in primary care in 39 countries: A cross-country comparative study. *European Journal of Public Health, 26*(6), 927–934.

Malakoff, D. (2017). A matter of fact. (Introduction to a featured Series of articles on evidence and its influence, role, and use in policy making). *Science, 355*(6325), 562–563.

Manchanda, P., & Honka, E. (2005). The effects and role of direct-to-physician marketing in the pharmaceutical industry: An integrative review. *Yale Journal of Health Policy, Law, and Ethics, 5*(2), article 8. Retrieved from http://digitalcommons.law.yale.edu/yjhple/vol5/iss2/8

Marker, C. D., Comer, J. S., Abramova, V., & Kendall, P. C. (2013). The reciprocal relationship between alliance and symptom improvement across the treatment of childhood anxiety. *Journal of Clinical Child & Adolescent Psychology, 42*(1), 22–33.

Marrast, L., Himmelstein, D. U., & Woolhandler, S. (2016). Racial and ethnic disparities in mental health care for children and young adults: A national study. *International Journal of Health Services: Planning, Administration, Evaluation, 46*(4), 810–824.

Marshall, C. R., Noor, A., Vincent, J. B., Lionel, A. C., Feuk, L., Skaug, J., . . . Thiruvahindrapduram, B. (2008). Structural variation of chromosomes in autism spectrum disorder. *American Journal of Human Genetics, 82*(2), 477–488.

Marteau, T. M., Hollands, G.J., & Kelly, M. P. (2015). Changing population behavior and reducing health disparities: Exploring the potential of "choice architecture" interventions. In R. M. Kaplan, M. L. Spittel, & D. M. David (Eds.), *Population health: Behavioral and social science insights* (pp. 105–126). AHRQ Publication No. 15-0002. Rockville, MD: Agency for Healthcare Research and Quality and Office of Behavioral and Social Science Research, National Institutes of Health.

Marti, P., Bacigalupo, M., Giusti, L., Mennecozzi, C., & Shibata, T. (2006). Socially assistive robotics in the treatment of behavioural and psychological symptoms of dementia. *First International Conference on Biomedical Robotics and Biomechatronics*, 483–488.

Martin, S. L., Macy, R. J., & Young, S. K. (2011). Health and economic consequences of sexual violence. In J. W. White, M. P. Koss, & A. E. Kazdin, (Eds.). *Violence against women and children: Volume I: Mapping the terrain* (pp. 173–195). Washington, DC: American Psychological Association.

Martini, M. G., Hewage, C. T., Nasralla, M. M., Smith, R., Jourdan, I., & Rockall, T. (2013, July). 3-D robotic tele-surgery and training over next generation wireless networks. In *Engineering in Medicine and Biology Society (EMBC), 2013 35th Annual International Conference of the IEEE*, 6244–6247.

Masuda, N., Kurahashi, I., & Onari, H. (2013). Suicide ideation of individuals in online social networks. *PLoS One*, *8*(4), e62262.

May, T. (2017, January 9). *The shared society*. Speech delivered at the annual meeting of the Charity Commission, Royal Society, London. Retrieved from http://blogs.spectator.co.uk/2017/01/full-text-theresa-mays-shared-society-speech/

McAleavey, A. A., & Castonguay, L. G. (2015). The process of change in psychotherapy: Common and unique factors. In O. C. G. Gelo, A. Pritz, & B. Rieken (Eds.), Psychotherapy research: Foundations, process, and outcome (pp. 293–310). Vienna: Springer Verlag.

McColl, D., & Nejat, G. (2014). Recognizing emotional body language displayed by a human-like social robot. *International Journal of Social Robotics*, *6*(2), 261–280.

McEvoy, P. M., Nathan, P., & Norton, P. J. (2009). Efficacy of transdiagnostic treatments: A review of published outcome studies and future research directions. *Journal of Cognitive Psychotherapy*, *23*(1), 20–33.

McEvoy, P. M., & Nathan, P. (2007). Effectiveness of cognitive behavior therapy for diagnostically heterogeneous groups: A benchmarking study. *Journal of Consulting and Clinical Psychology*, *75*(2), 344–350.

McEvoy, P. M., & Mahoney, A. E. J. (2012). To be sure, to be sure: Intolerance of uncertainty mediates symptoms of various anxiety disorders and depression, *Behavior Therapy*, *43*, 533–545.

McGowan, A. K., Lee, M. M., Meneses, C. M., Perkins, J., & Youdelman, M. (2016). Civil Rights Laws as tools to advance health in the twenty-first century. *Annual Review of Public Health*, *37*, 185–204.

McGuire, T. G., Alegria, M., Cook, B. L., Wells, K. B., & Zaslavsky, A. M. (2006). Implementing the Institute of Medicine definition of disparities: An application to mental health care. *Health Services Research*, *41*(5), 1979–2005.

McGuire, T. G., & Miranda, J. (2008). New evidence regarding racial and ethnic disparities in mental health: Policy implications. *Health Affairs*, *27*, 393–403.

McHugh, R. K., & Barlow, D. H. (2010). The dissemination and implementation of evidence-based psychological treatments: A review of current efforts. *American Psychologist*, *65*, 73–84.

McLaughlin, K. A., Koenen, K. C., Friedman, M. J., Ruscio, A. M., Karam, E. G., Shahly, V., . . . Kessler, R. C. (2015). Subthreshold posttraumatic stress disorder in the World Health Organization World Mental Health Surveys. *Biological Psychiatry*, *77*(4), 375–384.

McMartin, S. E., Jacka, F. N., & Colman, I. (2013). The association between fruit and vegetable consumption and mental health disorders: Evidence from five waves of a national survey of Canadians. *Preventive Medicine*, *56*(3), 225–230.

McMichael, A. J., & Butler, C. D. (2011). Promoting global population health while constraining the environmental footprint. *Annual Review of Public Health*, *32*, 179–197.

McMillan, K. A., Enns, M. W., Asmundson, G. J., & Sareen, J. (2010). The association between income and distress, mental disorders, and suicidal ideation and attempts: Findings from the collaborative psychiatric epidemiology surveys. *Journal of Clinical Psychiatry, 71*(9), 1168–1175.

McMorris, T., Tomporowski, P. D., & Audiffren, M. (2009). *Exercise and cognitive function*. New York, NY: John Wiley & Sons.

McMunn, A. M., Nazroo, J. Y., Marmot, M. G., Boreham, R., & Goodman, R. (2001). Children's emotional and behavioural well-being and the family environment: Findings from the Health Survey for England. *Social Science & Medicine, 53*(4), 423–440.

Moorhead, S. A., Hazlett, D. E., Harrison, L., Carroll, J. K., Irwin, A., & Hoving, C. (2013). A new dimension of health care: Systematic review of the uses, benefits, and limitations of social media for health communication. *Journal of Medical Internet Research, 15*(4), e85.

McWilliams, L. A., Goodwin, R. D., & Cox, B. J. (2004). Depression and anxiety associated with three pain conditions: Results from a nationally representative sample. *Pain, 111*(1), 77–83.

Medco. (2011). *America's state of mind*. Medco Health Solutions, Inc. http://apps.who.int/medicinedocs/documents/s19032en/s19032en.pdf

Medved, J. (2015, February). 33 Mental health experts on Twitter you need to follow. Capterra Medical Software Blog. Retrieved from http://blog.capterra.com/33-mental-health-experts-on-twitter-you-need-to-follow//

Meltzoff, J., & Kornreich, M. (1970). *Research in psychotherapy*. New York: Atherton.

Mendlowicz, M. V., & Stein, M. B. (2014). Quality of life in individuals with anxiety disorders. *American Journal of Psychiatry, 157*, 669–682.

Merikangas, K. R., He, J. P., Burstein, M., Swendsen, J., Avenevoli, S., Case, B., . . . Olfson, M. (2011). Service utilization for lifetime mental disorders in US adolescents: Results of the National Comorbidity Survey—Adolescent Supplement (NCS-A). *Journal of the American Academy of Child &Adolescent Psychiatry, 50*(1), 32–45.

Merrill, K. A., Tolbert, V. E., & Wade, W. A. (2003). Effectiveness of cognitive therapy for depression in a community mental health center: A benchmarking study. *Journal of Consulting and Clinical Psychology, 71*(2), 404–409.

Metcalf, D., Milliard, S. T., Gomez, M., & Schwartz, M. (2016). Wearables and the Internet of Things for health: Wearable, interconnected devices promise more efficient and comprehensive health care. *IEEE Pulse, 7*(5), 35–39.

Meyer-Lindenberg, A., & Tost, H. (2012). Neural mechanisms of social risk for psychiatric disorders. *Nature Neuroscience, 15*, 663–668.

Michael, C. (2014). *Exorcism: A Christian manual*. Online: Amazon Digital Services, LLC.

Milner, A., Sveticic, J., & De Leo, D. (2013). Suicide in the absence of mental disorder? A review of psychological autopsy studies across countries. *International Journal of Social Psychiatry, 59*, 545–554.

Minami, T., Wampold, B. E., Serlin, R. C., Hamilton, E. G., Brown, G. S., & Kircher, J. C. (2008). Benchmarking the effectiveness of psychotherapy treatment for adult depression in a managed care environment: A preliminary study. *Journal of Consulting and Clinical Psychology, 76*, 116–124.

Miranda, J., Bernal, G., Lau, A. S., Kohn, L., Hwang, W. C., & LaFromboise, T. (2005). State of the science on psychosocial interventions for ethnic minorities. *Annual Review of Clinical Psychology, 1*, 113–142.

Mitchell, S., Brian, J., Zwaigenbaum, L., Roberts, W., Szatmari, P., Smith, I., & Bryson, S. (2006). Early language and communication development of infants later diagnosed with autism spectrum disorder. *Journal of Developmental & Behavioral Pediatrics, 27*(2), S69–S78.

Modinos, G., Mechelli, A., Pettersson-Yeo, W., Allen, P., McGuire, P., & Aleman, A. (2013). Pattern classification of brain activation during emotional processing in subclinical depression: Psychosis proneness as potential confounding factor. *PeerJ, 1*, e42.

Moffitt, T. E., Caspi, A., Taylor, A., Kokaua, J., Milne, B. J., Polanczyk, G., & Poulton, R. (2010). How common are common mental disorders? Evidence that lifetime prevalence rates are doubled by prospective versus retrospective ascertainment. *Psychological Medicine, 40*, 899–909.

Mohr, D. D. (2014). The IntelliCare Apps. Center for Behavioral Intervention Technologies,: Northwestern University. Retrieved from https://intellicare.cbits.northwestern.edu/

Mojtabai, R., Olfson, M., Sampson, N. A., Jin, R., Druss, B., Wang, P. S., . . . Kessler, R. C. (2011). Barriers to mental health treatment: Results from the National Comorbidity Survey Replication. *Psychological Medicine, 41*(08), 1751–1761.

Montreuil, B. (2011). Toward a physical internet: Meeting the global logistics sustainability grand challenge. *Logistics Research, 3*(2–3), 71–87.

Morris, G., Berk, M., Klein, H., Walder, K., Galecki, P., & Maes, M. (2016). Nitrosative stress, hypernitrosylation, and autoimmune responses to nitrosylated proteins: New pathways in neuroprogressive disorders including depression and chronic fatigue syndrome. *Molecular Neurobiology*, 1–21. Retrieved from http://link.springer.com/article/10.1007/s12035-016-9975-2

Morris, L. G. T., Veeriah, S., & Chan, T. A. (2010). Genetic determinants at the interface of cancer and neurodegenerative disease. *Oncogene, 29*(24), 3453–3464.

Morse, R. M., & Flavin, D. K. (1992, August 26). The definition of alcoholism. The Joint Committee of the National Council on Alcoholism and Drug Dependence and the American Society of Addiction Medicine to Study the Definition and Criteria for the Diagnosis of Alcoholism. *JAMA, 268*(8), 1012–1014.

Moyle, W., Cooke, M., Beattie, E., Jones, C., Klein, B., Cook, G., & Gray, C. (2013). Exploring the effect of companion robots on emotional expression in older adults with dementia: A pilot randomized controlled trial. *Journal of Gerontological Nursing, 39*(5), 46–53.

Mueller, A. S., Abrutyn, S., & Stockton, C. (2015). Can social ties be harmful? Examining the spread of suicide in early adulthood. *Sociological Perspectives, 58*(2), 204–222.

Mueller, C. (2014, December). Newtown receives $775K grant for mental health services. Connecticut Post. Retrieved from www.ctpost.com/local/article/Newtown-receives-775K-grant-for-mental-health-5954505.php

Mueller, D. P. (1980). Social networks: A promising direction for research on the relationship of the social environment to psychiatric disorder. *Social Science & Medicine. Part A: Medical Psychology & Medical Sociology, 14*(2), 147–161.

Muñoz, R. F., Bunge, E. L., Chen, K., Schueller, S. M., Bravin, J. I., Shaughnessy, E. A., & Pérez-Stable, E. J. (2016). Massive open online interventions a novel model for delivering behavioral-health services worldwide. *Clinical Psychological Science, 4*, 194–205.

Murphy, S., Irving, C. B., Adams, C. E., & Driver, R. (2012). Crisis intervention for people with severe mental illnesses. The Cochrane Library. *Cochrane Database Systematic Review, 5*, CD001087.

Murray, C. J., & Frenk, J. (2008). Health metrics and evaluation: Strengthening the science. *Lancet, 371*(9619), 1191–1199.

Murray, C. J., Abraham, J., Ali, M. K., Alvarado, M., Atkinson, C., Baddour, L. M., . . . Bolliger, I. (2013). The state of US health, 1990–2010: Burden of diseases, injuries, and risk factors. *JAMA, 310*(6), 591–606.

Murray, L. K., & Dorsey, S. (2013). *Common Elements Treatment Approach (CETA): Counselor manual* (Thailand version). Baltimore: Bloomberg School of Public Health, Johns Hopkins University.

Murray, L. K., Dorsey, S., Haroz, E., Lee, C., Alsiary, M. M., Haydary, A., . . . Bolton, P. (2014). A common elements treatment approach for adult mental health problems in low-and middle-income countries. *Cognitive and Behavioral Practice, 21*(2), 111–123.

Nadkarni, A., Weobong, B., Weiss, H. A., McCambridge, J., Bhat, B., Katti, B., . . . Patel, V. (2016). Counselling for Alcohol Problems (CAP), a lay counsellor-delivered brief psychological treatment for harmful drinking in men, in primary care in India: A randomised controlled trial. *Lancet, 389*(10065), 186–195.

Nakhleh, M. K., Amal, H., Jeries, R., Broza, Y. Y., Aboud, M., Gharra, A., . . . Glass-Marmor, L. (2016). Diagnosis and classification of 17 diseases from 1404 subjects via pattern analysis of exhaled molecules. *ACS Nano*. Retrieved from http://pubs.acs.org/doi/abs/10.1021/acsnano.6b04930

Nathan, P. E., & Gorman, J. M. (Eds.). (2015). *Treatments that work* (4th ed.). New York: Oxford University Press.

National Academies of Sciences, Engineering, and Medicine. (2016). *Hearing health care for adults: Priorities for improving access and affordability*. Washington, DC: National Academies Press.

National Academies of Sciences, Engineering, and Medicine. (2017). *Making eye health a population health imperative: Vision for tomorrow*. Washington, DC: National Academies Press.

National Center for Chronic Disease Prevention and Health Promotion. (2011). *Can lifestyle modifications using therapeutic lifestyle changes (TLC) reduce weight and the risk for chronic disease?* Retrieved from https://www.cdc.gov/nutrition/downloads/r2p_life_change.pdf

National Institute for Health and Care Excellence. (2009). *Depression: Treatment and management of depression in adults. Clinical guideline 90*. London: NICE.

National Institutes of Health, National Center for Complementary and Integrative Health. (2015, August). NIH analysis shows Americans are in pain. US Department of Health and Human Services. Retrieved from https://nccih.nih.gov/news/press/08112015

National Physical Activity Plan Alliance. (2016). *National physical activity plan*. Retrieved from http://physicalactivityplan.org/docs/2016NPAP_Finalforwebsite.pdf

Nelson, A. R., Smedley, B. D., & Stith, A. Y. (Eds.). (2002). *Unequal treatment: Confronting racial and ethnic disparities in health care*. Washington, DC: National Academies Press.

Nelson, T. D., & Steele, R. G. (2006). Beyond efficacy and effectiveness: A multifaceted approach to treatment evaluation. *Professional Psychology: Research and Practice, 37*(4), 389–397.

Nemeroff, C. B., & Goldschmidt-Clermont, P. J. (2012). Heartache and heartbreak: The link between depression and cardiovascular disease. *Nature Reviews Cardiology*, *9*(9), 526–539.

Neuner, F., Onyut, P. L., Ertl, V., Odenwald, M., Schauer, E., & Elbert, T. (2008). Treatment of posttraumatic stress disorder by trained lay counselors in an African refugee settlement: A randomized controlled trial. *Journal of Consulting and Clinical Psychology*, *76*(4), 686–694.

Newby, J. M., McKinnon, A., Kuyken, W., Gilbody, S., & Dalgleish, T. (2015). Systematic review and meta-analysis of transdiagnostic psychological treatments for anxiety and depressive disorders in adulthood. *Clinical Psychology Review*, *40*, 91–110.

Newman, F. L., & Howard, K. I. (1986). Therapeutic effort, treatment outcome, and national health policy. *American Psychologist*, *41*, 181–187.

Ng, M. Y., & Weisz, J. R. (2017). Personalizing evidence-based psychotherapy for children and adolescents in clinical care. In J. R. Weisz & A. E. Kazdin (Eds.), *Evidence-based psychotherapies for children and adolescents* (3rd ed.). New York: Guilford Publications.

Nguyen, H. (2014). Buddhism-based exorcism and spirit-calling as a form of healing for mental problems: Stories from Vietnam. *Journal of Religion & Spirituality in Social Work: Social Thought*, *33*(1), 33–48.

Noertjojo, K., Maberley, D., Bassett, K., & Courtright, P. (2006). Awareness of eye diseases and risk factors: Identifying needs for health education and promotion in Canada. *Canadian Journal of Ophthalmology/Journal Canadien d'Ophtalmologie*, *41*(5), 617–623.

Norcross, J. C. (1999). Collegially validated limitations of empirically validated treatments. *Clinical Psychology: Science and Practice*, *6*(4), 472–476.

Norcross, J. C., VandenBos, G. R., & Freedheim, D. K. (2011). *History of psychotherapy: Continuity and change*. Washington, DC: American Psychological Association.

Nordentoft, M., Wahlbeck, K., Hällgren, J., Westman, J., Osby, U., Alinaghizadeh, H., . . . Laursen, T. M. (2013). Excess mortality, causes of death and life expectancy in 270,770 patients with recent onset of mental disorders in Denmark, Finland and Sweden. *PLoS One*, *8*, e55176.

Nordt, C., Rössler, W., & Lauber, C. (2006). Attitudes of mental health professionals toward people with schizophrenia and major depression. *Schizophrenia Bulletin*, *32*(4), 709–714.

North American Quitline Consortium. (2016a). *A promising practices report. Quitlines and priority populations: An update on our progress to reach and serve those most impacted by tobacco's harm*. Phoenix, Arizona. Retrieved from http://c.ymcdn.com/sites/www.naquitline.org/resource/resmgr/links/QuitlinesandPriorityPopulati.pdf

North American Quitline Consortium. (2016b). *Quitline services: Current practice and evidence base, 2016*. Phoenix, Arizona. Retrieved from http://c.ymcdn.com/sites/www.naquitline.org/resource/resmgr/issue_papers/Quitline_Services_issue_pape.pdf

Norton, P. J. (2012). A randomized clinical trial of transdiagnostic cognitive-behavioral treatments for anxiety disorder by comparison to relaxation training. *Behavior Therapy*, *43*(3), 506–517.

Novins, D. K., Green, A. E., Legha, R. K., & Aarons, G. A. (2013). Dissemination and implementation of evidence-based practices for child and adolescent mental health: A systematic review. *Journal of the American Academy of Child & Adolescent Psychiatry, 52*(10), 1009–1025.

O'Donohue, W. T., & Cucciare, M. A. (2005). Pathways to Medi Cal service utilization. *Journal of Clinical Psychology in Medical Settings, 12*, 185–197.

O'Neil, A., Quirk, S. E., Housden, S., Brennan, S. L., Williams, L. J., Pasco, J. A., . . . Jacka, F. N. (2014). Relationship between diet and mental health in children and adolescents: A systematic review. *American Journal of Public Health, 104*(10), e31–e42.

Office of the Surgeon General. (2000). *Oral health in America: A report of the Surgeon General*. National Institute of Dental and Craniofacial Research and National Institutes of Health, Rockville, MD: USSDHHS. Retrieved from www.nidcr.nih.gov/DataStatistics/SurgeonGeneral/Documents/hck1ocv.@www.surgeon.fullrpt.pdf

Office of the Surgeon General. (2016). *Facing addiction in America: The Surgeon General's report on alcohol, drugs, and health*. Washington, DC: USSDHHS. Retrieved from http://addiction.surgeongeneral.gov

Office of the Surgeon General and National Action Alliance for Suicide Prevention. (2012). *National strategy for suicide prevention: Goals and objectives for action*. Washington, DC: USDHHS.

Olatunji, B. O., Cisler, J. M., & Deacon, B. J. (2010). Efficacy of cognitive behavioral therapy for anxiety disorders: A review of meta-analytic findings. *Psychiatric Clinics of North America, 33*(3), 557–577.

Olfson, M., Blanco, C., & Marcus, S. C. (2016). Treatment of adult depression in the United States. *JAMA Internal Medicine, 176*(10), 1482–1491.

Opriş, D., Pintea, S., García-Palacios, A., Botella, C., Szamosközi, Ş., & David, D. (2012). Virtual reality exposure therapy in anxiety disorders: A quantitative meta-analysis. *Depression and Anxiety, 29*(2), 85–93.

Orlinsky, D. E., RØnnestad, M. H., & Willutzki, U. (2004). Fifty years of psychotherapy process-outcome research: Continuity and change. In M. J. Lambert (Ed.), *Bergin and Garfield's handbook of psychotherapy and behavior change* (5th ed., pp. 307–389). New York: Wiley & Sons.

Otto, F. (2015). A "check-up from the neck up": Mental health screening kiosks at Drexel. Drexel Now (January 7, 2015). Retrieved from http://drexel.edu/now/archive/2015/January/Mental_Health_Screening_Kiosks/

Oudin, A., Bråbäck, L., Åström, D. O., Strömgren, M., & Forsberg, B. (2016). Association between neighbourhood air pollution concentrations and dispensed medication for psychiatric disorders in a large longitudinal cohort of Swedish children and adolescents. *BMJ Open, 6*(6), e010004.

Ougrin, D. (2011). Efficacy of exposure versus cognitive therapy in anxiety disorders: Systematic review and meta-analysis. *BMC Psychiatry, 11*(1), 1.

Padhy, S. K., Sarkar, S., Panigrahi, M., & Paul, S. (2015). Mental health effects of climate change. *Indian Journal of Occupational and Environmental Medicine, 19*(1), 3–7.

Pagliari, C., Burton, C., McKinstry, B., Szentatotai, A., David, D., Serrano-Blanco, A., . . . Wolters, M. K. (2012). Psychosocial implications of avatar use in supporting therapy for depression. *Annual Review of Cybertherapy and Telemedicine, 181*, 329–333.

Pallavicini, F., Algeri, D., Repetto, C., Gorini, A., & Giuseppe Riva, G. (2009). Biofeedback, virtual reality and mobile phones in the treatment of generalized anxiety disorder (GAD): A phase-2 controlled clinical trial. *Journal of Cyber Therapy and Rehabilitation, 2*, 315–327.

Palpacuer, C., Gallet, L., Drapier, D., Reymann, J. M., Falissard, B., & Naudet, F. (2017). Specific and non-specific effects of psychotherapeutic interventions for depression: Results from a meta-analysis of 84 studies. *Journal of Psychiatric Research, 87*, 95–104.

Paniagua, F. A., & Yamada, A. M. (Eds.). (2013). *Handbook of multicultural mental health: Assessment and treatment of diverse populations* (2nd ed.). San Diego, CA: Academic Press.

Parhami, I., Mojtabai, R., Rosenthal, R. J., Afifi, T. O., & Fong, T. W. (2014). Gambling and the onset of comorbid mental disorders: A longitudinal study evaluating severity and specific symptoms. *Journal of Psychiatric Practice, 20*(3), 207–219.

Patel, V., & Kleinman, A. (2003). Poverty and common mental disorders in developing countries. *Bulletin of the World Health Organization, 81*(8), 609–615.

Patel, V., Chowdhary, N., Rahman, A., & Verdeli, H. (2011). Improving access to psychological treatments: Lessons learned from developing countries. *Behaviour Research and Therapy, 49*, 523–528.

Patel, V., Weiss, H. A., Chowdhary, N., Naik, S., Pednekar, S., Chatterjee, S., . . . Kirkwood, B. R. (2010). Effectiveness of an intervention led by lay health counsellors for depressive and anxiety disorders in primary care in Goa, India (MANAS): A cluster randomised controlled trial. *Lancet, 376*, 2086–2095.

Patel, V., Weiss, H. A., Chowdhary, N., Naik, S., Pednekar, S., Chatterjee, S., . . . Kirkwood, B. R. (2011). Lay health worker led intervention for depressive and anxiety disorders in India: Impact on clinical and disability outcomes over 12 months. *British Journal of Psychiatry, 199*, 459–466.

Patel, V., Weobong, B., Weiss, H. A., Anand, A., Bhat, B., Katti, B., . . . Fairburn, C. G. (2016). The Healthy Activity Program (HAP). A lay counsellor-delivered brief psychological treatment for severe depression, in primary care in India: A randomised controlled trial. *Lancet, 389*(10065), 176–185.

PatientView. (2016). The myhealthapps directory 2015-2016 of health apps. London: PatientView. Retrieved from http://www.patient-view.com/

Patwardhan, A., Davis, J., Murphy, P., & Ryan, S. F. (2012). After-hours access of convenient care clinics and cost savings associated with avoidance of higher-cost sites of care. *Journal of Primary Care & Community Health, 3*(4), 243–245.

Peckham, C. (2016). *Medscape physician compensation report 2016*. Retrieved from www.medscape.com/features/slideshow/compensation/2016/public/overview

Pekarik, G., & Wolff, C. B. (1996). Relationship of satisfaction to symptom change, follow-up adjustment, and clinical significance. *Professional Psychology: Research and Practice, 27*, 202–208.

Pennebaker, J., Mehl, M., & Niederhoffer, K. (2003). Psychological aspects of natural language use: Our words, ourselves. *Annual Review of Psychology, 54*, 547–577.

Perry, Y., Petrie, K., Buckley, H., Cavanagh, L., Clarke, D., Winslade, M., . . . Christensen, H. (2014). Effects of a classroom-based educational resource on adolescent mental health literacy: A cluster randomised controlled trial. *Journal of Adolescence, 37*(7), 1143–1151.

Perry-Parrish, C., Copeland-Linder, N., Webb, L., Shields, A. H., & Sibinga, E. M. (2016). Improving self-regulation in adolescents: Current evidence for the role of mindfulness-based cognitive therapy. *Adolescent Health, Medicine and Therapeutics, 7*, 101–108.

Pescosolido, B. A. (2013). The public stigma of mental illness: What do we think; what do we know; what can we prove? *Journal of Health and Social Behavior, 54*(1), 1–21.

Pescosolido, B. A., Martin, J. K., Long, J. S., Medina, T. R., Phelan, J. C., & Link, B. G. (2010). "A disease like any other"? A decade of change in public reactions to schizophrenia, depression, and Kaplan, A. M., & Haenlein, M. (2010). Users of the world, unite! The challenges and opportunities of Social Media. *Business Horizons, 53*(1), 59–68.

Pew Research Center. (2015). Cell phones in Africa: Communication lifeline. Washington, DC: Pew Research Center. Retrieved from http://www.pewglobal.org/2015/04/15/cell-phones-in-africa-communication-lifeline/

Phelan, J. C. (2005). Geneticization of deviant behavior and consequences for stigma: The case of mental illness. *Journal of Health and Social Behavior, 46*(4), 307–322.

Piepoli, M. F., Hoes, A. W., Agewall, S., Albus, C., Brotons, C., Catapano, A. L., . . . Graham, I. (2016). 2016 European Guidelines on cardiovascular disease prevention in clinical practice. *European Heart Journal, 37*, 2315–2381.

Pine, D. S., Cohen, E., Cohen, P., & Brook, J. (1999). Adolescent depressive symptoms as predictors of adult depression: Moodiness or mood disorder? *American Journal of Psychiatry, 156*, 133–135.

Pitman, A., Osborn, D., King, M., & Erlangsen, A. (2014). Effects of suicide bereavement on mental health and suicide risk. *Lancet Psychiatry, 1*(1), 86–94.

Poirier, J., & Cobb, N. K. (2012). Social influence as a driver of engagement in a web-based health intervention. *Journal of Medical Internet Research, 14*(1).

Pompili, M., Sher, L., Serafini, G., Forte, A., Innamorati, M., Dominici, G., . . . Girardi, P. (2013). Posttraumatic stress disorder and suicide risk among veterans: A literature review. *Journal of Nervous and Mental Disease, 201*(9), 802–812.

Porto, P. R., Oliveira, L., Mari, J., Volchan, E., Figueira, I., & Ventura, P. (2009). Does cognitive behavioral therapy change the brain? A systematic review of neuroimaging in anxiety disorders. *Journal of Neuropsychiatry and Clinical Neurosciences, 21*, 114–125.

Poser, E. G. (1966). The effect of therapists' training on group therapeutic outcome. *Journal of Consulting Psychology, 30*(4), 283–289.

Poston, J. M., & Hanson, W. E. (2010). Meta-analysis of psychological assessment as a therapeutic intervention. *Psychological Assessment, 22*(2), 203–212.

Powell, L. M., Chriqui, J. F., Khan, T., Wada, R., & Chaloupka, F. J. (2013). Assessing the potential effectiveness of food and beverage taxes and subsidies for improving public health: A systematic review of prices, demand and body weight outcomes. *Obesity Reviews, 14*(2), 110–128.

Prange, G. B., Jannink, M. J., Groothuis-Oudshoorn, C. G., Hermens, H. J., & IJzerman, M. J. (2006). Systematic review of the effect of robot-aided therapy on recovery of the hemiparetic arm after stroke. *Journal of Rehabilitation Research and Development, 43*, 171–183.

Pratt, K. (2012). A constructive critique of public health arguments for anti-obesity soda Taxes and Food taxes. *Tulane Law Review, 87*(73), Loyola-LA Legal Studies Paper No. 2012–44. Retrieved from http://ssrn.com/abstract=2171493

Pratt, S. R. (2010). Barriers to hearing health care: Current status and a glimpse at the future. *American Journal of Audiology, 19*(1), 1–2.

Predny, M. L., & Relf, D. (2004). Horticulture therapy activities for preschool children, elderly adults, and intergenerational groups. *Activities, Adaptation & Aging, 28*(3), 1–18.

Preschl, B., Maercker, A., & Wagner, B. (2011). The working alliance in a randomized controlled trial comparing online with face-to-face cognitive-behavioral therapy for depression. *BMC Psychiatry*, *11*(1), 189. Retrieved from https://bmcpsychiatry.biomedcentral.com/articles/10.1186/1471-244X-11-189

President's New Freedom Commission on Mental Health. (2003). *Achieving the promise: Transforming mental health care in America*. Washington, DC: White House.

Press, W. H. (2015, April 30). Scientists must communicate both of science's "story lines." The William B. Carey Lecture Presented at the 40th annual AAAS Forum on Science and Technology Policy, Washington, DC. Retrieved from www.aaas.org/news/william-press-scientists-must-communicate-both-science-s-story-lines

Price, M., Yuen, E. K., Goetter, E. M., Herbert, J. D., Forman, E. M., Acierno, R., & Ruggiero, K. J. (2014). mHealth: A mechanism to deliver more accessible, more effective mental health care. *Clinical Psychology & Psychotherapy*, *21*(5), 427–436.

Prince, M., Patel, V., Saxena, S., Maj, M., Maselko, J., Phillips, M. R., & Rahman, A. (2007). No health without mental health. *Lancet*, *370*, 859–877.

Proctor, E. K., Landsverk, J., Aarons, G., Chambers, D., Glisson, C., & Mittman, B. (2009). Implementation research in mental health services: An emerging science with conceptual, methodological, and training challenges. *Administration and Policy in Mental Health and Mental Health Services Research*, *36*(1), 24–34.

Quidé, Y., Witteveen, A. B., El-Hage, W., Veltman, D. J., & Olff, M. (2012). Differences between effects of psychological versus pharmacological treatments on functional and morphological brain alterations in anxiety disorders and major depressive disorder: A systematic review. *Neuroscience and Biobehavioral Reviews*, *36*, 626–644.

Rabbitt, S. M., Kazdin, A. E., & Hong, J. H. (2015). Acceptability of robot-assisted therapy for disruptive behavior problems in children. *Archives of Scientific Psychology*, *3*, 101–110.

Rabbitt, S. M., Kazdin, A. E., & Scassellati, B. (2015). Integrating socially assistive robotics into mental healthcare interventions: Applications and recommendations for expanded use. *Clinical Psychology Review*, *35*, 35–46.

Rahman, A., Hamdani, S. U., Awan, N. R., Bryant, R. A., Dawson, K. S., Khan, M. F., . . . van Ommeren M. (2016). Effect of a multicomponent behavioral intervention in adults impaired by psychological distress in a conflict-affected area of Pakistan: A randomized clinical trial. *JAMA*, *316*, 2609–2617.

Rahman, A., Malik, A., Sikander, S., Roberts, C., & Creed, F. (2008). Cognitive behaviour therapy–based intervention by community health workers for mothers with depression and their infants in rural Pakistan: A cluster-randomised controlled trial. *Lancet*, *372*, 902–909.

Ramanathan, V., & Feng, Y. (2009). Air pollution, greenhouse gases and climate change: Global and regional perspectives. *Atmospheric Environment*, *43*(1), 37–50.

Ranck, J. (2012). The wearable computing market: A global analysis. *Gigaom Pro*. Retrieved from http://static1.squarespace.com/static/516c369de4b00b44ca2bcdce/t/527fee38e4b0217581602d6e/1384115768724/wearable-computing-the-next-big-thing-in-tech.pdf

Ratnayake, U., Quinn, T., Walker, D., & Dickinson, H. (2013). Cytokines and the neurodevelopmental basis of mental illness. *Frontiers in Neuroscience*, *7*, 180. Retrieved from http://journal.frontiersin.org/article/10.3389/fnins.2013.00180/full

Ray, L. B., & Travis, J. (2016). On the clock. Special Section on Sleep. *Science*, *354*(6315), 987–1015.

Reavley, N. J., Mackinnon, A. J., Morgan, A. J., & Jorm, A. F. (2014). Stigmatising attitudes towards people with mental disorders: A comparison of Australian health professionals with the general community. *Australian and New Zealand Journal of Psychiatry, 48*, 433–441.

Reavley, N. J., McCann, T. V., Cvetkovski, S., & Jorm, A. F. (2014). A multifaceted intervention to improve mental health literacy in students of a multicampus university: A cluster randomised trial. *Social Psychiatry and Psychiatric Epidemiology, 49*(10), 1655–1666.

Reeves, W. C., Strine, T. W., Pratt, L. A., Thompson, W., Ahluwalia, I., Dhingra, S. S., . . . Morrow, B. (2011). Mental illness surveillance among adults in the United States. *Morbidity and Mortality Weekly Report, Surveillance Summit, 60*(Suppl 3), 1–29.

RelaxLine. (2010). *Bellybio interactive breathing*. Retrieved from http://itunes.apple.com/us/app/bellybio-interactive-breathing/id353763955?mt=8

Rice, V. H., & Stead, L. F. (2008) Nursing interventions for smoking cessation. *Cochrane Database of Systematic Reviews*, (1), CD001188.

Richards, D., & Richardson, T. (2012). Computer-based psychological treatments for depression: A systematic review and meta-analysis. *Clinical Psychology Review, 32*(4), 329–342.

Rimer, J., Dwan, K., Lawlor, D. A., Greig, C. A., McMurdo, M., Morley, W., & Mead, G. E. (2012, July 11). Exercise for depression. *Cochrane Database of Systematic Reviews, 7*.

Riper, H., & Cuijpers, P. J. (2016). Telepsychology and eHealth. In J. C. Norcross, G. R. VandenBos, D. K. Freedheim, & R. Krishnamurthy (Eds.) *APA handbook of clinical psychology: Applications and methods* (Vol. 3, pp. 451–463). Washington, DC: American Psychological Association.

Rippentrop, A. E., Altmaier, E. M., Chen, J. J., Found, E. M., & Keffala, V. J. (2005). The relationship between religion/spirituality and physical health, mental health, and pain in a chronic pain population. *Pain, 116*(3), 311–321.

Rittel, H. W. J., & Webber, M. M. (1973). Dilemmas in a general theory of planning. *Policy Sciences, 4*, 155–169.

Riva, G. (2005). Virtual reality in psychotherapy: Review. *Cyberpsychology and Behavior, 8*, 220–240.

Rivard, J. C., & Butler, A. S. (2017). *Lessons learned from diverse efforts to change social norms and opportunities and strategies to promote behavior change in behavioral health: Proceedings of two workshops*. Washington, DC: The National Academies Press.

Rizzo, A., Difede, J., Rothbaum, B. O., Reger, G., Spitalnick, J., Cukor, J., & Mclay, R. (2010). Development and early evaluation of the virtual Iraq/Afghanistan exposure therapy system for combat-related PTSD. *Annals of the New York Academy of Sciences, 1208*, 114–125.

Robinson, A. (2015, September). Meet Ellie, the machine that can detect depression. *The Guardian*, September 17, 2015. Retrieved from www.theguardian.com/sustainable-business/2015/sep/17/ellie-machine-that-can-detect-depression

Robinson, H., MacDonald, B., Kerse, N., & Broadbent, E. (2013). The psychosocial effects of a companion robot: A randomized controlled trial. *Journal of the American Medical Directors Association, 14*, 661–667.

Robst, J., & Weinberg, C. (2010). Childhood behavioral problems and dropping out of school. *Eastern Economic Journal, 36*(4), 523–538.

Rockett, I. R., & Caine, E. D. (2015). Self-injury is the eighth leading cause of death in the United States: It is time to pay attention. *JAMA Psychiatry, 72*(11), 1069–1070.

Rodríguez, M. R., Nuevo, R., Chatterji, S., & Ayuso-Mateos, J. L. (2012). Definitions and factors associated with subthreshold depressive conditions: A systematic review. *BMC Psychiatry, 12*(1), 181. Retrieved from www.biomedcentral.com/1471-244X/12/181

Roffman, J. L., Marci, C. M., Glick, D. M., Dougherty, D. D., &. Rauch, S. L. (2005). Neuroimaging and the functional neuroanatomy of psychotherapy. *Psychological Medicine, 35*, 1385–1398.

Rogers, C. R., & Dymond, R. F. (Ed.) (1954). *Psychotherapy and personality change.* Chicago, IL: University of Chicago Press.

Rogers, E. M. (2003). *Diffusion of innovations* (5th ed.). New York: Free Press.

Rogers, E. S., & Swarbrick, M. (2016). Editorial (Introduction to a Special Series). Peer-delivered services: Current trends and innovations. *Psychiatric Rehabilitation Journal, 39*(3), 193–196.

Roine, R., Ohinmaa, A., & Hailey, D. (2001). Assessing telemedicine: A systematic review of the literature. *Canadian Medical Association Journal, 165*, 765–771.

Roman, P. M., & Blum, T. C. (1996). Alcohol: A review of the impact of worksite interventions on health and behavioral outcomes. *American Journal of Health Promotion, 11*, 136–149.

Rones, M., & Hoagwood, K. (2000). School-based mental health services: A research review. *Clinical Child and Family Psychology Review, 4*, 223–241.

Rosenbaum, S., Tiedemann, A., Sherrington, C., Curtis, J., & Ward, P. B. (2014). Physical activity interventions for people with mental illness: A systematic review and meta-analysis. *Journal of Clinical Psychiatry, 75*(9), 964–974.

Rosenquist, J. N., Fowler, J. H., & Christakis, N. A. (2011). Social network determinants of depression. *Molecular Psychiatry, 16*(3), 273–281.

Rosenzweig, S. (1936). Some implicit common factors in diverse methods of psychotherapy. *American Journal of Orthopsychiatry, 6*(3), 412–415.

Rotaru, T. Ş., & Rusu, A. (2016). A meta-analysis for the efficacy of hypnotherapy in alleviating PTSD symptoms. *International Journal of Clinical and Experimental Hypnosis, 64*(1), 116–136.

Rotheram-Borus, M. J., Swendeman, D., & Chorpita, B. F. (2012). Disruptive innovations for designing and diffusing evidence-based interventions. *American Psychologist, 67*(6), 463–476.

Rothman, A. J., & Salovey, P. (1997). Shaping perceptions to motivate healthy behavior: The role of message framing. *Psychological Bulletin, 121*(1), 3–19.

Rousseau, C. (2017). Illinois law enlists hairstylists to prevent domestic abuse. Associated Press, January 1, 2017. Retrieved from www.yahoo.com/news/illinois-law-enlists-hairstylists-prevent-domestic-abuse-142846982.html

Rubenstein, E. A., & Parloff, M. B. (Eds.). (1962). *Research in psychotherapy* (Vol. I). Washington, DC: American Psychological Association.

Rucklidge, J. J., & Kaplan, B. J. (2013). Broad-spectrum micronutrient formulas for the treatment of psychiatric symptoms: A systematic review. *Expert Review of Neurotherapeutics, 13*(1), 49–73.

Rudd, R. A., Paulozzi, L. J., Bauer, M. J., Burleson, R. W., Carlson, R. E., Dao, D., . . . Fondario, A. (2014). Increases in heroin overdose deaths—28 States, 2010 to 2012. *Morbidity and Mortality Weekly Report, 63*(39), 849–854.

Rural Education Action Project. (2012). *Best buy tool kit for health.* Retrieved from http://reap.stanford.edu/research/best_buy_toolkit_for_health

Rutledge, T., & Loh, C. (2004). Effect sizes and statistical testing in the determination of clinical significance in behavioral medicine research. *Annals of Behavioral Medicine, 27*(2), 138–145.

Ryder, D. (1988). Minimal intervention: A little quality for a lot of quantity. *Behaviour Change, 5*, 100–107.

Sabry, W. M., & Vohra, A. (2013). Role of Islam in the management of psychiatric disorders. *Indian Journal of Psychiatry, 55*(Suppl 2), S205.

Sacher, D. (2000). Eliminating global health disparities. *JAMA, 284*(22), 2864.

Sachs, S. (2016, May). *BACtrack® wins Wearable Alcohol Biosensor Challenge.* Issued through National Institutes of Health (NIH). Retrieved from www.bactrack.com/pages/bactrack-skyn-wearable-alcohol-monitor

Sadler, G., Thomas, A. G., Gebrekristos, B., Dhanjal, S. K., & Mugo, J. (2000). Black cosmetologists promoting health program: Pilot study outcomes. *Journal of Cancer Education, 15*, 33–37.

Salter, A. (1952). *The case against psychoanalysis.* New York: Holt.

Sattler, K. M., & Deane, F. P. (2016). Hairdressers' preparedness to be informal helpers for their clients. *Journal of Community Psychology, 44*(6), 687–694.

Scharf, D. M., Eberhart, N. K., Schmidt, N., Vaughan, C. A., Dutta, T., Pincus, H. A., & Burnam, M. A. (2013). Integrating primary care into community behavioral health settings: Programs and early implementation experiences. *Psychiatric Services, 64*(7), 660–665.

Schinka, K. C., van Dulmen, M. H., Mata, A. D., Bossarte, R., & Swahn, M. (2013). Psychosocial predictors and outcomes of loneliness trajectories from childhood to early adolescence. *Journal of Adolescence, 36*(6), 1251–1260.

Schmidt, C. W. (2012). Trending now: Using social media to predict and track disease outbreaks. *Environmental Health Perspectives, 120*, a30–a33.

Schnittker, J. (2008). An uncertain revolution: Why the rise of a genetic model of mental illness has not increased tolerance. *Social Science & Medicine, 67*(9), 1370–1381.

Schoenwald, S. K., & Hoagwood, K. (2001). Effectiveness, transportability, and dissemination of interventions: What matters when? *Psychiatric Services, 52*(9), 1190–1197.

Schultz, P. W., Nolan, J. M., Cialdini, R. B., Goldstein, N. J., & Griskevicius, V. (2007). The constructive, destructive, and reconstructive power of social norms. *Psychological Science, 18*(5), 429–434.

Scott, A. J., Webb, T. L., & Rowse, G. (2015). Self-help interventions for psychosis: A meta-analysis. *Clinical Psychology Review, 39*, 96–112.

Scott, K. M., Lim, C., Al-Hamzawi, A., Alonso, J., Bruffaerts, R., Caldas-de-Almeida, J. M., . . . Kawakami, N. (2016). Association of mental disorders with subsequent chronic physical conditions: World mental health surveys from 17 countries. *JAMA Psychiatry, 73*(2), 150–158.

Scull, A. (2015). *Madness in civilization: A cultural history of insanity, from the Bible to Freud, from the madhouse to modern medicine.* Princeton, NJ: Princeton University Press.

Sechrest, L., White, S. O., & Brown, E. D. (1979). *The rehabilitation of criminal offenders: Problems and prospects.* Washington, DC: National Academy of Sciences.

Segerstrom, S. C., & Miller, G. E. (2004). Psychological stress and the human immune system: A meta-analytic study of 30 years of inquiry. *Psychological Bulletin, 130*(4), 601–630.

Sen, S., Duman, R., & Sanacora, G. (2008). Serum brain-derived neurotrophic factor, depression, and antidepressant medications: Meta-analyses and implications. *Biological Psychiatry, 64*, 527–532.

Sentissi, O., Bartolomei, J., Moeglin, C., Baeriswyl-Cottin, R., & Philippe, R. (2014). The Geneva Model of crisis intervention: A retrospective study. *Journal of Psychology & Psychotherapy, 4*(4), 1–7.

Shalev, I., Moffitt, T. E., Sugden, K., Williams, B., Houts, R. M., Danese, A., . . . Caspi, A. (2013). Exposure to violence during childhood is associated with telomere erosion from 5 to 10 years of age: A longitudinal study. *Molecular Psychiatry, 18*(5), 576–581.

Shannahan, R., & Fields, S. (2016). Services in support of community living for youth with serious behavioral health challenges: Mobile crisis response and stabilization services. Prepared for the National Technical Assistance Network for Children's Behavioral Health. Retrieved from www.cbhda.org/wp-content/uploads/2014/12/SAMHSA_Brief_Services_in_Support_of_Comm._Living_May2016_5-31-16.pdf

Shapiro, A. K., & Morris, L. A. (1978). The placebo effect in medical and psychological therapies. In S. L. Garfield & A. E. Bergin (Eds.), *Handbook of psychotherapy and behavior change: An empirical analysis* (2nd ed., pp. 369–409). New York: John Wiley & Sons.

Sharan, P., Gallo, C., Gureje, O., Lamberte, E., Mari, J. J., Mazzotti, G., . . . Saxena, S. (2009). Mental health research priorities in low- and middle-income countries of Africa, Asia, Latin America and the Caribbean. *British Journal of Psychiatry, 195*, 354–363.

Sharpe, M., Walker, J., Hansen, C. H., Martin, P., Symeonides, S., Gourley, C., . . . Murray, G. (2014). Integrated collaborative care for comorbid major depression in patients with cancer (SMaRT Oncology-2): A multicentre randomised controlled effectiveness trial. *Lancet, 384*(9948), 1099–1108.

Sheehan, D. V. (1983). *The anxiety disease*. New York: Charles Scribner and Sons.

Sheehan, K. H., & Sheehan, D. V. (2008). Assessing treatment effects in clinical trials with the discan metric of the Sheehan Disability Scale. *International Clinical Psychopharmacology, 23*(2), 70–83.

Shibata, T. (2012). Therapeutic seal robot as biofeedback medical device: Qualitative and quantitative evaluations of robot therapy in dementia care. *Proceedings of the IEEE, 100*, 2527–2538.

Shibata, T., & Wada, K. (2010). Robot therapy: A new approach for mental health care of the elderly: A mini-review. *Gerontology, 57*, 378–386.

Shih, M., Yang, Y. H., & Koo, M. (2009). A meta-analysis of hypnosis in the treatment of depressive symptoms: A brief communication. *International Journal of Clinical and Experimental Hypnosis, 57*(4), 431–442.

Shirayama, Y., Andrew, C. H., Chen, S. N., Russell, D. S., & Duman, R. S. (2002). Brain-derived neurotrophic factor produces antidepressant effects in behavioral models of depression. *Journal of Neuroscience, 2*, 3251–3261.

Shiue, I. (2015). Neighborhood epidemiological monitoring and adult mental health: European Quality of Life Survey, 2007–2012. *Environmental Science and Pollution Research, 22*(8), 6095–6103.

Shlien, J. M. (Ed.). (1968). *Research in psychotherapy* (Vol. III). Washington DC: American Psychological Association.

Shoham-Salomon, V., & Rosenthal, R. (1987). Paradoxical interventions: A meta-analysis. *Journal of Consulting and Clinical Psychology, 55*(1), 22–28.

Sidhu, K., Vandana, P., & Balon, R. (2009). Exercise prescription: A practical effective therapy for depression. *Current Psychiatry, 8*, 39–51.

Signorini, A., Segre, A. M., & Polgreen, P. M. (2011). The use of Twitter to track levels of disease activity and public concern in the U.S. during the influenza A H1N1 pandemic. *PLoS ONE, 6*, e19467.

Silverman, W. K., & Hinshaw, S. P. (Eds.) (2008). Evidence-based psychosocial treatments for children and adolescents: A ten year update [Special Issue]. *Journal of Clinical Child & Adolescent Psychology, 37*, 1–301.

Singh, M. (2014, March). Therapists' apps aim to help with mental health issues. Spot: Medical News from NPR. Retrieved from www.npr.org/blogs/health/2014/03/26/294374936/therapists-apps-aim-to-help-with-mental-health-issues

Singhal, A., Cody, M. J., Rogers, E. M., & Sabido, M. (Eds.). (2004). *Entertainment-education and social change: History, research, and practice*. Mahwah, NJ: Lawrence Erlbaum Associates.

Singhal, A., & Rogers, E. M. (1999). *Entertainment-education: A communication strategy for social change*. Mahwah, NJ: Erlbaum.

Singla, D. R., Kohrt, B., Murray, L. K., Anand, A., Chorpita, B. F., & Patel, V. (2017). Psychological treatments for the world: Lessons from low-and middle-income countries. *Annual Review of Clinical Psychology, 13*(1), 149–181.

Sisti, D. A., Segal, A. G., & Emanuel, E. J. (2015). Improving long-term psychiatric care: Bring back the asylum. *JAMA, 313*(3), 243–244.

Smedley, B. D., Stith, A. Y., & Nelson, A. R. (2003). *Unequal treatment: Confronting racial and ethnic disparities in health care.* Institute of Medicine. Washington DC: National Academies Press.

Smit, Y., Huibers, M. J., Ioannidis, J. P., van Dyck, R., van Tilburg, W., & Arntz, A. (2012). The effectiveness of long-term psychoanalytic psychotherapy: A meta-analysis of randomized controlled trials. *Clinical Psychology Review, 32*(2), 81–92.

Smith, H., Sawyer, D. A., & Way, B. B. (2002). Central New York psychiatric center: An approach to the treatment of co-occurring disorders in the New York State correctional mental health system. *Behavioral Sciences and the Law, 20*, 523–534.

Smith, M. L., & Glass, G. V. (1977). Meta-analysis of psychotherapy outcome studies. *American Psychologist, 32*, 752–760.

Smith, M. L., Glass, G. V., & Miller, T. I. (1980). *The benefits of psychotherapy*. Baltimore, MD: Johns Hopkins University Press.

Smith, P. H., Mazure, C. M., & McKee, S. A. (2014). Smoking and mental illness in the US population. *Tobacco Control, 23*(e2), e147–e153.

Smith, T. B., Bartz, J., & Richards, P. S. (2007). Outcomes of religious and spiritual adaptations to psychotherapy: A meta-analytic review. *Psychotherapy Research, 17*(6), 643–655.

Smoller, J. W., Craddock, N., Kendler, K., Lee, P. H., Neale, B. M., Nurnberger, J. I., . . . Sullivan, P. F. (2013). Identification of risk loci with shared effects on five major psychiatric disorders: A genome-wide analysis. *Lancet, 381*, 1371–1379.

Snyder, D. K., & Halford, W. K. (2012). Evidence-based couple therapy: Current status and future directions. *Journal of Family Therapy, 34*(3), 229–249.

Snyder, L. B., Hamilton, M. A., Mitchell, E. W., Kiwanuka-Tondo, J., Fleming-Milici, F., & Proctor, D. (2004). A meta-analysis of the effect of mediated health communication campaigns on behavior change in the United States. *Journal of Health Communication*, 9(S1), 71–96.

Social Security Administration. (2011). *Annual Performance plan for fiscal year 2012*. US Government. Retrieved from https://www.ssa.gov/performance/2012/APP%20 2012%20508%20PDF.pdf

Society of Clinical Psychology, American Psychological Association. (2013). Psychological treatments. Retrieved from www.div12.org/psychological-treatments/ treatments/

Sokhom, B., Okpo, E., Tonna, I., & Poobalan, A. (2015). does quality of care differ when HIV patients are treated by non-specialist and specialist HIV healthcare providers in developed countries? A systematic narrative review. *World Journal of AIDS*, *5*(03), 161–174.

Solomon, F. M., Linnan, L. A., Wasilewski, Y., Lee, A. M., Katz, M. L., & Yang, J. (2004). Observational study of ten beauty salons: Results informing development of the North Carolina BEAUTY and Health Project. *Health Education and Behavior*, *31*, 790–807.

Soni, A. (2015a, April). *Trends in the five most costly conditions among the U.S. civilian noninstitutionalized populations, 2002 and 2012*. Statistical Brief #470. Agency for Healthcare Research and Quality, Rockville, MD. Available at https://meps.ahrq.gov/ data_files/publications/st470/stat470.shtml

Soni, A. (2015b, April). *Top five most costly conditions among children, ages 0-17, 2012. Estimates for the U.S. civilian noninstitutionalized populations*. Statistical Brief #472. Agency for Healthcare Research and Quality, Rockville, MD. Available at https:// meps.ahrq.gov/data_files/publications/st472/stat472.shtml

Sorenson, R. L., Gorsuch, R. L., & Mintz, J. (1985). Moving targets: Patients' changing complaints during psychotherapy. *Journal of Consulting and Clinical Psychology*, *53*, 49–54.

Spek, V., Cuijpers, P. I. M., Nyklícek, I., Riper, H., Keyzer, J., & Pop, V. (2007). Internet-based cognitive behaviour therapy for symptoms of depression and anxiety: A meta-analysis. *Psychological Medicine*, *37*, 319–328.

Spielmans, G. I., Gatlin, E. T., & McFall, J. P. (2010). The efficacy of evidence-based psychotherapies versus usual care for youths: Controlling confounds in a meta-reanalysis. *Psychotherapy Research*, *20*(2), 234–246.

Standley, J. M. (2002). A meta-analysis of the efficacy of music therapy for premature infants. *Journal of Pediatric Nursing*, *17*(2), 107–113.

Stankovic, J. A. (2014). Research directions for the internet of things. *IEEE Internet of Things Journal*, *1*(1), 3–9.

Stanley, M. A., Wilson, N. L., Amspoker, A. B., Kraus-Schuman, C., Wagener, P. D., Calleo, J. S., . . . Masozera, N. (2014). Lay providers can deliver effective cognitive behavior therapy for older adults with generalized anxiety disorder: A randomized trial. *Depression and Anxiety*, *31*(5), 391–401.

Stanton, C. A., Moadel, A. B., Kim, R. S., Weinberger, A. H., & Shuter, J. (2015). Loneliness in HIV-infected smokers. *AIDS Care*, *27*(2), 268–272.

Starfield, B. (1992). *Primary care: Concept, evaluation, and policy*. New York: Oxford University Press.

Statistics Portal. (2016). *Statistics and facts about social networks*. Retrieved from www.statista.com/topics/1164/social-networks/

Staufenbiel, S. M., Penninx, B. W., Spijker, A. T., Elzinga, B. M., & van Rossum, E. F. (2013). Hair cortisol, stress exposure, and mental health in humans: A systematic review. *Psychoneuroendocrinology, 38*(8), 1220–1235.

Stead, L. F., Bergson, G., & Lancaster, T. (2008). Physician advice for smoking cessation. *Cochrane Database of Systematic Reviews*, CD000165.

Steel, Z., Chey, T., Silove, D., Marnane, C., Bryant, R. A., & Van Ommeren, M. (2009). Association of torture and other potentially traumatic events with mental health outcomes among populations exposed to mass conflict and displacement: A systematic review and meta-analysis. *JAMA, 302*(5), 537–549.

Steel, Z., Marnane, C., Iranpour, C., Chey, T., Jackson, J. W., Patel, V., & Silove, D. (2014). The global prevalence of common mental disorders: A systematic review and meta-analysis 1980–2013. *International Journal of Epidemiology, 43*(2), 476–493.

Steptoe, A. (Ed.). (2007). *Depression and physical illness*. Cambridge, UK: Cambridge University Press.

Stewart, M. O., Karlin, B. E., Murphy, J. L., Raffa, S. D., Miller, S. A., McKellar, J., & Kerns, R. D. (2015). National dissemination of cognitive-behavioral therapy for chronic pain in Veterans: Therapist and patient-level outcomes. *Clinical Journal of Pain, 31*(8), 722–729.

Stravynski, A., & Boyer, R. (2001). Loneliness in relation to suicide ideation and parasuicide: A population-wide study. *Suicide and Life-Threatening Behavior, 31*(1), 32–40.

StressEraser. (2012). *Portable biofeedback device*. Retrieved from http://stresseraser.com/

Strine, T. W., Mokdad, A. H., Balluz, L. S., Gonzalez, O., Crider, R., Berry, J. T., & Kroenke, K. (2015). Depression and anxiety in the United States: Findings from the 2006 behavioral risk factor surveillance system. *Psychiatric Services, 59*(12), 1383–1390.

Ströhle, A. (2009). Physical activity, exercise, depression and anxiety disorders. *Journal of Neural Transmission, 116*, 777–784.

Stuart, H., Arboleda-Flórez, J., & Santorius, N. (2012). *Paradigms lost: Fighting stigma and the lessons learned*. New York: Oxford University Press.

Substance Abuse and Mental Health Services Administration. (2012). *SAMHSA's working definition of recovery: 10 guiding principles*. Rockville, MD: SAMHSA.

Substance Abuse and Mental Health Services Administration. (2013). *Report to Congress on the nation's substance abuse and mental health workforce issues*. Rockville, MD: SAMHSA. Retrieved from https://store.samhsa.gov/shin/content/PEP13-RTC-BHWORK/PEP13-RTC-BHWORK.pdf

Substance Abuse and Mental Health Services Administration. (2016). *SAMHSA's suicide prevention efforts*. Rockville, MD: SAMHSA. Retrieved from www.samhsa.gov/suicide-prevention/samhsas-efforts.

Substance Abuse and Mental Health Services. (2017a). Center for Integrated Health Solutions. Rockville, MD: SAMHSA. Retrieved from www.integration.samhsa.gov/about-us/what-is-integrated-care

Substance Abuse and Mental Health Services Administration. (2017b). *National registry of evidence-based programs and practices*. Rockville, MD: SAMHSA. Retrieved from http://nrepp.samhsa.gov/01_landing.aspx

Sun, S., Pan, W., & Wang, L. L. (2010). A comprehensive review of effect size reporting and interpreting practices in academic journals in education and psychology. *Journal of Educational Psychology, 102*(4), 989–1004.

Sundström, G., Fransson, E., Malmberg, B., & Davey, A. (2009). Loneliness among older Europeans. *European Journal of Ageing*, *6*(4), 267–275.

Suppli, N. F. P., Johansen, C., Kessing, L. V., Nielsen, A. T., Kroman, N. T., Ewertz, M., & Dalton, S. (2016). Survival after early-stage breast cancer of women previously treated for depression: A nationwide Danish cohort study. *Journal of Clinical Oncology*. Retrieved from http://ascopubs.org/doi/abs/10.1200/JCO.2016.68.8358

Swarbrick, M., Tunner, T. P., Miller, D. W., Werner, P., & Tiegreen, W. W. (2016). Promoting health and wellness through peer-delivered services: Three innovative state examples. *Psychiatric Rehabilitation Journal*, *39*(3), 204–210.

Sweeney, A. M., & Moyer, A. (2015). Self-affirmation and responses to health messages: A meta-analysis on intentions and behavior. *Health Psychology*, *34*(2), 149–159.

Szasz, T. (1972). Bad habits are not diseases: A refutation of the claim that alcoholism is a disease. *Lancet*, *300*(7767), 83–84.

Tanenbaum, S. J. (2005). Evidence-based practice as mental health policy: Three controversies and a caveat. *Health Affairs*, *24*(1), 163–173.

Tay, L., Tan, K., Diener, E., & Gonzalez, E. (2013). Social relations, health behaviors, and health outcomes: A survey and synthesis. *Applied Psychology: Health and Well-Being*, *5*(1), 28–78.

Taylor, E. M., Yanni, E. A., Pezzi, C., Guterbock, M., Rothney, E., Harton, E., . . . Burke, H. (2014). Physical and mental health status of Iraqi refugees resettled in the United States. *Journal of Immigrant and Minority Health*, *16*(6), 1130–1137.

Telecare Corporation. (2015). Mental Health Urgent Care Center, Long Beach, CA. Retrieved from http://www.telecarecorp.com/mental-health-urgent-care-center/

ten Have, M., de Graaf, R., Ormel, J., Vilagut, G., Kovess, V., Alonso, J., & ESEMeD/MHEDEA 2000 Investigators. (2010). Are attitudes towards mental health help-seeking associated with service use? Results from the European Study of Epidemiology of Mental Disorders. *Social Psychiatry and Psychiatric Epidemiology*, *45*(2), 153–163.

Thakur, M., Dofe, R., & Jadhav, S. (2014). Flexible electronic skin. *International Journal of Current Engineering and Technology*, *4*(6), 4041–4046.

Thaler, R. H., & Sunstein, C. R. (2008). *Nudge: Improving decisions about health, wealth, and happiness*. New Haven, CT: Yale University Press.

Thompson, A., Issakidis, C., & Hunt, C. (2008). Delay to seek treatment for anxiety and mood disorders in an Australian clinical sample. *Behaviour Change*, *25*, 71–84.

Thornicroft, G. (2011). Physical health disparities and mental illness: The scandal of premature mortality. *British Journal of Psychiatry*, *199*(6), 441–442.

Thow, A. M., Downs, S., & Jan, S. (2014). A systematic review of the effectiveness of food taxes and subsidies to improve diets: Understanding the recent evidence. *Nutrition Reviews*, *72*(9), 551–565.

Titov, N., Dear, B. F., Staples, L. G., Bennett-Levy, J., Klein, B., Rapee, R. M., . . . Purtell, C. (2015). MindSpot clinic: An accessible, efficient, and effective online treatment service for anxiety and depression. *Psychiatric Services*, *66*(10), 1043–1050.

Tkachuk, G. A., & Martin, G. L. (1999). Exercise therapy for patients with psychiatric disorders: Research and clinical implications. *Professional Psychology: Research and Practice*, *30*, 275–282.

Tolin, D. F. (2010). Is cognitive-behavioral therapy more effective than other therapies? A meta-analytic review. *Clinical Psychology Review*, *30*(6), 710–720.

Torrey, E. F., Kennard, A. D., Eslinger, D., Lamb, R., & Pavle, J. (2010). *More mentally ill persons are in jails and prisons than hospitals: A survey of the States*. Arlington, VA: Treatment Advocacy Center.

Touchette, E., Henegar, A., Godart, N. T., Pryor, L., Falissard, B., Tremblay, R. E., & Côté, S. M. (2011). Subclinical eating disorders and their comorbidity with mood and anxiety disorders in adolescent girls. *Psychiatry Research*, *185*(1), 185–192.

Treat Depression. (2013, September). *Top 40 mental health accounts to follow on Twitter*. Retrieved from http://treat-depression.com/top-mental-health-accounts-to-follow-on-twitter

Trockel, M., Karlin, B. E., Taylor, C. B., Brown, G. K., & Manber, R. (2015). Effects of cognitive behavioral therapy for insomnia on suicidal ideation in veterans. *Sleep*, *38*(2), 259–265.

Tung, J., Barreiro, L. B., Johnson, Z. P., Hansen, K. D., Michopoulos, V., Toufexis, D., . . . Gilad, Y. (2012). Social environment is associated with gene regulatory variation in the rhesus macaque immune system. *Proceedings of the National Academy of Sciences*, *109*(17), 6490–6495.

Turner, W. A., & Casey, L. M. (2014). Outcomes associated with virtual reality in psychological interventions: Where are we now? *Clinical Psychology Review*, *34*(8), 634–644.

Uchino, B. N. (2006). Social support and health: A review of physiological processes potentially underlying links to disease outcomes. *Journal of Behavioral Medicine*, *29*(4), 377–387.

United Nations Development Program. (1992). *1992 Human development report*. New York: Oxford University Press.

United Nations. (2000, September). *Resolution adopted by the General Assembly: United Nations Millennium Declaration*. Retrieved from www.un.org/millennium/declaration/ares552e.pdf

US Department of Health and Human Services. (2000, November). *Healthy People 2010: Understanding and improving health* (2nd ed.) Washington, DC: US Government Printing Office. Retrieved from http://www.healthypeople.gov/2010/Document/pdf/uih/2010uih.pdf

US Department of Health and Human Services. (2001). *Mental health: Culture, race, and ethnicity—A supplement to mental health: A Report of the Surgeon General*. Rockville, MD: USDHHS, Substance Abuse and Mental Health Services Administration, Center for Mental Health Services.

US Department of Health and Human Services. (2010). Centers for Disease Control and Prevention National Center for Health Statistics. *National Health Interview Survey: The principal source of information on the health of the US population*. Atlanta, GA: USDHHS. Retrieved from www.cdc.gov/nchs/data/nhis/brochure2010january.pdf

US Department of Health and Human Services. (2017). *National survey on drug use and health*. Substance Abuse and Mental Health Services Administration. Washington, DC: USDHHS. Retrieved from www.datafiles.samhsa.gov/study-series/national-survey-drug-use-and-health-nsduh-nid13517

US Department of Veterans Affairs. (2015, June). *Help your fellow veterans live life to the fullest*. Washington, DC: US Department of Veterans Affairs. Retrieved from www.vacareers.va.gov/peer-to-peer/faqs.asp

Valente, T. W. (2010). *Social networks and health: Models, methods, and applications*. New York: Oxford University Press.

Valente, T. W. (2012). Network interventions. *Science*, *337*(6090), 49–53.

Valente, T. W., Ritt-Olson, A., Stacy, A., Unger, J. B., Okamoto, J., & Sussman, S. (2007). Peer acceleration: Effects of a social network tailored substance abuse prevention program among high-risk adolescents. *Addiction, 102*, 1804–1815.

Van Boekel, L. C., Brouwers, E. P., Van Weeghel, J., & Garretsen, H. F. (2013). Stigma among health professionals towards patients with substance use disorders and its consequences for healthcare delivery: Systematic review. *Drug and Alcohol Dependence, 131*(1), 23–35.

Vanderborght, B., Simut, R., Saldien, J., Pop, C., Rusu, A. S., Pineta, S., & David, D. O. (2012). Using the social robot Probo as a social story telling agent for children with ASD. *Interaction Studies, 13*, 348–372.

Vargas, S., & Camilli, G. (1999). A meta-analysis of research on sensory integration treatment. *American Journal of Occupational Therapy, 53*(2), 189–198.

Varmus, H., Klausner, R., Zerhouni, E., Acharya, T., Daar, A. S., & Singer, P. A. (2003). Grand challenges in global health. *Science, 302*(5644), 398–399.

Vasan, A., Ellner, A., Lawn, S. D., Gove, S., Anatole, M., Gupta, N., . . . Farmer, P. E. (2014). Integrated care as a means to improve primary care delivery for adults and adolescents in the developing world: A critical analysis of Integrated Management of Adolescent and Adult Illness (IMAI). *BMC Medicine, 12*(6). Retrieved from https://bmcmedicine.biomedcentral.com/articles/10.1186/1741-7015-12-6

Vaughan, W., Rogers, E. M., Singhal, A., Ramadhan, M., & Swalehe, P. (2000). Entertainment-education and HIV/AIDS prevention: A field experiment in Tanzania. *Journal of Health Communication, 5*(Suppl. 1), 81–100.

Victor, C. R., & Yang, K. (2012). The prevalence of loneliness among adults: A case study of the United Kingdom. *Journal of Psychology, 146*(1-2), 85–104.

Virués-Ortega, J., Pastor-Barriuso, R., Castellote, J. M., Población, A., & de Pedro-Cuesta, J. (2012). Effect of animal-assisted therapy on the psychological and functional status of elderly populations and patients with psychiatric disorders: A meta-analysis. *Health Psychology Review, 6*(2), 197–221.

Visweswara, R., & Hua Gan, S. (2015). Recent advances in nanotechnology-based diagnosis and treatments of diabetes. *Current Drug Metabolism, 16*(5), 371–375.

Vivek, H., & Murthy, M. D. (2016). Office of the Surgeon General. *Facing addiction in America: The Surgeon General's report on alcohol, drugs, and health.* Washington, DC: USDHHS; November 2016. Retrieved from http://addiction.surgeongeneral.gov (https://addiction.surgeongeneral.gov/)

Vriniotis, M., Barber, C., Frank, E., Demicco, R., & the New Hampshire Firearm Safety Coalition. (2015). A suicide prevention campaign for firearm dealers in New Hampshire. *Suicide and Life-Threatening Behavior, 45*, 157–163.

Wada, K., & Shibata, T. (2006). Robot therapy in a care house: Its sociopsychological and physiological effects on the residents. *Proceedings of the IEEE International Conference on Robotics and Automation*, 3966–3971.

Wada, K., & Shibata, T. (2007, August). Robot therapy in a care house: Change of relationship among the residents and seal robot during a 2-month long study. 16th IEEE International Symposium. *Robot and Human Interactive Communication, RO-MAN*, 107–112.

Wada, K., Shibata, T., Saito, T., Sakamoto, K., & Tanie, K. (2005, April). Psychological and social effects of one year robot assisted activity on elderly people at a health service facility for the aged. Proceedings of the 2005 IEEE International Conference. *Robotics and Automation*, 2785–2790.

Wadman, M. (2016). For chronic fatigue syndrome, a "shifting tide" at NIH. *Science, 354*(6313), 691–692.

Waller, G., & Turner, H. (2016). Therapist drift redux: Why well-meaning clinicians fail to deliver evidence-based therapy, and how to get back on track. *Behaviour Research and Therapy, 77*, 129–137.

Walrond-Skinner, S. (1986). *Dictionary of psychotherapy.* London: Routledge & Kegan Paul.

Walsh, A., Ndubani, P., Simbaya, J., Dicker, P., & Brugha1, R. (2010). Task sharing in Zambia: HIV service scale-up compounds the human resource crisis. *Bio Medical Central Health Services Research, 10*, 272.

Walsh, R. (2011). Lifestyle and mental health. *American Psychologist, 66*, 579–592.

Wampold, B. E., Budge, S. L., Laska, K. M., Del Re, A. C., Baardseth, T. P., . . . Gunn, W. (2011). Evidence-based interventions for depression and anxiety versus intervention-as usual: A meta-analysis of direct comparisons. *Clinical Psychology Review, 31*, 1304–1312.

Wampold, B. E., & Imel, Z. E. (2015). *The great psychotherapy debate: The evidence for what makes psychotherapy work.* New York: Routledge.

Wampold, B. E., Minami, T., Tierney, S. C., Baskin, T. W., & Bhati, K. S. (2005). The placebo is powerful: Estimating placebo effects in medicine and psychotherapy from randomized clinical trials. *Journal of Clinical Psychology, 61*(7), 835–854.

Wang, P. S., Angermeyer, M., Borges, G., Bruffaerts, R., Chiu, W. T., de Girolamo, G., . . . Ustun, T. B. (2007). Delay and failure in treatment seeking after first onset of mental disorders in the World Health Organization's World Mental Health Survey Initiative. *World Psychiatry, 6*, 177–185.

Wang, P. S., Lane, M., Olfson, M., Pincus, H. A., Wells, K. B., & Kessler, R. C. (2005). Twelve-month use of mental health services in the United States: Results from the National Comorbidity Survey Replication. *Archives of General Psychiatry, 62*(6), 629–640.

Wei, M., Russell, D. W., & Zakalik, R. A. (2005). Adult attachment, social self-efficacy, self-disclosure, loneliness, and subsequent depression for freshman college students: A longitudinal study. *Journal of Counseling Psychology, 52*(4), 602–614.

Weinberg, M. (2009). Reforming patient assistance programs: Perfect world meets real world. *Health Affairs, 28*(3), 839–842.

Weinick, R. M., Burns, R. M., & Mehrotra, A. (2010). Many emergency department visits could be managed at urgent care centers and retail clinics. *Health Affairs, 29*(9), 1630–1636.

Weiss, W. M., Murray, L. K., Zangana, G. A. S., Mahmooth, Z., Kaysen, D., Dorsey, S., . . . Bolton, P. (2015). Community-based mental health treatments for survivors of torture and militant attacks in Southern Iraq: A randomized control trial. *BMC Psychiatry, 15*(1), 1.

Weisz, J. R., Chorpita, B. F., Palinkas, L. A., Schoenwald, S. K., Miranda, J., Bearman, S. K., . . . the Research Network on Youth Mental Health. (2012). Testing standard and modular designs for psychotherapy treating depression, anxiety, and conduct problems in youth: A randomized effectiveness trial. *Archives of General Psychiatry, 69*, 274–282.

Weisz, J. R., & Kazdin, A. E. (Eds.) (2017). *Evidence-based psychotherapies for children and adolescents* (3rd ed.). New York: Guilford Press.

Weisz, J. R., Krumholz, L. S., Santucci, L., Thomassin, K., & Ng, M. Y. (2015). Shrinking the gap between research and practice: Tailoring and testing youth psychotherapies in clinical care contexts. *Annual Review of Clinical Psychology, 11*, 139–163.

Weisz, J. R., Kuppens, S., Eckshtain, D., Ugueto, A. M., Hawley, K. M., & Jensen-Doss, A. (2013). Performance of evidence-based youth psychotherapies compared with usual clinical care: A multilevel meta-analysis. *JAMA Psychiatry, 70*(7), 750–761.

Weisz, J. R., Ng, M. Y., & Bearman, S. K. (2014). Odd couple? Re-envisioning the relation between science and practice in the dissemination and implementation era. *Clinical Psychological Science, 2*, 58–74.

Weisz, J. R., Ugueto, A. M., Cheron, D. M., & Herren, J. (2013). Evidence-based youth psychotherapy in the mental health ecosystem. *Journal of Clinical Child & Adolescent Psychology, 42*(2), 274–286.

Weitoft, G. R., Hjern, A., Haglund, B., & Rosén, M. (2003). Mortality, severe morbidity, and injury in children living with single parents in Sweden: A population-based study. *Lancet, 361*(9354), 289–295.

Wells, K., Klap, R., Koike, A., & Sherbourne, C. (2001). Ethnic disparities in unmet need for alcoholism, drug abuse, and mental health care. *American Journal of Psychiatry, 158*, 2027–2032.

Westen, D., & Bradley, R. (2005). Empirically supported complexity rethinking evidence-based practice in psychotherapy. *Current Directions in Psychological Science, 14*(5), 266–271.

Westen, D., Novotny, C. M., & Thompson-Brenner, H. (2004). The empirical status of empirically supported psychotherapies: Assumptions, findings, and reporting in controlled clinical trials. *Psychological Bulletin, 130*, 631–663.

Wheaton, B., & Montazer, S. (2010). Stressors, stress, and distress. In T. L. Scheid & T. N. Brown (Eds.), *A handbook for the study of mental health: Social contexts, theories, and systems* (2nd ed., pp. 171–199). Cambridge, UK: Cambridge University Press.

Whiteford, H. A., Degenhardt, L., Rehm, J., Baxter, A. J., Ferrari, A. J., Erskine, H. E., . . . Vos, T. (2013). Global burden of disease attributable to mental and substance use disorders: Findings from the Global Burden of Disease Study 2010. *Lancet, 382*(9904), 1575–1586.

Wible, B., Mervis, J., & Wigginton, N. S. (2014, June). Rethinking the global supply chain. *Science, 344*(6188), 1100–1103.

Wichstrøm, L., Berg-Nielsen, T. S., Angold, A., Egger, H. L., Solheim, E., & Sveen, T. H. (2012). Prevalence of psychiatric disorders in preschoolers. *Journal of Child Psychology and Psychiatry, 53*(6), 695–705.

Wiechers, I. R., Leslie, D. L., & Rosenheck, R. A. (2013). Prescribing of psychotropic medications to patients without a psychiatric diagnosis. *Psychiatric Services, 64*(12), 1243–1248.

Wilson, T. E., Fraser-White, M., Feldman, J., Homel, P., Wright, S., King, G., . . . Browne, R. (2008). Hair salon stylists as breast cancer prevention lay health advisors for African American and Afro-Caribbean women. *Journal of Health Care for the Poor and Underserved, 19*, 216–226.

Wittchen, H. U., Jacobi, F., Rehm, J., Gustavsson, A., Svensson, M., Jönsson, B., . . . Steinhausen, H. C. (2011). The size and burden of mental disorders and other disorders of the brain in Europe 2010. *European Neuropsychopharmacology, 21*(9), 655–679.

Wittchen, H. U., Muhlig, S., & Beesdo, K. (2003). Mental disorders in primary care. *Dialogues in Clinical Neuroscience, 5*, 115–128.

Wolf, M. M. (1978). Social validity: The case of subjective measurement or how applied behavior analysis is finding its heart. *Journal of Applied Behavior Analysis, 11*, 203–214.

Wolff, E., Gaudlitz, K., von Lindenberger, B. L., Plag, J., Heinz, A., & Ströhle, A. (2011). Exercise and physical activity in mental disorders. *European Archives of Psychiatry and Clinical Neuroscience, 261*(2), 186–191.

Wolitzky-Taylor, K., Dour, H., Zinbarg, R., Mineka, S., Vrshek-Schallhorn, S., Epstein, A., . . . Craske, M. G. (2014). Experiencing core symptoms of anxiety and unipolar mood disorders in late adolescence predicts disorder onset in early adulthood. *Depression and Anxiety, 31*(3), 207–213.

Wong, K. K., Engelman, J. A., & Cantley, L. C. (2010). Targeting the PI3K signaling pathway in cancer. *Current Opinion in Genetics & Development, 20*(1), 87–90.

Wood, C. (2014). Loneliness: A silent epidemic. *Independent Nurse. 2013* (6). Retrieved from www.magonlinelibrary.com/doi/10.12968/indn.2013.17.6.99114

Wood, J. J., Ehrenreich-May, J., Alessandri, M., Fujii, C., Renno, P., Laugeson, E., . . . Storch, E. A. (2015). Cognitive behavioral therapy for early adolescents with autism spectrum disorders and clinical anxiety: A randomized, controlled trial. *Behavior Therapy, 46*, 7–19.

Woolf, S. W. (2008). The meaning of translational research and why it matters. *Journal of the American Medical Association, 299*(2), 211–213.

Wooton, R. (Ed.). (2003). *Telepsychiatry and e-mental health*. London: Royal Society of Medicine Press.

World Federation for Mental Health. (2011). *The great push: Investing in mental health.* Baltimore: World Federation for Mental Health.

World Health Organization. (1978). *Primary health care: Report of the International Conference on Primary Health Care*. Geneva: WHO.

World Health Organization. (2001a). *International Classification of Functioning, Disability and Health* (ICF). Geneva: WHO.

World Health Organization. (2001b). *The World Health Report 2001. Mental health: New understanding, new hope*. Geneva: WHO.

World Health Organization. (2003). *WHO framework convention on tobacco control, 2005*. Geneva: WHO.

World Health Organization. (2004a). *Composite international diagnostic interview*. Geneva, WHO. Retrieved from www.hcp.med.harvard.edu/wmhcidi/about-the-who-wmh-cidi/

World Health Organization. (2004b). *Global burden of disease 2004 update: Disability weights for diseases and conditions*. Geneva, WHO. Retrieved from www.who.int/healthinfo/global_burden_disease/GBD2004_DisabilityWeights.pdf?ua=1

World Health Organization. (2005). *Mental health: Facing the challenges, building solutions*. Report from the WHO European Ministerial Conference. Regional Office for Europe, Copenhagen: WHO.

World Health Organization. (2006). *The World Health Report 2006: Working together for health*. Geneva: WHO.

World Health Organization. (2008a). *Task shifting: Global recommendations and guidelines*. Geneva: WHO.

World Health Organization. (2008b). *The global burden of disease: 2004 update*. Geneva: WHO.

World Health Organization. (2009). *Telemedicine: Opportunities and developments. Report on the second global survey on eHealth Global Observatory for eHealth series* (Vol. 2). Geneva: WHO.

World Health Organization. (2010). *International classification of diseases—10* (4th ed.). Geneva: WHO.

World Health Organization. (2011a, April). *Prevention and control of NCDS: Summary*. Paper presented at the First Global Ministerial Conference on Healthy Lifestyles and Noncommunicable Disease Control, Moscow, Russia.

World Health Organization. (2011b). *Scaling up action against non-communicable diseases: How much will it cost?* Geneva: WHO.

World Health Organization. (2013). Metrics: Disability-adjusted life year (DALY): Quantifying the burden of disease from mortality and morbidity. Retrieved from www.who.int/healthinfo/global_burden_disease/metrics_daly/en/

World Health Organization. (2014a). *Measuring health and disability: Manual for the WHO Disability Assessment Schedule*. Geneva: WHO.

World Health Organization. (2014b). *Preventing suicide: A global imperative.* Geneva: WHO.

World Health Organization. (2016). *Fiscal policies for diet and the prevention of noncommunicable diseases.* Geneva: WHO.

World Mental Health Survey Consortium. (2004). Prevalence, severity, and unmet need for treatment of mental disorders in the World Health Organization World Mental Health Surveys. *JAMA, 291*(21), 2581–2590.

Wu, A. C., Donnelly-McLay, D., Weisskopfl, M. G., McNeely, E., Betancourt, T. S., & Allen, J. G. (2016). Airplane pilot mental health and suicidal thoughts: A cross-sectional descriptive study via anonymous web-based survey. *Environmental Health, 15*, 121–133.

Wu, Y., Zhang, D., & Kang, S. (2013). Physical activity and risk of breast cancer: A meta-analysis of prospective studies. *Breast Cancer Research and Treatment, 137*(3), 869–882.

Yuen, E. K., Herbert, J. D., Forman, E. M., Goetter, E. M., Comer, R., & Bradley, J. C. (2013). Treatment of social anxiety disorder using online virtual environments in second life. *Behavior Therapy, 44*(1), 51–61.

Zane, N., Sue, S., Chang, J., Huang, L., Huang, J., Lowe, S., . . . Lee, E. (2005). Beyond ethnic match: Effects of client-therapist cognitive match in problem perception, coping orientation, and therapy goals on treatment outcomes. *Journal of Community Psychology, 33*(5), 569–585.

Zhang, E. Y., & Cheok, A. D. (2016, October). Forming intimate human-robot relationships through a kissing machine. In *Proceedings of the Fourth International Conference on Human Agent Interaction*, 233–234.

Zhang, J., Shoham, D. A., Tesdahl, E., & Gesell, S. B. (2015). Network interventions on physical activity in an afterschool program: An agent-based social network study. *American Journal of Public Health, 105*(S2), S236–S243.

Zhang, Z., Wu, H., Wang, W., & Wang, B. (2010, October). *A smartphone based respiratory biofeedback system.* Paper presented at the Third International Conference on Biomedical Engineering and Informatics, Yantai, China.

Zhu, S.-H., Wong, S., Stevens, C., Nakashima, D., & Gamst, A. (2010). Use of a smokers' quitline by Asian language speakers: Results from 15 years of operation in California. *American Journal of Public Health, 100*, 846–852.

Zivin, K., Yosef, M., Miller, E. M., Valenstein, M., Duffy, S., Kales, H. C., . . . Kim, H. M. (2015). Associations between depression and all-cause and cause-specific risk of death: A retrospective cohort study in the Veterans Health Administration. *Journal of Psychosomatic Research, 78*(4), 324–331.

Zoogman, S., Goldberg, S. B., Hoyt, W. T., & Miller, L. (2015). Mindfulness interventions with youth: A meta-analysis. *Mindfulness, 6*(2), 290–302.

ABOUT THE AUTHOR

Alan E. Kazdin (PhD, Northwestern University) is the Sterling Professor of Psychology and Child Psychiatry at Yale University and Director of the Yale Parenting Center, an outpatient treatment service for children and families. Before coming to Yale, he was on the faculty of the Pennsylvania State University and the University of Pittsburgh School of Medicine. At Yale he has been Chairman of the Psychology Department, Director and Chair of the Yale Child Study Center at the Yale School of Medicine, and Director of Child Psychiatric Services at Yale–New Haven Hospital. In 2008, he was President of the American Psychological Association.

Kazdin is a licensed clinical psychologist, a Diplomate of the American Board of Professional Psychology (ABPP), and a Fellow of the Association for the Advancement of Science, the American Psychological Association (APA), and the Association for Psychological Science. His honors include Research Scientist Career and MERIT Awards from the National Institute of Mental Health (NIMH) and Awards for Distinguished Scientific Contribution to Clinical Psychology and Distinguished Professional Contribution to Clinical Child Psychology (APA), Outstanding Research Contribution by an Individual (Association for Behavioral and Cognitive Therapies), Joseph Zubin Award for Lifetime Contributions to Understanding Psychopathology (Society for Research in Psychopathology), and Awards for Lifetime Contributions to Psychology (APA; Connecticut Psychological Association). He has served as editor of six professional journals: *Journal of Consulting and Clinical Psychology, Psychological Assessment, Behavior Therapy, Clinical Psychology: Science and Practice, Current Directions in Psychological Science,* and *Clinical Psychological Science.*

His main areas of research are on the development and evaluation of psychosocial interventions, especially in relation to the treatment of oppositional, aggressive, and antisocial behavior among children and adolescents. Kazdin's 750+ publications include 49 books that focus on evidence-based interventions, parenting and childrearing, methodology and research design, and interpersonal violence. His work on parenting and childrearing has been featured on NPR, PBS, BBC, and CNN, and he has appeared on the Today Show, Good Morning America, ABC News, 20/20, and Dr. Phil.

His other books with Oxford University Press include:

Kazdin, A. E. (2000). *Psychotherapy for children and adolescents: Directions for research and practice.*

Kazdin, A. E. (Ed.) (2000). *The encyclopedia of psychology* (Vols. 1–8).

Kazdin, A. E. (2005). *Parent management training: Treatment for oppositional, aggressive, and antisocial behavior in children and adolescents.*

Kazdin, A. E. (2011). *Single-case research designs: Methods for clinical and applied settings* (2nd ed.).

INDEX